T0182123

Diagnosis of Aging Skin Diseases

Robert A. Norman
Editor

Diagnosis of Aging Skin Diseases

Foreword by Albert M. Kligman, MD

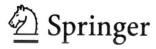 Springer

Robert A. Norman, DO, MPH, FAAIM
Associate Professor, Nova Southeastern Medical School
President and CEO, Dermatology Healthcare, Tampa, Florida
President and CEO, Dermatology and Skin Cancer Centers of Florida
President and Founder, International Society of Geriatric Dermatology

British Library Cataloguing in Publication Data

Diagnosis of aging skin diseases
    1. Skin – Diseases – Diagnosis 2. Older people – Diseases –
    Diagnosis 3. Age factors in disease
    I. Norman, Robert A.
    618.9'765075

ISBN-13: 9781846286773

A catalogue record for this book is available from the British Library

Library of Congress Control Number: 2008927301

ISBN: 978-1-84628-677-3   e-ISBN: 978-1-84628-678-0

Printed on acid-free paper

© Springer-Verlag London Limited 2008

9 8 7 6 5 4 3 2 1

Springer Science+Business Media

springer.com

Foreword

The population is aging rapidly, even faster than demographers envisioned two decades ago. Longevity, especially for women, has nearly doubled, since the beginning of the twentieth century, now approaching 85. People over 80 are the fastest growing segment in the aging epidemic. Remarkably every day now 1,000 Americans will celebrate their 100th birthday!

Today, many 70-year-old persons, who have aged successfully, have about the same degree of health and vigor as people 50 years old, a generation ago.

Despite these gains, it is an inescapable truism that increasing age is associated with increasing physiologic losses, which negatively affect the quality of life. Persons in their eighties and nineties may be taking as many as 10 different medicines daily to control and moderate age-dependent disorders such as arthritis, diabetes, hypertension, heart disease, Alzheimer's.

Textbooks of geriatric medicine recognize and give each of these the space they deserve.

By contrast, age-associated cutaneous disorders are given short shrift in geriatric texts. Skin disorders, when mentioned at all, are inadequately presented. This downgrading of cutaneous disorders occurs despite the findings of national health surveys which showed that people over 70 years of age had at least one skin disorder worthy of medical attention. Startlingly, the same rigorously conducted epidemiologic survey showed that the number and diversity of skin problems increased proportionately with advancing age. Some older persons had as many as 10 problems which were deemed to be worthy of medical attention.

This marginalizing of skin disorders in geriatric textbooks is usually attributed to the fact that skin diseases are not life-threatening, a blinkered, benighted description. The skin disorders of old age rarely kill, but they certainly can ruin the quality of life and, when chronic as they so often are, can make people miserable, depressed, and even suicidal.

Dr Robert Norman's book is designed to correct that gap and to provide practitioners a practical guide for diagnosing and treating cutaneous disorders of the elderly. This treatise is the first of its kind to make non-specialists aware of the powerful therapeutic resources that have come online through the growth of scientific dermatologic knowledge.

Dr Norman's book is especially timely and valuable because most medical school graduates do not receive adequate training about dermatologic subjects and are thereafter ill-prepared to provide optimal treatment. As the population grows ever older, an increasing number will spend their remaining years in nursing and retirement homes where expert dermatologic services are limited or non-existent, leaving it to untrained nursing personnel to take care of the numerous and multifarious skin problems which affect the elderly.

All too often skin problems suffer from the perception that they are merely nuisances or trivial cosmetic concerns that older people simply have to live with. This is a serious misconception.

For example, all persons over 70 will suffer from dry, scaly skin, often associated with pruritus. Itching skin can be maddening. It interferes with sleep and leads to relentless scratching and excoriations which may lead to bacterial infections. What is less well known is that dry, cracked, scaly skin may be the first sign of a major problem in nursing homes, namely, pressure sores which not only are difficult to treat but may even be fatal. The skin is also susceptible to bacterial infections of *Staphylococcus aureus* and *β-hemolytic streptococci*, which are likely to go unrecognized because older persons do not readily mount an inflammatory response with fever, redness, and edema, signifying an impending cellulitis.

Nutritional problems are easily over-looked in the old-old, especially vitamin deficiencies, whose daily requirements may be much greater than in the young. Scurvy and pellagra, rare in the young, are not uncommon in the malnourished elderly and have recognizable clinical manifestations to the experienced eye.

Common skin disorders such as psoriasis and lichen planus have different expressions in the old and are frequently misdiagnosed and are accordingly mistreated.

It is a common belief too that common skin disorders regress and disappear spontaneously in the elderly. This is not always the case and again leads to misdiagnosis. Rosacea is a case in point, vividly described by R. Marks in this volume.

Just as children are not simply similar adults, the elderly are not simply older adults. Geriatricians are generally not well acquainted with the special needs of the elderly, especially with regard to cutaneous disorders.

This comprehensive text should be in easy reach of medical practitioners who will find it an enlightening, very useful and credible source of the latest information regarding the diagnosis and treatment of the cutaneous disorders of our aging population.

Albert M. Kligman, MD

Preface

As "baby-boomers" begin to enter into senior citizenship and the elderly get older, an increased emphasis in geriatric medicine is inevitable. Those 65 years and older are increasing in numerical strength and therefore, along with the common problems prevalent in an aging population, will also have new dermatological problems related to wear and tear, the effects of sun exposure, as well as pharmacologically induced problems arising from treating other conditions. This trend is expected to continue well into the twenty-first century. Additionally, the population of those aged 80+ is rapidly increasing.

Geriatric dermatology is a specialty that is receiving increasing attention. Among the topics and diseases reviewed here are pruritus and xerosis, eczematous dermatitis, psychosomatic maladies, infections of the skin, purpura, vascular compromise and chronic venous insufficiency, decubitus ulcers and bullous pemphigoid. Illnesses originating in other organ systems that are made manifest on the skin often complicate the diagnostic and therapeutic picture. Chronic diseases such as diabetes mellitus and HIV compound the diagnoses and treatment of geriatric dermatological problems. As the population of older adults live longer, chronic diseases will become more prevalent as will the diseases of the skin, and will require increasing attention by dermatologists, primary care physicians and other health professionals.

Many of the elderly will spend their time in nursing homes and assisted living facilities. Caregivers and medical personnel can help decrease or prevent the development of skin disorders in the elderly by addressing many factors, including the patient's nutritional state, medical history, current medications, allergies, physical limitations, mental state and personal hygiene.

Robert A. Norman

Acknowledgments

I thank the editors at Springer, especially Grant Weston and Hannah Wilson and also I thank the project manager, Ragavia Ramakrishnan, at Integra Software Services Pvt. Ltd., India. I have great appreciation for the authors that have contributed to this very important book and I know the readers and their patients will benefit greatly from the time and effort of these accomplished authors.

I encourage readers to keep current on advances within geriatrics and geriatric dermatology as the science presented in our meetings and literature will impact clinical dermatology in enormous ways in the coming decades.

Contents

Contributors

Margaret I. Aguwa, DO, MPH
Family and Community Medicine
College of Osteopathic
Medicine, Michigan State University
East Lansing, MI, USA

Cristiane Benvenuto-Andrade, MD
Sector of Dermatology and
Post-Graduation Course
HUCFF/UFRJ and
School of Medicine, Federal University
of Rio de Janeiro, Rio de
Janeiro, Brazil

Megan Bock, PA
"Dermatology Healthcare," Tampa
FL, USA

Charles Camisa, MD
Department of Dermatology
Cleveland Clinic Florida, Naples
FL, USA

Tania Ferreira Cestari, MD, PhD
Department of Dermatology,
HCPA/UFRGS and School
of Medicine, University of Rio
Grande do Sul, Porto Alegre
Rio Grande do Sul, Brazil

Arun Chakrabarty, MD
Solano Clinical Research, Davis
CA, USA

Sueli Coelho da Silva Carneiro, MD, PhD
Sector of Dermatology, HUPE-UERJ
and School of Medicine, State
University of Rio de Janeiro and
HUCFF-UFRJ and School of Medicine
Federal University of Rio de Janeiro
Rio de Janeiro, Brazil

Charles Dewberry, DO
Department of Dermatology, Randall
Dermatology, West Lalayette
IN, USA

T.S. Dharmarajan, MD, FACP, AGSF
Division of Geriatrics, Our Lady
of Mercy Medical Center, Bronx
NY, USA

Dirk M. Elston, MD
Geisinger Medical Center, Danville
PA, USA

Cynthia A. Fleck, MBA, BSN, RN, ET/WOCN, CWS, DNC, DAPWCA, FCCWS Advanced Wound and Skin
Care American Academy of Wound
Management, Association for the
Advancement of Wound Care
Saint Louis, MO, USA and Clinical
Marketing Medline Industries Inc.,
Mundelein, IL, USA

Robert R. Haight, MD, MSPH
Tampa, Florida

Amor Khachemoune, MD, CWS
Ronald O. Perelman Department
of Dermatology, New York
University School of Medicine
NY, USA

Erica Liverant, MD
Department of Medicine, Crozer
Chester Medical Center, Upland
PA, USA

Ronald Marks, FRCP, FRC Path
Department of Dermatology, Cutest
Systems Ltd, Heath, Cardiff
UK

Robyn Menendez, PA
Physician Assistant VA Hospital
Tampa, Florida

Anusuya A. Mokashi
New York Medical College
Montrose, Los Angeles
CA, USA

Michael B. Morgan, MD
Department of Pathology, Haley VA
Hospital, USF College of Medicine
Tampa, FL, USA

Claudio de Moura Jacques, MD
Sector of Dermatology, HUCFF-UFRJ
and School of Medicine
Federal University of Rio de Janeiro
Rio de Janeiro, Brazil

Diya F. Mutasim, MD
Department of Dermatology, University
of Cincinnati, Cincinnati
OH, USA

**Robert A. Norman, DO, MPH,
FAAIM**
"Dermatology Healthcare," Tampa
FL, USA

Tania J. Phillips, MD
Department of Dermatology
Boston University School of
Medicine, Boston
MA, USA

Marcia Ramos-e-Silva, MD, PhD
Sector of Dermatology, HUCFF-UFRJ
and School of Medicine
Universidade Federal do Rio de Janeiro
Rio de Janeiro, Brazil

Carlos F. Rodríguez, MD
University of Illinois, Chicago School
of Medicine, Chicago
IL, USA

Sadia Saeed, MD
Clinical Associate Dermotology UCSF
San Francisco

Elizabeth Sagatys, MD
Clinical Associate Pathology USFCOM
Tampa

Noah S. Scheinfeld, MD, JD
Department of Dermatology, St Luke's
Roosevelt Hospital Center
New York City
NY, USA

Marcy Street, MD
Doctor's Approach Dermatology and
Laser Center, Doctor's
Approach Skin and Hair Care
East Lansing
MI, USA

Athena Theodosatos, DO, MPH
Department of Family Medicine
Florida Hospital, Orlando
FL, USA

Justin R. Wasserman, BS
Clinical Associate Dermatology
University of Chicago

Chapter 1

The Demographic Imperative

Robert A. Norman

Introduction

The demographic imperative has reached the shores of dermatology. Those of us allowed the honor of treating our elderly have a great responsibility for our aging population in the years ahead.

After World War II we built more schools, trained more teachers, and created more playgrounds to gear up for the explosive birth rate. Not only does the post-World War II generation have more members than any other generation but will also live longer.

The vast majority of people older than 70 years of age have at least one bothersome skin condition, and approximately 10% have 3–4 dermatological problems.

Demographics

The world population of older adults is increasing significantly; by the year 2050, adults older than 65 years will comprise one-fifth of the global population [1]. The United States 2000 census suggests there are about 35 million individuals (or 13% of the population) aged 65 years and older [2] and by 2020 will comprise a fourth of the US population [1, 3]. The age group of 85 and older is the fastest growing segment of the population, and at present rates of growth, there will be more than 380,000 centenarians by the year 2030 [2]. A basic understanding of the aging process will enable health care providers to distinguish age-related physiological changes from disease-related pathological processes.

Definitions

While *aging* is an ongoing process, *senescence* refers to the "post-maturational processes that lead to diminished homeostasis and increased vulnerability of the organism." *Normal aging* involves inevitable changes related to physiological processes occurring at certain stages in life, e.g. menopause. *Usual aging* refers to

R.A. Norman (ed.), *Diagnosis of Aging Skin Diseases,*
© Springer-Verlag London Limited 2008

age-related diseases that typically occur in older individuals, e.g. coronary artery disease and hypertension. *Life expectancy* refers to the age reached by half a given population and varies with race, gender, and geographical influences. The *maximum life span potential* is the age attained by the longest-lived member of a given population [4]. The oldest properly documented human (Jeanne Calment) died at age 122 in 1997 [5]. In 1997, life expectancy at birth in the United States was 79.4 years for women and 73.6 years for men; at age 85, it was 6.6 and 5.5 years, respectively [2]. In general, the female outlives the male with reference to the human and most species.

The Graying of America
35 million Americans are senior citizens
2010–40 million
2020–53 million
2030–70 million
Those over 65 has increased 100 percent between 1960 and 1994
America's 65-and-over population will increase from one in eight to one in five people by 2050

Getting old is a new phenomenon. While there have always been some people who have lived into their 1980s and 1990s, the magnitude of this longevity today is a very recent development among the human species. If age at death is plotted for the human evolutionary line beginning about 3–5 million years ago, most hominids were dying in their teens and 1920s. By the time the first *Homo sapiens* of the Neanderthal subspecies were around, human life averaged about 30–38 years. The date was 100,000 years ago. By 50,000 years, the first *Homo sapiens sapiens* were present and lived into their late thirties and early forties as a group. It is true that some lived into their sixties, but only a few. By 10,000 years ago, humans had discovered how to grow plants and tend herd animals for an improved food supply. Yet, longevity stayed basically the same as it had been for the last 40,000 years. The probable cause for the ceiling effect on longevity was the lack of control over infectious disease.

It was not until the twentieth century that human longevity began to commonly climb to its current extent of 75-plus years for most people in technologically developed societies. In 1900 AD, the average age of death was 49 years, due primarily to problems of high infant mortality. However, by the mid-century mark, the rapid ascent of human longevity was well on its way. It has not yet stopped climbing. Today, medicine and public health is practiced in the face of an unprecedented demographic event marked by common and extreme longevity.

Over the past few years, the world's population has continued on its remarkable transition path from a state of high birth and death rates to one characterized by low birth and death rates. At the heart of that transition has been the growth in the number and proportion of older persons. Such a rapid, large and ubiquitous growth has never been seen in the history of civilization.

The current demographic revolution is predicted to continue well into the coming centuries. Its major features include the following.

One of every 10 persons is now 60 years or above; by 2050, one out of five will be 60 years or older; and by 2150, one out of three persons will be 60 years or older.

The older population itself is aging. The increase in the number of very old people (aged 80+ years): that group is projected to grow by a factor of 8–10 times on the global scale, between 1950 and 2050. Currently, the oldest old constitute 11 % of the population aged 60 and above. By 2150, about a third of the older population will be 80 years or older. The majority of older persons (55%) are women. Among the oldest old (80 years or older), 65% are women.

Striking differences exist between regions. More than 43% of the world's oldest old in 1996 lived in just four countries: The People's Republic of China, the United States, India, and Japan. One out of five Europeans, but 1 out of 20 Africans, is 60 years or older.

As the tempo of aging in developing countries is more rapid than in developed countries, developing countries will have less time than the developed countries to adapt to the consequences of population aging. In some African and Asian nations, the population age 75 and over constitutes less than 1% of total population. This contrasts sharply with the situation in Europe and North America, where the oldest old share reaches as high as 8.5% (Sweden). For example, over the next 50 years the elderly population will increase by 23% in the UK, but by 292% in Brazil, 324% in Mexico, and 414% in Indonesia [6].

Changes in the proportion of elderly in the total population have a different causal basis. The projections of a very high and increasing proportion of elderly from 2010 to 2030 are accounted for by three factors: (a) declining and low fertility in the past and the prospect of continuing low fertility up to 2030 (and beyond); (b) maturing of the baby-boom cohorts; and (c) sharp declines in mortality at the adult and older ages in the recent past and the prospect of continuing low mortality up to 2030 (and beyond). Once the baby-boom influx is over (i.e., has completely passed age 65) in 2030, the proportion of elderly in the total population stabilizes.

The figures for all race groups combined tend to reflect mainly the changes in the white elderly population. Blacks, Asian and Pacific Islanders, and Hispanics will share in the main trends described, but to a more intensive degree. Between 2010 and 2030, the size of these racial/ethnic groups will increase dramatically. Similarly, dramatic increases are projected between 2030 and 2050 for the 85-and-over age group. The rates of growth for Asian and Pacific Islanders (the main component of the "other races" group) and Hispanics far exceed those for whites in all periods [6].

Our time has come. It is our duty to care for the aging boomers. We are in enormous need of increasing our skills to respond to this unprecedented demographic shift. Over the last several decades, we have enjoyed a sustained achievement in our basic scientific knowledge and proven effectiveness of clinical interventions. We need to be at the top in providing comprehensive health care delivery for older adults. We must be at the forefront of prevention and treatment of skin diseases and be able to recognize the dermatologic signs of chronic systemic disease so often noted in our elderly.

Many diseases, including psoriasis and onychomycosis, have been the subject of great interest of the pharmaceutical industry, and the time from discovery of new therapies to clinical application has become relatively short. All therapeutic costs and benefits must be weighed, of course, with the patient in mind. The ethical standards and actions of treating our elderly directly reflect our great profession's character. Perhaps nowhere can this be seen to a greater extent than with the rise in cosmetic enhancements that our elderly population has demanded of us as practitioners.

References

1. Jackson SA. The epidemiology of aging. In Hazzard WR, Blass JP, Ettinger WH Jr, Halter JB, Ouslander JG, eds. Principles of Geriatric Medicine and Gerontology, 4th ed. New York: McGraw-Hill, 1999, pp. 203–25.
2. Federal Interagency Forum on Aging-Related Statistics. Older Americans 2000: Key Indicators of Well-Being. Federal Interagency Forum on Aging-Related Statistics, Washington, DC: US Government Printing Office, August 2000.
3. Furner SE, Brody JA, Jankowski LM. Epidemiology and Aging. In Cassel CK, Cohen HJ, Larson EB, Meier DE, Resnick NM, Rubenstein LZ, Sorenson LB, eds. Geriatric Medicine, 3rd ed. New York: Springer, 1997, pp. 37–43.
4. Troen BR, Cristofalo VJ, eds. The biology of aging. In Cobbs EL, Duthie EH Jr, Murphy JB, eds. Geriatrics Review Syllabus, 4th ed. Iowa: Kendall/Hunt Publishing Co., 1999, pp. 5–10.
5. Perls T, Kunkel LM, Puca A. The genetics of exceptional human longevity. JAGS 2002; 50: 359–68.
6. Kinsella K, Velfoff V. An Aging World: 2001. US Census Bureau. Series P95/01-1. Washington, DC: US Government Printing Office, 2001.

Chapter 2

Structure and Function of Aging Skin

Robert A. Norman and Robyn Menendez

Introduction

Numerous changes occur in our bodies as we age. Our skin is no exception. There are both natural and environmental factors that will shape aging human skin. Cell replacement, barrier function, chemical clearance, mechanical protection, immune responsiveness, wound healing, thermoregulation, DNA repair, sweat and sebum production, and vitamin D production are intrinsic alterations in the aging process (see Table 2.1). Exposure to the sun will also cause an array of changes in our skin. It is important to know the basic structure and function of aging skin in order to better understand the processes that will occur in our skin as our bodies develop.

Structure of the Skin

The skin is divided into two main layers, the dermis and the epidermis (see Table 2.2). Subcutaneous fat lies directly beneath these layers. The epidermis is keratinizing stratified squamous epithelium. Within this epithelium are epidermal dendritic cells and appendages. There are four defined layers of the epidermis which are (a) basal cell, (b) prickle cell, (c) granular cell, and (d) keratin [1]. The epidermal dendritic cells are the melanocytes and Langerhans cells. Melanocytes give the skin its color by producing melanin. They also protect against UV radiation. Langerhans cells are derived from bone marrow and play a role in immunology. Merkel cells are found in the epidermis; however, they can also be found within the dermis and play a role with peripheral nerve endings. Sebaceous glands, apocrine glands, eccrine glands, hair, and nails are considered appendages in the epidermis. The major function of the sebaceous glands is waterproofing. They control water loss and protect the skin from fungi and bacteria. The function of the apocrine glands is uncertain. Both sebaceous and apocrine glands become larger after puberty. Eccrine sweat glands help to provide thermoregulation. The hair and nails offer good skin protection as well [1].

The dermis lies beneath the epidermis and consists of collagen, elastin, and ground substance. It has two layers: the papillary, which gives us fingerprints, and

R.A. Norman (ed.), *Diagnosis of Aging Skin Diseases,*
© Springer-Verlag London Limited 2008

Table 2.1 Alterations of aging skin

Cell replacement	Wound healing
Barrier function	Thermoregulation
Chemical clearance	DNA repair
Mechanical protection	Sweat and sebum production
Immune responsiveness	Vitamin D production

Table 2.2 Epidermis and dermis

Epidermis	Dermis
Four layers	Two layers
Basal	Papillary
Prickle	Reticular
Granular	Consists of:
Keratin	Collagen
Dendritic cells	Elastin
Melanocytes	Ground substance
Langerhans	
Appendages	
Sebaceous glands	
Apocrine glands	
Eccrine glands	
Hair	
Nails	

the reticular layer that provides the lines of cleavage [1]. There is a rich blood and nerve supply found in the dermis. Collagen is a complex protein made in numerous cells. Its purpose in the skin is to provide the framework which helps the skin to maintain its shape [2]. Elastin provides the skin with retractability. Ground substance helps to transport water and electrolytes.

Skin and the Aging Process

The main functions of the skin that decrease with age are cell replacement, barrier function, chemical clearance, mechanical protection, immune responsiveness, wound healing, thermoregulation, DNA repair, sweat and sebum production, and Vitamin D production.

Cell Replacement

Numerous cells responsible for proper skin function decline as we age. These include fibroblasts, melanocytes, keratinocytes, Langerhans cells, mast cells, nerves, eccrine and apocrine sweat glands, hair follicles, and nail. There is also a decreased response to growth inhibitors. A decrease in subcutaneous fat is also noted on the face and distal extremities but on the waist of men and thighs of women there is an increase.

Barrier Function

With aging, our barrier function is compromised at each level in our skin (see Table 2.3). The epidermal layer has decreased cell replacement and turnover rates. It begins to lose its rete ridges and dermal papillae retract [3]. The thickness of the stratum corneum (keratin) does not change with age but there is an increase in the corneocyte area. Lipid formation is gradually lessened which can lead to compromise at this level of the stratum corneum. Sebaceous gland size increases but their function of producing sebum declines in response to androgen levels [4]. Alopecia may also occur due to aging and other factors. Hairs also turn gray due to decreased synthesis of melanin. Size and number of hair follicles decline due to a decrease in capillary vasculature as well as chronic inflammation [5]. Hair thinning is due to decreased number of follicles, slower growth rate, and decreased diameter of the hair. The anagen phase of hair growth decreases and therefore growth rate decreases. The rate of nail growth is reduced by 50%.

The dermoepidermal junction is lessened which may lead to more shear-type injuries and bullae formation [6]. The dermis thins with age as there is loss of collagen and proteoglycan. Elastic fibers are also more irregular. Subcutaneous fat is thinner in the face, particularly in the cheeks, and in the distal extremities as well as in the plantar aspect of the foot [6].

Mechanical Protection

Due to decreases especially in melanocytes and the dermis, there is a disruption in the mechanical protection served by the skin (see Table 2.4). The enzymatically active melanocytes decrease which allows for UV penetration and damage. The dermoepidermal junction flattens, possibly leading to loss of communication and decreased nutrient transfer [7]. The overall dermal thickness is reduced. Reductions in collagen can be found and at a rate of approximately

Table 2.3 Compromise of the barrier function

Stratum corneum thickness remains the same but corneocyte area increases
Less lipid formation at the stratum corneum level
Sebaceous gland size increases but sebum production is less
Hair loss and graying hair
Dermoepidermal junction flattens
Dermal thinning
Areas of less subcutaneous fat

Table 2.4 Compromises of mechanical protection

Melanocyte cell replacement decreases
Dermoepidermal junction flattens
Dermal thickness decreases
Decreased collagen

1% annually throughout adulthood [6]. The fibers, however, increase in stiffness and become less soluble. The decreases in the dermal layer leads to decreased elasticity, increased laxity, decreased recovery from indention pressure, decreased torsion extensibility, and decreased turgor [8].

Wound Healing

With aging, the wound repair of the skin can be delayed. There is a decreased IgE hypersensitivity. Dermal collagenase increases while elastin is broken down. The replenishment of the vasculature is also delayed. The subcutaneous fat distribution changes and alters pressure diffusion. Various growth factors, altered early inflammatory response associated with the upregulation of matrix metalloproteinases, reproductive hormones such as estrogen, and growth factors are also believed to be involved in the breakdown of tissue, impaired wound healing, and a possible predisposition to chronic wounds in the elderly.

Immune Responsiveness

Immune response is not rapid in the elderly skin. Langerhans cells decrease their antigen-presenting capacity when exposed to UV radiation [1]. With age alone, Langerhans cells are decreased by 20–50% [7]. The function of T cells and IgE titers declines. There is an increase in autoantibodies IgA and IgG leading to beta cell dysfunction. Acute inflammatory reactions are less noticeable.

Thermoregulation

As one ages, sweat glands, nerve, vasculature, and sebaceous gland secretions all decrease. These changes lead to an overall decrease in thermoregulation. Sweat glands are highly active at puberty as they are androgen dependent, then they peak at adolescence and are constant throughout adulthood until menopause in women and when testosterone decreases in men [9]. The actual sebaceous gland will increase in size in the elderly but the activity declines. As sweat gland secretions are reduced, so is body odor and perspiration. Changes in perspiration therefore lead to a change in the thermoregulation process. Lower thresholds for pain perception and reaction develop as the nerves change. Meissners corpuscles decrease in number but the free nerve endings remain the same [3]. Vasculature losses lead to pallor and a lower skin temperature. The lumen of the blood vessels begins to thicken and the number of capillary vessels decreases. The epidermis is instead supplied proper nutrients by vessels in the dermal papillae [10]. Lastly, subcutaneous fat decreases in certain areas that can also make a change in thermoregulation.

Sweat and Sebum Production

There is a gradual decline, although not very noticeable, in the eccrine, apocrine, and sebaceous glands, which also results in decreased sweat and sebum production. The decrease does not become apparent until menopause in women and about 80 years of age in men when the testosterone levels decline. Yaar attributes this decline in all of the glands partially to decreased vasculature. The sebaceous gland does not vary noticeably in size although the secretions are markedly reduced. In opposition, the eccrine and apocrine glands do decrease in size and function. With the decreased eccrine gland there is less sweat produced, therefore less body odor and a change in thermoregulation.

Vitamin D Production

Vitamin D production is essential for calcium regulation. Decreases in calcium can lead to osteomalacia. The 7-dehydrocholesterol is activated by UV radiation at less than 320 nm to make previtamin D3 which is then thermally isomerized to form vitamin D3. D3 binds in the capillaries to vitamin D binding proteins [7]. During the stages of adulthood, the level of epidermal 7-dehydrocholesterol per unit of skin surface area declines linearly by approximately 75% [7]. This decrease begins in the second decade of life [6].

DNA Repair

DNA has changes that occur with aging. Somatic cells begin to have more mutations. Decreased proteins lead to some of these mutations.

Cutaneous Aging: Chronologic versus Photoaging

Intrinsic or chronically aged skin is the normal physiologic changes that occur in our skin throughout life. Photo aging is the process by which sunlight changes our skin. UVA radiation is between 315 and 400 nm. Connective tissue and fibroblasts sustain the majority of UVA radiation while there is little to no effect on the collagen [10]. UVB radiation is between 290 and 315 nm. UVB radiation can lead to DNA damage, skin cancers, and erythroderma [10].

Keratinocytes are different depending on intrinsic or photo aging. With intrinsically aged skin the stratum corneum and number of horny cell layers remain unchanged. There is a decrease in epidermal filaggrin making the skin dry [10]. In photo-aged skin, the distribution of the stratum corneum is varied. Vitamin D production is decreased intrinsically. Not only does Vitamin D decrease due to the decreased level of 7-dehydrocholesterol per unit of skin surface area but there can also be a lack of sun exposure or a poor diet deficient in dairy products [9]. This can be the case also with photo-aged skin as they are subject to all of the same intrinsic depletions or if they should decide to limit their sun exposure.

Elastic tissue also changes depending on intrinsic or photo factors. There is hyperplasia of the elastic tissue in the photo aged and atrophy of the collagen [10]. Lavker distinguishes different phases in elastic fibers depending upon the skin being chronically aged or photo aged. In intrinsically aged skin, the first phase is hyperplasia where there is an increase in the number and thickness of normal elastic fibers. Phase two is elastolysis which results in the loss of fine vertical fibers that insert into the basal lamina. Numerous holes appear in these fibers and give the loss of elasticity we see with age. With photo aging, the first phase consists of elastogenesis followed by actinic degeneration which leads to loss of resilience. Mast cells are also more abundant in photo-aged skin, which can cause damage and produce inflammatory mediators. The vasculature also decreases. In intrinsically aged skin, the vessels thicken and become more dilated and tortuous which leads to telangiectasias [10]. In photo-aged vasculature, the wall thickens as well but is also surrounded by inflammatory cells particularly lymphocytes, then histiocytes and mast cells, which is not the case in intrinsic microvasculature.

References

1. Elder D. Lever's Histopathology of the Skin, 8th ed. Philadelphia: Lippincott-Raven, 1997.
2. Kohn R, Schnider S. Collagen changes in aging skin, Chap. 6. In Balin AL, Kligman AM, eds. Aging and the Skin. New York: Raven Press, 1989.
3. Kligman A, Balin A. Aging of Human Skin, Chap. 1. New York: Raven Press, 1989.
4. Young EM, Newcomer VD, Kligman AM. Geriatric dermatology: Color Atlas and Practitioner's Guide. Williams & Wilkins, 1992.
5. Marks R, Dunitz M. Structure and function of aged skin. Skin Disease in Old Age, 2nd ed. United Kingdom, 1987.
6. Fenske NA, Lober CW. Structural and functional changes of normal aging skin. J. Am. Acad. Dermatol. 1986; 15(4 Part 1): 571–585.
7. Yaar M, Gilchrest B. Skin aging. Clin. Geriatr. Med. 2001; 17(4): 617–30.
8. McKee P. Pathology of the Skin. Philadelphia: JB Lippincott, 1989.
9. Berkow R, Beers MH. Merck Manual of Geriatrics, Chap. 122. In Mark H, Beers MD, Berkow RMD, eds. Aging and the Skin. Merck, 2000.
10. Marks R. Epidermal aging, Chap. 13. Aging and the Skin. New York: Raven Press, 1989.

Chapter 3
Photoaging

Anusuya A. Mokashi and Noah S. Scheinfeld

Introduction

The composition, structure, and organization of the skin change with age. This skin aging is a result of the combination of intrinsic and extrinsic factors (external insults). Intrinsic factors are related to the natural aging process. Grossly, intrinsically aged skin is smooth, pale, and finely wrinkled. The most important extrinsic factor in increasing the aged appearance of the skin (so called photoaging) is the ultraviolet (UV) radiation contained in sunlight. This chapter discusses the effects of solar radiation on the skin including photoaging.

Historical Aspects of Skin Exposure to Solar Radiation

The concept of environmental factors as a cause of skin damage was first empirically recognized in the late nineteenth century by Unna and Dubreuilh. Unna and Dubreuilh observed that farmers and sailors, who spent most of their time in the sun, developed "Seemannshaut," or "sailor's skin." It was later observed in the early 1900s that farmers showed an increased incidence of skin cancer [1–3].

Epidemiology

UV radiation is thought to be the mechanism by which the sun causes skin damage as well as skin cancer. The most important mechanism in this regard is the generation of single strand defects due to UVB. The equator is where the UV intensity is greatest, and where the highest mortality from melanoma is observed. The extent of UV damage experienced by an individual also depends on skin color. Even in similar geographic locations, the incidence of melanomas in light-skinned individuals is several times higher than darker skinned individuals [4]

The influence of the sun is also highly dependent on the subject's age. There is an association of increasing age and sun exposure with the development of cutaneous elastosis and telangiectasias [5]. In one study, sun related aging of skin was observed

R.A. Norman (ed.), *Diagnosis of Aging Skin Diseases,*
© Springer-Verlag London Limited 2008

to increase proportionally with age up to a certain point. For example, at age 12, sun exposure influences were determined to account for 2% of variation in skin pattern versus 17.6% in persons at the age of 16, possibly due to a cumulative effect of sun exposure. By a mean age of 71 however, in a study by Leung et al., a cumulative effect due specifically to sun exposure was no longer measurable. This may be due to the overwhelming influence of genetic factors at this age. Genetic influence on skin pattern deterioration initially is inversely proportional to age, and later in life is a dominant factor. For example, in one study, genetic factors were shown to have 86% influence on skin pattern at age 12, but 62% influence at age 47 [6].

Elastosis and telangiectasia development, characteristics of aging skin, also depend on age and gender. Telangiectasia development is strongly associated more with men than women. Elastosis as a marker of sun-damage is strongly associated in persons below age 60, however the association disappears above the age of 60. Explanation of this relative association can be explained by intrinsic age related increase of elastosis. (Fig. 3.1) For example, when analyzing the skin of persons in a similar age group below the age of 60, a wide range of the appearance of aged skin is observed depending on skin type and amount of exposure to extrinsic influences. With increasing age, however, the standard deviation of the appearance of aging skin narrows, and by age 90, most of the skin looks similar, regardless of extrinsic influences. After the age of 60, the baseline percentage of elastosis due to intrinsic causes has increased to an extent that makes it difficult to distinguish between low and high

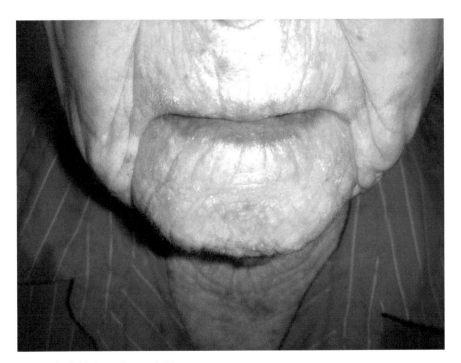

Fig. 3.1 Wrinkled sun-damaged skin

sun exposure. Telangiectasia development due to sun exposure in contrast is only apparent in persons above the age of 50. A possible explanation of this association has been attributed to the increased atrophy of aging skin, making telangiectasia more visible (Table 3.1) [7].

Ultraviolet Light

The ultraviolet A and B light in sunlight promote photoaging. These effects vary proportionally to the intensity, duration, and frequency of exposure, and range from

Table 3.1 Skin types

	Sun history	Skin appearance	Eye appearance	Hair color	Example
Type I	Always burns in the sun/never gets tan/extremely sensitive skin	Fair skin/freckles	Blue/light colored	Usually blonde or red	Celtic, Irish-Scots
Type II	Almost always burns, sometimes turns into a tan/tans minimally/very sensitive skin	Fair skin	Light–dark colored	Light brown hair to brown	Caucasians
Type III	Usually tans/sometimes burns/sun sensitive	Medium skin	Medium–dark colored	Light brown to brown	Caucasians, Asians
Type IV	Seldom burns/moderate tan	Olive skin	Dark	Brown or black	Mediterranean Caucasians, Asian, or Hispanic
Type V	Almost never burns/tans well	Dark skin	Dark eyes	Dark hair	Mediterranean, Hispanic, light skin African-American
Type VI	Never burns/deeply pigmented, sun insensitive skin	Very dark skin	Dark eyes	Usually black hair	African-Americans

the acute effects such as erythema, photosensitivity, and immunologic reactions to long-term effects of photoaging and carcinogenesis [8]. Exposure to sunlight has a cumulative effect on skin changes and is referred to as photoaging or photo-damage. Both the epidermal and dermal layers of the skin are affected by sun exposure, thus accounting for the development of melanoma, squamous cell carcinomas, actinic keratoses, multiple sclerosis, and basal cell carcinomas (Fig. 3.2) and seborrheic keratoses (Fig. 3.3).

This energy travels via radiation in various frequencies and wavelengths and is known as electromagnetic energy. The entire scope of electromagnetic energy is known as the electromagnetic spectrum. Regions of spectrum in the order of increasing wavelength and decreasing frequency are as follows: gamma rays, x-rays, UV, visible light, infrared, microwaves, and radio waves.

The electromagnetic spectrum is classified as either ionizing or non-ionizing radiation depending on their frequency and energy. While ionizing radiation create ionization (positively or negatively charged molecules or atoms) by breaking atomic bonds, non-ionizing radiation have photon energy too weak to break atomic bonds. The solar spectrum encompasses a large portion of the electromagnetic spectrum including mostly a small amount of UV light, all visible light, and some infrared and is classified as non-ionizing radiation. The energy of a photon of non-ionizing radiation is inversely proportional to its wavelength and defines its ability to interact with a given molecule. Photon energy exerts its effect on biologic systems by being absorbed by molecules that are involved in complex cellular interactions. For example, a molecule that absorbs photon energy is raised to an excited state, and in the process of dissipating this energy to return to its resting state, creates a chemical change which can result in biologic alterations.

Specifically UVB (290–320 nm) is responsible for sunburn that results after acute overexposure to sunlight. A sun burn represents damage to the epidermal and dermal

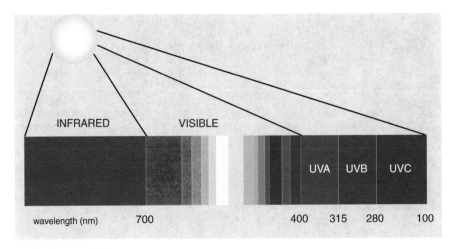

Fig. 3.2 Types of light

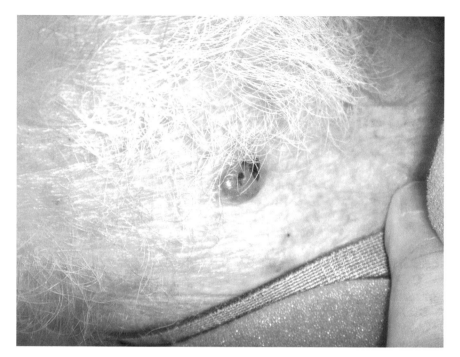

Fig. 3.3 Basal cell carcinoma

layers of the skin including dermal blood vessels and sweat glands. Thermoregulatory components, and cellular changes also occur that are not visible. The cellular changes include damage to the membrane and impaired DNA, RNA, and protein. In addition, cytokines and inflammatory mediators are released.. Visibly, after sun exposure, clinical affects are apparent within 2–6 h that manifests as erythema, and becomes maximal within 24 h. If damage is sufficient enough, skin peeling can occur within 48 h. In milder reactions, skin peeling occurs later.

Biological damage as a result of UVR include: DNA photo-damage, infiltration of inflammatory cells, induction of photoaging-associated proteolytic enzymes, keratinocyte proliferation, and immune suppression [9].

After UV exposure significant to cause a sunburn, inflammatory cells infiltrate the skin and neutrophilic granulocytes are present [10]. Neutrophils produce proteolytic enzymes, such as neutrophil elastase and matrix metalloproteinase 9, which are capable of causing extracellular matrix damage. MMP-1 is produced by karatinocytes and fibroblasts and is most often associated with extracellular matrix damage in the pathogenesis of photoaging. UV radiation can activate keratinocytes hand induce hyperproliferation in vivo resulting in increased epidermal thickness, possibly adaptive by creating a more effective physical barrier.

Usually when photoaging is discussed, the population most often referred to are Caucasians or lighter skinned people. Due to a higher melanin content and a different melanosomal dispersion pattern in the epidermis, black skin has been observed to be more resistant to the deleterious effects of UV radiation. This topic is discussed further under the subheading of melanin.

Cancer

The most common etiological factor towards the development of skin cancer is UVR exposure, evidenced by a 2.4-fold increase in incidence of SCC among people who live close to the equator compared to those in higher altitudes. DNA damage and cellular disruption from UVB (290–320 nm), UVA (320–400 nm), UVA1 (340–400 nm), and UVC (200–290 nm) can result in NMSC and melanoma. The ozone layer absorbs UVC, and therefore at present is not important in inducing skin cancer from sunlight.

UVB causes mutations, immunosuppressive and immunomodulatory affects all which contribute to photocarcinogenesis. These include, affecting the regulation of apoptosis, the expression of cell-surface receptors, and the production of soluble mediators. The most important event in the initiation of skin tumors however is that UVB induces DNA damage that disrupts oncogene and tumor suppressor gene expression.

UVB causes a very specific mutation in that it is absorbed by pyrimidine bases in DNA and induces cis–syn diasteroemer formation of cyclobutant-type pyrimidine dimmers and pyrimidine pyrimidone lesions and their alkali-iable Dewar valence isomers [11]. The result is the covalent association of adjacent pyrimidines and usually occur in areas of consecutive pyrimidine residues. The placement and frequency of mutations depend on the nucleotide flanking the mutation and are three times more likely to result in the formation of pyrimidine dimmers compared to the cylcobutane dimmers. The primary event in the induction of most skin cancer is the formation of thymidine dimmers and photoproducts including SCC and BCC. Although this mechanism has not been documented in the induction of melanoma, it is also thought to be a factor.

These pyrimidine dimmers occasionally remain unrepaired or are incorrectly repaired leading to mutations very specific to UVB damage. Such errors are when a cytosine is incorrectly changed to thymine and occur often when two cytosines are adjacent or a cytosine is adjacent to a thymine.

Another form of UVB damage involve the production of reactive oxygen species (ROS), such as hydrogen peroxide, superoxide anions and singlet oxygens. ROS damage results in single strand breaks in DNA, purine base modifications, and alkai-labile sites. Evidence of ROS damage have been found in cells from skin cancer-prone patients with dysplastic nevus syndrome and basal cell nevus syndrome [12–15].

Immunosuppression is also a result of UVR that occurs locally as well as systemically. A demonstration of the local immunosuppression that occurs is the loss of hypersensitivity to a sensitizing dose of a hapten that occurs after UVR is given. Langerhans cells are observed to fall in number while T-suppressor lymphocytes increase in number. UVR can also directly affect lymphocytes by (a) the induction of apoptosis, (b) altering the expression of cell-surface receptors, and (c) leading to the production of soluble mediators which can lead to changes in their function and distribution. It has been noted that systemic effects of UVB can interfere with a natural host control mechanism and result in cancer at distant sites. IL-10 is the cytokine responsible for UV-induced immunosuppression. Inflammatory cells that produce IL-10 infiltrate the epidermis after erythemogenic doses of UV, and may be involved in skin carcinogenesis.

Other areas of UVB damage include the stimulation of phospholipase A (1 or 2) and lysophospholipase production which in turn has profound effects of UVB-induced inflammation and control of cell growth in human skin and may play a role in the promotion stage of carcinogenesis.

UVA is also carcinogenic, and although it makes up 90–95% of the UVR that reaches human skin, is not as efficient probably by orders of magnitude. UVA radiation affects both epidermal and dermal chromophores [16]. UVA-mediated damage can occur indirectly absorption by non-DNA endogenous sensitizers, generating ROS, which can cause further damage as mentioned above with UVB. The DNA product associated with UVA damage is 8-hydroxyguanine, which is highly mutagenic.

Other effects of UVA include phospholipase activation, stimulation of arachadonic acid release and cylooxygenase activity and protein kinase C activity. UVA also can transiently disrupt gap junctional communications in keratinocytes. The ROS-related point mutations (e.g., G–T) that occur from UVB and UVA damage can result in genetic changes and frame-shifts.

Photo-sensitizers such as oral psoralen and methotrexate can compound UVA damage and increase the likelihood of the induction of skin cancer.

UVA and UVB damage play a role in carcinogenesis largely by their effect on tumor suppressor gene p53, the most commonly mutated tumor suppressor gene. P53 mutations are present in more than 50% of breast, lung and colon cancer and more than 90% of SCC and in most basal cell carcinomas. P53 mutations are also found in most actinic keratoses. BCC often correlate with PTCH mutations in addition to p53 defects.

Melanin

Higher epidermal melanin content and different melanosomal dispersion pattern is thought to function as a barrier to sun damage, protecting basal keratinocytes and the dermis beneath. Melanin is concentrated at the apical pole of basal keratinocytes, and photo-damage above this layer are equal in whites and blacks, however dermal cells in black-skinned individuals are far better protected [15].

For example, the appearance of thymine dimers was shown to be significantly greater in the upper dermis of white skin compared to black skin after the same amount of sun-simulating radiation (SSR) exposure. In addition after, equal exposure of SSR, neutrophil elastase MMP-9 and MMP-1 was detected in white skin and not in black skin. In black skin there was an absence of neutrophilic infiltrate and MMP-9 and MMP-1 cells, while they were abundant in white skin irradiated with equal or lower SSR dose [15].

It has also been noted that erythemogenic doses are required to induce neutrophils and MMP-9 and MMP-1, and much higher doses of SSR are required to induce erythema in black skin, possibly explaining the increased resistance to photoaging in black skin. Higher doses of SSR are necessary to induce infiltrating neutrophils, which release active proteolytic enzymes contributing to photoaging [15].

Skin changes after exposure to SSR of 12,000–10,000 mJ/cm^2 in white skin were DNA photo-damage in the epidermis and dermis; infiltrating neutrophils; the presence of enzymatically active neutrophil elastase, MMP-0 or MMP-1; activation of keratinocytes, and IL-10 positive cells in the epidermis. In black skin DNA damage was limited to the supra-basal epidermis and no other changes were observed [15].

Immunosuppression as a result of UV exposure correlates to the degree of erythemal reactivity. Lighter skin shows increased erythemal response, while darker skin demonstrates weak or no erythemal response. Those that do not have an erythemal response do not show signs of immunosuppression.

Thus a lack of IL-10 producing inflammatory cells in the epidermis was noted in black skin after SSR that did not produce erythema in black skin, but did in white skin [15].

Hyperproliferative keratinocytes, as induced by UV exposure, express different set of cytokeratins from basal and differentiating keratinocytes, enabling evaluation by immunochemical staining. The hyperproliferative keratinocytes express cytokeratins K6, K16, and K17; while basal express K5, K14; and differentiating display K1, K2, and K10. It was noted that hyperproliferation was noted in white skin, however absent in black skin after equal SSR exposure.

Genetics

Environmental influence acts on genetic predisposition. Shekar et al. conclude from a study performed on 332 monozygotic twins and 488 dizygotic twin pairs that sun exposure contributed to only 3.4% of variation in skin pattern, while genetic factors explained up to 86% of variation in skin pattern [6].

Factors of aging thought to be controlled by genetic endowment include hemoglobin levels and melanin content, and have been shown to be protective factors and is inversely proportional to the progression of aging skin [6].

Additive and Non-additive Effects of Genetics

The MC1R gene is associated with phenotypic traits such as red hair, fair skin, and lack of tanning ability and is a recessive trait, accounting for non-additive genetic effect of skin color. Additive genetic effects on skin color are thought to be because of genes for melanocyte formation, and thus the melanin content. Melanin may also harbor protective effects on its possible association with dermal elastosis. Of genetic factors on skin pattern, 26% is thought to be explained by skin color at age 12, versus

2.2% correlation with sun exposure. Dermal elastosis is thought to factor between 4 and 21% of skin pattern variation.

It is hypothesized that the protective influence of melanin on the progression of skin aging arises from structural differences in melanosomes. In addition, melanin has been shown to demonstrate free radical scavenging properties also contributing to its photo-protective effects. In dark skin persons, a 100-fold increased photo-protective effect against non-melanoma skin cancer has been noted.

Histology

Photo-damage is analyzed by six histological signs based on the Beagley–Gibson rating. These patterns are based on the evenness, clarity, and depth of primary and secondary lines of the skin [17]. The resulting conditions of photo-damaged skin include actinic keratoses, solar elastosis, and non-melanotic skin cancer.

The epidermal layer of the skin is primarily composed of melanocytes and keratinocytes. It has been hypothesized that the rate of skin pattern deterioration may be due to histological differences in melanocytes and melanosomes.

Chronically aged skin results in a reduced synthesis of collagen types I and III. This feature is magnified in photo-damaged skin. UV radiation results in the up-regulation of collagen-degrading matrix metalloproteinases (MMPs) at a faster rate than aging alone. In addition to the destruction of collagen compared to sun-protected skin, there is decreased collagen synthesis. When compared to young skin (age 18–29), type I procollagen, a marker of ongoing collagen synthesis, was decreased by 68% in older skin (80+ years). In addition, when comparing collagen structure between aged and young skin, fiber bundles were observed to be thicker with less open space within and between bundles in the papillary dermis of young skin. Aged skin showed open spaces interspersed with criss-crossing, tangled, thin fibers in the papillary dermis. Fiber bundle orientation was mostly lost. Cell shape in young skin is noted to be more spread. Similar results are seen through the layers of the dermis including the deeper layers of the (reticular) dermis as well. It has also been observed two-dimensionally that fibroblasts had greater surface area contact with collagen fibrils than old skin [18].

Solar elastosis, also known as dermal elastosis (the accumulation of elastotic material in the dermis) is the histological feature specific to photoaging. The elastotic material includes changes in elastin (the principal component of the elastic fibers), and extracellular-matrix components normally present in the skin. In photo-damaged skin, there is a disturbance of the organization of these structures and their function. Photo-damaged skin shows increased activation of the elastin gene. It is thought that this may be due to transcriptional activation of the gene as a result of the influence of cytokines, such as transforming growth factor β and various interleukin [19].

It has recently been shown in a study by Battistuta et al. that skin surface topography grading assessed by silicone impressions correlates with dermal elastosis and can be used as a tool for assessing photoaging [20].

Increased sun exposure also leads to an increased incidence of skin cancer. Epidemiologic studies correlating chronic sun exposure with skin cancer in the twentieth century showed that skin cancer correlated with chronic sun exposure, specifically through UVR damage. UVR was found to cause immunologic changes, cellular changes, and molecular events, all which lead to UVR induced skin carcinogenesis.

The effects of photo-damage vary depending on race and gender. Both Caucasians and Koreans feature wrinkling as a major manifestation of photoaging. It has been empirically observed however that dyspigmentation patterns differ between Korean sexes. While seborrheic keratosis is the major lesion in Korean men, hyperpigmented macules predominate in Korean women [21]. Although wrinkling is a sign of photo-damage in Asians, the appearance of skin wrinkling is not readily apparent until about age 50, and the degree is less than in Caucasian skin. In addition wrinkling patterns in Asians appear different than Caucasians. While caucasians show fine wrinkles on cheeks and crow's feet area, Asians have coarser, thicker and deeper wrinkles concentrated on the forehead, perioral, and Crow's feet areas [22].

Elderly of Different Racial Groups

In the United States, Caucasians have 50-fold higher rates of basal and squamous cell carcinomas than African Americans and a 13-fold higher incidence of melanoma than African Americans [23, 24]. Susceptibility differences among ethnicities have been observed, and in a study by Tadokoro et al., differences of UV-induced damage in six different ethnicities were studied. It was found that levels of DNA damage after equivalent UV radiation was in descending order as follows: White skin, Asian skin, Hispanic skin, Black or African American skin. This was shown to inversely correlate with melanin content amongst the different ethnicities. Interestingly, melanin was fourfold higher in Black skin than White skin, although DNA damage was seven to eightfold lower in Black skin than White skin; suggesting that in addition to absolute melanin content, other factors such as melanin distribution play a factor in susceptibility to photo-damage. For example, it was noted that while an African American individual visually appeared to have pigmentation differences by over 20-fold than a White individual, the actual melanin content difference between the two individuals was only sevenfold.This was contributed to different pigment distribution patterns.

Another factor important to photo-carcinogenesis is the efficiency of DNA repair. It is of note that no association was noted between DNA repair rates and skin type. There were no differences in DNA repair between melanocytes that were highly pigmented compared to those that were less pigmented [23].

Manifestations of Photoaging

Photoaging manifest as prematurely aged skin in sun-exposed areas of the skin. A simple manifestation of this phenomenon is that non-sun-exposed areas of the arms are invariably more pale, less wrinkled, and less populated by skin lesions than the sun-exposed areas of the arm. Photoaging is the result of UVB damage to the epidermis and UVA damage to the middle layers of the dermis, and preferentially affect those with fair skin. The result of photo-damage is the appearance of severe wrinkles, dyspigmentation, such as solar lentigos and mottled pigmentation, and textural changes.

A thinning of the epidermis occurs and becomes more susceptible to blistering, tears, and grazes. Skin also loses its ability to hold water and becomes dry. Damage to elastin protein results in tangled masses of damaged elastin protein that create elastosis, or thickened bumps. Additionally, repeated inflammation as a result of sunburn causes increased dermal collagen and a loss of dermal elasticity, creating weaker skin.

UV radiation produces visible skin changes such as texture changes (solar elastosis), blood vessel changes (telengiectasias), pigment changes (solar lentigo), skin bumps, and skin cancer.

Idiopathic guttate hypomelanosis are 2–5 mm flat white spots of unknown cause. Although their origins are not proven, it is known that they appear with age and are possibly caused by photo-damage. They most commonly are found on shins and sun-exposed parts of the forearms, however can appear on the face, neck, and shoulders. They commonly appear in persons over 40 years of age, and are more common in women. There may be some genetic factors and they appear to be more common amongst family members. They also have been observed to occur at an earlier age in fair-skinned women. While the etiology of idiopathic guttate hypomelanosis is still controversial, one study showed that a woman developed the lesion after UVB treatment for mycosis fungoides, correlating the etiology with photo-damage [25].

Hypopigmented areas greater than 5 mm are called macular hypomelanosis and can be less white and less well demarcated. The two disorders are thought to be related along a spectrum of depigmentation [26].

Another hypopigmented characteristic of photoaged skin is the occurrence of stellate pseudoscars. Stellate pseudoscars (Fig. 3.4) are linear scars that occur from tearing of fragile photo-damaged skin and are commonly seen with senile purpura. Solar damage also results in belphrochalasis and lid laxity that can have a yellow color. Just as the skin thins and becomes fragile, aging also results in blood vessels that are easily disrupted causing senile purpura.

It has been empirically observed that persons over 25–30 years of age express with each decade of aging 10–20% fewer enzymatically active melanocytes are present, although sun-exposed skin was seen as having approximately twice as many pigment cells as unexposed skin. It is theorized that sun exposure may stimulate the melanocyte system resulting in hyperpigmented areas of the skin. The

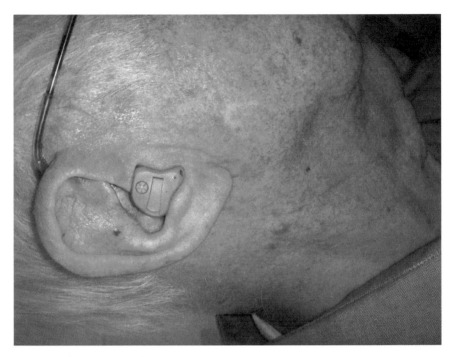

Fig. 3.4 White Stellate Pseudoscar

latter coupled with the decrease in melanocytes may explain the resulting hetero-geneous pigment distribution in areas of exposed skin. Hyperpigmented lesions of sun-exposed skin include ephelides, actinic lentigo, pigmented solar keratosis and seborrheoic keratoses, and lentigo maligna. Poikiloderma of Civatte (Fig. 3.5) has also been observed in photo-damaged skin (Table 3.2). Its etiology is unknown however, although theories of contributing factors include fair skin, accumulated sun exposure, photo-sensitizing components of cosmetics and toiletries especially perfumes, and hormonal factors. Affected skin appears red–brown with prominent hair follicles and occurs and the sides and front of the neck sparing the sun-protected area under the chin. The skin is thin, and often has telengiectasias. It occurs most commonly in fair-skinned females and effects middle aged and elderly individuals.

In addition to texture, blood vessels, and pigment changes caused by the sun, flesh colored cutaneous papules (skin bumps) are also caused by the sun. Precancerous lesions called actinic keratosis are small crusty bumps that develop on the face, ears, and backs of hands. One in hundred cases per year develop into squamous cell carcinoma. Seborrheic keratoses, also a result of UV radi-ation, are not precancerous and are warty lesions that appear to be "stuck" on the skin.

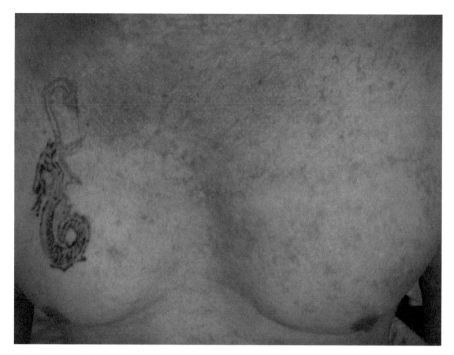

Fig. 3.5 Poilkiloderma of Civettee

Table 3.2 Visual changes in skin in the aging process

Intrinsic process	Extrinsic process	Attributable to both
Smooth, pale and fine wrinkled skin	Ephelides, actinic lentigo, pigmented solar keratosis and seborrhoeic keratoses, and coarsely wrinkled and associated with dyspigmentation and telengiectasias. Senile or solar purpura	Poikiloderma of civatte Idiopathic guttate hypomelanosis

Conclusion

Skin aging is a result of two clinically and biologically processes that occur simultaneously. The first process, innate or intrinsic aging occurs to skin just as it occurs to all organs, by a slow irreversible degeneration of tissue and occurs all over the skin Extrinsic aging, or photoaging is the second process and is primarily a result of UV irradiation. The photoaging process compounds damage from innate aging, and occurs in areas exposed to the sun, such as the face and the backs of hands.

It has been suggested that as much as 80% of facial aging can be attributable to sun exposure [27].

Effects of the sun on the skin include visible as well as microscopic changes in the skin. Visible changes in the skin include texture changes, blood vessel changes, pigment changes, skin bumps, and skin cancer.

Mechanisms of DNA damage induced by UV radiation has been shown to be critical in skin photo-carcinogenesis, and racial/ethnic origin plays a role in susceptibility to UV damage. There is an inverse relationship between melanin content the extent of DNA damage after UV radiation. The relationship between DNA damage/repair and melanin content and distribution in individuals of different ethnicities varies and plays a role in the manifestations of photo-damage [28].

References

1. Urbach F, Forbes PD, Davies RE, Berger D. Cutaneoush photobiology: past, present and future. J. Invest. Dermatol. 1976; 67: 209–24.
2. Unna PG. Die Histopathologie der Hauptkrankheiten. Berling: August Hirschwald, 1894.
3. Hyde JN, On the influence of light in the production of skin cancer. Am. J. Med. Sci. 1906; 1311: 1–22.
4. Farmer KC, Naylor MF. Sun exposure, sunscreens, and skin cancer prevention: a year-round concern. Ann. Pharmacother. 1996; 30: 662–73.
5. Yaar M, Eller MS, Gilchrest BA. Fifty years of skin aging. J. Invest. Dermatol. Symp. Proc. 2002; 7: 51–8.
6. Shekar SN, Luciano M, Duffy DL, Marin NG. Genetic and environmental influences on skin pattern deterioration. J. Invest. Dermatol. 2005; 125: 1119–29.
7. Kennedy C, Bastiaens MT, Bajdik CD. Effect of smoking and sun on the aging skin. J. Invest. Dermatol. 2003; Apr 120(4): 548–54.
8. Taylor CR, Sober AJ. Sun exposure and skin disease. Annu. Rev. Med. 1996; 47: 181–91.
9. Rijken F, Bruijnzeel PLB, Weelden Hv, Kiekens RCM. Responses of Black and white skin to solar-stimulating radiation: differences in DNA photodamage, infiltrating neutrophils, proteolytic enzymes induced, keratinocyte activation, and IL-10 Expression. J. Invest. Dermatol. 2004; 122: 1448–55.
10. McGregor B, Pfitzner J, Zhu G, et al. Genetic and environmental contributions to size, color, shape, and other characteristics of melanocytic naevi in a sample of adolescent twins. Genet. Epidemiol. 1999; 16: 40–53.
11. Peak MJ, Peak JG, Carnes BA. Induction of direct and indirect single-strand breaks in human cell DNA by far- and near-ultraviolet radiations: action spectrum and mechanisms. Photochem. Photobiol. 1987; 45: 381–7.
12. Runger TM, Epe B, Moller K. Processing of directly and indirectly ultraviolet-induced DNA damage in human cells. Recent Results Cancer Res. 1995; 139: 31–42.
13. Danpure HJ, Tyrrell RM. Oxygen-dependence of newar UV (365 NM) lethality and the interaction of near UV and X-rays in two mammalian cell lines. Photochem. Photobiol. 1976; 23: 171–7.
14. Runger TM, Epe B, Moller K, Dekant B, Hellfritsch D. Repair of directly and indirectly UV-induced dysplastic nevus syndrome or basal cell nevus syndrome. Recent Results Cancer Res. 1997; 143: 337–51.
15. Simeonova PP, Luster MI. Mechanisms of arsenic carcinogenicity: genetic or epigenetic mechanisms? J. Environ. Pathol. Toxicol. Oncol. 2000; 19: 281–6.
16. Krutman J. Photocarcinogenesis. Schweiz. Rundsch. Med. Prax. 2001; 90: 297–9.

17. Holman CD, Armstrong BK, Evans PR, et al. Relationship of solar keratosis and history of skin cancer to objective measures of actinic skin damage. Br. J. Dermatol. 1984; 110: 129–38.
18. Varani J, Dame MK, Rittie L. Decreased collagen production in chronologically aged skin: roles of age-dependent alteration in fibroblast function and defective mechanical stimulation. Am. J. Path. 2006; 168(6): 1861–1868.
19. Uitto J. Understanding premature skin aging. N. Engl. J. Med. 1997; 337: 1463–65.
20. Battistuta D, Pandeya N, Strutton GM. Skin surface topography grading is a valid measure of skin photoaging. Photodermatol. Photoimmunol. Photomed. 2006; 22: 39–45.
21. Chung JH, Lee SH, Youn CS, Park BJ, Kim KH, Park KC, Cho KH, Eun HC. Cutaneous photodamage in Koreans: influence of sex, sun exposure, smoking, and skin color. Arch. Dermatol. 2001; 137: 1043–51.
22. Chung JH. Photoaging in Asians. Photodermatol. Photoimmunol. Photomed. 2003; 19: 109–21. Review.
23. Tadokoro T, Kobayashi N, Zmudzka BZ, Ito S, Wakamatsu K, Yamaguchi Y, Korossy KS, Miller SA, Beer JZ, Hearing VJ. UV-induced DNA damage and melanin content in human skin differing in racial/ethnic origin. FASEB J. 2003; 17: 1177–9.
24. Halder RM, Bridgeman-Shah S. Skin cancer in African Americans. Cancer 1995; 75(2 Suppl.): 667–73.
25. Kaya TI, Yazici AC, Tursen U, Ikizoglu G. Idiopathic guttate hypomelanosis: idiopathic or ultraviolet induced? Photodermatol. Photoimmunol. Photomed. 2005; 21: 270–1.
26. Pagnoni A, Kligman AM, Sadiq I, Stoudemayer T. Hypopigmented macules of photodamaged skin and their treatment with topical tretinoin. Acta Derm. Venereol. 1999; 79: 305–10.
27. Kadunce DP, Burr R, Gress R, Kanner R, Lyon JL, Zone JJ. Cigarette smoking: risk factor for premature facial wrinkling. Ann. Intern. Med. 1991; 114: 840–4.
28. Ortonne JP. The effects of ultraviolet exposure on skin melanin pigmentation. J. Int. Med. Res. 1990; 18(Suppl. 3): 8C–17C.

Chapter 4

Aging and the Skin: The Geriatrician's Perspective

T. S. Dharmarajan

Introduction: An Aging Society

With changes in life expectancy in the last century, individuals tend to live longer. The life expectancy of a female born today in the United States is more than 80 years and that of a male is more than 74 years. The life expectancy is even higher in Italy, Sweden and Greece. Over the next 30 years, projections in the United States and Europe indicate that the over 65-year age group would be double the number of today. With aging of the population, there will also be widening of the disease spectrum, with the skin being no exception. Longevity, coupled with the development of illnesses, deficiency states—exposure to drugs, toxins and environmental insults provides a perfect backdrop for the most exposed organ of the aging individual, the skin, to deteriorate. Skin disorders may be most obvious or not apparent at all, and may be innocuous or suggest a fatal disease. Skin disease may impair quality of life and inflict social consequences.

While one should not be surprised at the many skin disorders likely to be encountered in the geriatric population, one wonders about the role of the primary health provider or geriatrician who takes care of older individuals over decades. Most primary providers are no experts in the diagnosis of dermatological illness, leave alone develop a meaningful differential diagnosis. All too often, the tendency is to ignore a lesion or refer the individual to a dermatologist. The following provides a broad perspective and general considerations that may be borne in mind when evaluating a geriatric patient with skin abnormalities; it is no replacement for many excellent narratives that are available, and some referenced here.

Aging in general is accompanied by changes in all organs including the skin. A simple way of expressing the physiological changes with age is the use of a 1% percent rule, with most organ functions peaking in the twenties and thirties, and a gradual decline of 1% occurring each year. This decline is easily measurable with certain organs such as the estimation of creatinine clearance for renal function. Changes in the body with age also include a decline in the water compartment, an increase in lipid stores, decline in muscle mass (sarcopenia) and bone mass (osteoporosis) besides declines in other organs. These physiological changes and decline in reserves are usually compounded by disease processes or comorbidity [1]. The

R.A. Norman (ed.), *Diagnosis of Aging Skin Diseases,*
© Springer-Verlag London Limited 2008

skin is no exception to physiological deterioration. Alterations in function form a basis for changes in the manner that the body handles medications (kinetics) and drug effect on the receptors (dynamics) [2].

The Aging Skin

Skin changes occur with age and as a result of numerous insults it is exposed to from within and from the environment over time. Most of the visible changes in the skin are in response to sunlight exposure rather than from chronological age per se [3]. The most consistent changes with age are flattening of the dermo-epidermal junction with the stratum corneum remaining intact. Alterations in lipid content compromise the barrier function. A decline in mast cells, fibroblasts, melanocytes and Langerhans cells as also glandular function (involving both sweat and sebaceous glands) occur. Cell replacement, barrier function and sensory perception decline with age. The slow epidermal turnover contributes to delay in wound healing [4], [5]. Immune function is compromised because of decline in activity of Langerhans cells and kertinocytes [5]. Loss of melanocytes leads to susceptibility to UV irradiation and DNA damage [5] (Table 4.1).

Atrophy and heterogeneity are features of aging; variations result from changes in anatomy and function of blood and lymphatic vessels, from insults during life.

Table 4.1 Age-related skin changes

Alterations in skin structure and function
Flattening of the dermo-epidermal junction
Decline in sweat and sebaceous gland activity (result dryness)
Decline in melanin production (melanocyte function)
Decline in immune function (Langerhan cells)
Decline in fibroblasts
Decline in mast cells and activity
Decline in elasticity of skin
Delay in wound healing
Altered barrier function due to changes in lipid content
Decline in production of vitamin D with age
May relate to amount of sunlight exposure
Influenced by pigmentation, clothing, sunscreens, age
Consequence in bone, muscle, elsewhere
Estrogen deficiency related (menopause)
Changes involve skin, mucous membrane, vagina, vulva, urethra, hair
Alterations in wound healing
Hair count, texture and loss (age or disease?)
Hair density maximum at birth, diminishes to half by third decade
Hair loss may be idiopathic, local or systemic process, medication effect
Hirsutism (increase in hair) common with age, more noticeable in women
Graying of hair a normal event, occurs in men and women
Onset of graying variable with race

Responses to injury are complex and involve cytokines, growth factors and immune surveillance systems [6].

Changes may occur as a result of intrinsic aging and photo-aging; the latter refers to premature skin changes cause by chronic exposure to solar ultraviolet (UV) radiation. Ultra violet A and B can be present in artificial sources besides sunlight; unlike UVB, UVA is transmitted through glass [7]. Photo-aging is characterized by wrinkles, pigmentation and rough texture along with functional changes. Cigarette smoking exacerbates both forms of skin change, resulting in wrinkling and discoloration, but also increases the prevalence of skin cancer [5]. Alterations with age from photo-aging can be minimized by decreasing UV exposure, and use of sunscreens, estrogens, antioxidants, all-transretinoic and alpha-hydroxy acids [5].

Aging is accompanied by alterations in barrier functions involving dryness, scaling and abnormal drug delivery through the skin; changes may also relate to inflammatory insults [8]. Intrinsic aging is aggravated by superimposed photo-aging [8]. Pruritus and dry skin are extremely common with age. A decline in sebaceous and sweat gland activity in the older skin predisposes to dryness, and is termed xerosis; the problem is worse in winter and predisposes to cracking and infections. The condition can be partially ameliorated by the use of ammonium lactate [9]. Other preventive measures include the use of humidifiers, control of environmental temperature, use of lotions after showers, and minimizing use of hot, long showers and irritant soaps [9].

Postmenopausal skin elasticity was noted to decline annually by 0.55% in a Japanese study; this alteration was negated by hormone replacement therapy, using conjugated estrogen and medroxyprogesterone acetate, a combination which increased elasticity by 5.2% over a year [10]. Interestingly, age also appears to influence the presence of perioral wrinkles, furrows, dryness and even dimensions of the lips. The postmenopausal skin is characterized by dry hair, alopecia, thinning and decline in lubrication, all changes reversible with estrogen. Sebum production also declines in the postmenopausal state [11] although it is not clear that the use of estrogen alters this decline. The effects of estrogen on the skin are interesting but not substantiated in large studies.

Aging is accompanied by a decline in vitamin D synthesis, demonstrated in experiments involving older skin [12]. Most body requirements for vitamin D are derived from synthesis in the skin rather than through diet or fortified food. On exposure to sunlight, 7-dehydrocholesterol in the skin is converted to cholecalciferol, which is then hydroxylated in the liver. Vitamin D synthesis is influenced by several factors, including exposure to sunlight, duration of exposure and time of day, degree of pigmentation (darker skin less effective), amount of clothing worn and extent of skin exposure, use of sunscreens and latitude, among other factors [13]. This is one condition where dermatological manifestations are not evident, but deficiency is detrimental. One such consequence affects quality of life, causing gait and balance disorders and falls, resulting in fractures. A recent study in our geriatric clinic demonstrated that half the older adults with gait disorder and falls had unrecognized vitamin D deficiency until tested for the study!

Hair Loss and Aging

Hair loss from aging or otherwise often attracts attention, and usually bothersome to the patient. The human scalp contains about 100,000 hairs and about half the amount is required to be lost to manifest alopecia (hair loss). Human hair may be large and visible (terminal hair) or small and fine (vellus hair). Hair growth occurs in 3 phases, termed the anagen (growing), transitional (catagen) and preshedding (telogen) phases. Most of the hair is in the anagen phase. Resting hairs are retained for about 100 days; hair loss is replaced by new hair, with about 50 hairs shed daily. An increase in loss to double the amount becomes noticeable. Hair cycles are regulated by many factors, aside from hormonal [14]. While local hair loss indicates injury or infection, it may also be a male pattern of alopecia. Generalized loss may result from systemic disease (e.g. hypothyroidism), adverse drug effect, malnutrition, local or systemic infection, malignant processes, inflammation, or psychiatric disease, all of which are seen in the elderly [15]. Hair density is highest at birth and declines after 1 year to further drop to half the original amount by the third decade. Unwanted and excessive hair growth may also occur with age, involving more than half the older women, with the hair tending to be coarse and wiry, and needing a mechanism for removal [14].

Graying of hair is a universal phenomenon, equally seen in men and women, but onset appears to differ somewhat with race. It begins earlier in the thirties in whites and later in blacks. Graying begins in the scalp to start with and involves the eyebrows, axillary and pubic hair much later [14]. Hair coloring products are an extremely popular industry and are well utilized by the baby boomers of today.

The Lower Limbs and Skin Disorders

In particular, periodic examination of the feet and legs helps detect the presence of infections, ulcerations, vascular changes (arterial or venous) and pre-malignant and malignant changes. Improper footwear may cause structural changes of the foot or nails, and consequent gait abnormalities, little indicating the origin of the problem [9]. The lower limbs are often the location for fungal and bacterial infections, stasis dermatitis, xerosis and venous, arterial, neuropathic or pressure ulcers. Nail changes are particularly common but overlooked. Stasis dermatitis is a consequence of xerosis, pruritus and venous stasis in the lower limbs and one basis for edema; diuretics produce poor results for stasis dermatitis. Infection and inflammation are concurrent; treatment should be directed to methods to counter venous insufficiency and treat infection [9] (Table 4.2).

The differential diagnosis of ulcers in the lower extremities includes pressure ulcer, neuropathic ulcer and vascular (arterial or venous) lesions; management differs with etiology [16]. Venous disease is a common basis [17]; arterial ulcers are the least common but far more painful [16]. The presence of skin ulcers warrants a complete physical examination for connective tissue disease, diabetes, vascular

Table 4.2 Skin disorders involving the legs in the elderly

Leg ulcers
Venous ulcers: most common basis
Neuropathic ulcers: next most likely
Arterial ulcers: least common, but most painful
Pressure ulcers: increased pressure a requirement with restricted mobility
Evaluation includes
Exclude systemic disease (connective tissue, diabetes, etc)
Check the ankle brachial index
Is an unusual infection present, e.g. osteomyelitis?
Is a neoplastic basis possible?
Consider the need for referral to a wound care expert
Skin deformities and nail changes
Relating to foot wear or gait abnormalities?
Brittle nails, tend to break
Fungal infections of nails require treatment for weeks
Attention addressed for moisture and hygiene; keep skin dry
Infections and infestations
Viral, e.g. herpes zoster, herpes simplex
Bacterial: e.g. streptoccal and staphylococcal
Fungal, e.g. candida
Parasitic, e.g. scabies
Skin manifestations may suggest underlying
Malignancy
Diabetes mellitus and other endocrine disorders
Cardiac or pulmonary disease (cyanosis, clubbing)
Connective tissue disorders such as systemic lupus or scleroderma
Bilateral lesions suggest possible medication effect
Nutritional deficiency (A, C, B vitamins or zinc)

and neurological disease. In addition to the pulses, the ankle brachial index is calculated by dividing the systolic pressure in the ankle by the systolic pressure in the arm; the former is higher than the latter, with an acceptable value of 1.1 [17]. A nonhealing ulcer may be indicative of a neoplastic basis, especially when vascular or neuropathic etiolgy appears unlikely. In any case, uncontrolled pain, failure to heal or the presence of persistent pain are reasons for referral to a wound care expert.

The majority of older individuals demonstrate nail changes, if looked for. Nails in the finger soften with age, whereas toe nails become tougher. Trauma contributes to some of these changes; nails may be best trimmed regularly and kept clean. Ingrowing toe nails and onychomycosis (fungal infection) are common. Treatment of fungal infections may be local or systemic antifungals and surgery [18]. Oral antifungals agents require to be used for several months in the treatment of onychomysosis, longer for toe nails than finger nails [19].

Aside from the above, deformities such as hallux valgus and limitus, hammer toes, bunions, mallet toes and claw toes are all noticeable in the geriatric age group.

Wound Healing

Although not universally accepted [20], wound healing and repair undergo delay with advancing age; prevention of injury is hence paramount in the aged. More than age itself, delayed healing may be associated with a variety of factors, including but not restricted to nutrient deficiencies, infections, restricted mobility and systemic illness [21]. Pressure ulcers take months to heal, especially stage 3 or 4 ulcers and entail huge expenses to providers; there is no better example where prevention is better than cure. Healing may be optimized by the use of topical growth factors that promote proliferation and migration of cells in the wound and the use of support surfaces that mitigate the effects of pressure, a key in the development or prevention of pressure ulcers [21]. Age-related delay in cutaneous wound healing has been also linked to decline in estrogen levels following menopause, impairing cytokine signal induction and altering protein balance [22]. Although morbid obesity is much more an issue in younger individuals, excessive weight may be an issue at any age and another dimension that promotes infections and wound dehiscence [23].

One view is that the aging factor causing delay in healing of acute wounds is small; poor healing is a bigger problem for chronic wounds and here the effect is truly related to comorbid processes than the age itself [3]. The impact of delay in wound healing in older adults is relevant in surgical wounds, including timing for removal of sutures; premature removal can cause wound dehiscence. Although historically, healing is said to be impaired in the older subject, it is nevertheless believed that in spite of some delay, the final result is qualitatively as good as in the young [24].

Endocrine Abnormalities

The presence of skin lesions sometimes enable a provider to consider a diagnosis of diabetes. Diabetes has a prevalence of about 25% in older adults; as people live longer eventual pancreatic burnout manifests as diabetes, with type 2 diabetes accounting for the majority of cases. Skin lesions include ulcerations of neuropathic or vascular etiology, xanthomas secondary to hyperlipidemia and classic bilateral symmetrical, pigmented circumscribed lesions over the shin of the tibia; a background of nontraumatic amputations is often apparent [25]. Diabetic xanthomas are red or yellow inflammatory papules seen over the buttocks or elbows; necrobiosis lipoidica are waxy, violaceous patches over the anterior legs that may manifest telengiectasia and ulcerations [25]. Acanthosis nigricans is a velvety dark hyperpigmentation seen in several disorders and not specific to diabetes.

Both hypothyroidism and hyperthyroidism are encountered with aging. The classic, moist warm skin is typical of hyperthyroidism, but less apparent in the elderly, as also the typical ophthalmopathy. Pretibial myxedema, is a form of bilateral, symmetric nonpitting edema seen in hyperthyroidism; it is the most common dermopathy

Table 4.3 Endocrine disorders and skin lesions

Diabetes mellitus:
Acanthosis nigricans
Xanthalesma and xanthomas
Necrobiosis lipoidica
Ulcers: arterial, neuropathic or mixed, pressure ulcers
Infections (bacterial, candida)
Other: drug eruptions, blisters, lipohypertrophy etc
Thyroid disease
Hyperthyroidism:
Classic eye changes and skin changes less common in the elderly
Nonpitting pretibial myxedema
Hypothyrodism
Features mimic or may be superimposed on normal aging
Typical facies, coarse dry skin and hair loss mimics the aged
Adrenal disorders
Hyperadrenalism
Purpura, striae, telengiectasia, bruisability, supraclavicular fat pads
Hypoadrenalism
Pigmentation predominantly in creases, scars, nipples

in this disorder and commonly associated with ophthalmopathy [26]. The facies of aging is sometimes hard to differentiate from hypothyroidism, as both manifest dry, rough skin with coarse, brittle hair and thinning of the eyebrows; aging certainly coexists with hpothyroidism!

The increasing opportunity and indications for use of steroids as one ages, in addition to Cushing's syndrome account for manifestations resulting from excessive cortisol in the body. Aside from the classic manifestations, striae, bruisability, telengiectasia and poor wound healing result from hyperadrenalism and may mimic aging. On the other hand skin and mucosal pigmentation, dominantly in skin creases and scars are consistent with Addison's disease (Table 4.3).

The Skin and Systemic Disease

Several dermatological manifestations of systemic disease have been discussed in other sections. Cutaneous vasculitis not uncommon, but a poorly understood topic. Palpable purpura is a common presentation for necrotizing vasculitis, a feature of inflammatory, malignant or autoimmune processes. Cutaneous manifestations in systemic disease may also represent a paraneoplastic syndrome or gastrointestinal disorder, especially inflammatory bowel disease. Rarely in the elderly, lesions indicate the presence of a neuro-cutaneous disorder involving nervous system and the skin. Cardiac and pulmonary disease, both increasingly common with age can be signaled by the presence of cyanosis, flushing or clubbing.

Nutritional deficiencies are known to present with dermatolgical manifestations, but escape recognition till late stages. Malnutrition is common in the elderly and based on the setting, may be prevalent in up to 50% (A6). While the manifestations of deficiency in vitamins A (coarse dry skin), ascorbic acid (bruisability, bleeding, poor healing), nicotinic acid (dermatitis in sunlight exposed areas) and zinc (alopacea, dermatitis in extremities, poor wound healing) are well described, some micronutrient deficiencies manifest no skin abnormalities. Such is the case of vitamin D deficiency, where the consequences are widespread and go beyond the bone and muscle, but spare the skin although it is the site of vitamin D synthesis [27].

Anemia is extremely common with aging; a third of the anemias in the over 65 age group are nutritional in origin and a third secondary to chronic disease [28, 29]. Pallor, icterus and findings such as purpura or petichae depend on the degree of anemia and its etiology; for example, vitamin B12 deficiency is associated with thrombocytopenia and hemolysis [30]. Recognition of anemia is important in view of the associated morbidity and mortality.

Pruritus or itch is recognized by some to be the most common symptom of skin disorders [31]. The unpleasant symptom, which affects quality of life, is transmitted through unmyelinated C fibers located between dermis and epidermis, and mediated by histamine, serotonin and a host of neuropeptides, cytokines and prostaglandins [31]. Disorders that cause pruritus may be systemic illness, malignancy and hematological disorders, age, psychogenic factors, infections or infestations and medications, and will require additional evaluation to arrive at a diagnosis. Management involves general measures (emollients, cool environment, avoiding long and warm showers, excessive soap) and a variety of topical or systemic therapies [31]. In this regard, drugs such as antihistamines or antidepressants should be used with caution for fear of impairing cognitive function and increasing propensity to falls or accidents.

Infections and Infestations

Older individuals are susceptible to infections and infestations because of alterations in their immune systems. Herpes zoster (shingles) manifests as pain, skin lesions (blisters) or both and occur typically in nerve root distribution. Lesions form over several days; pain can persist (postherpetic neuralgia), a problem that is worse in older age [32]. Prompt use of acyclovir, famciclovir or valacyclovir may decrease the neuralgia, while results with prednisone are inconsistent [32]. Staphylococcal impetigo and streptococcal cellulites are common infections treatable with antibiotics.

Scabies, an infestation due to *Sarcoptes* scabiei, is both under-diagnosed and over-diagnosed; it is common in institutions and spreads through infected linen or skin to skin transmission. Besides the classic sites of involvement (web of the fingers, wrist, genitalia, buttocks), diagnosis involves observing scrapings for the mite. Itching does not occur for weeks as cellular immunity takes time to develop [32]. The immune compromised older adults tend to get crusted scabies, a form of hyperinfection. Effective topical treatment involves use of 5% permethrin, safe and with little toxicity.

Candida intertrigo is a beefy red, painful, erosive patch in the inframammary, gluteal, inguinal and axillary folds due to Candida species thriving in moist environment, especially in the obese or diabetic settings; keeping the skin dry with the use of nystatin or chlortrimazole powder or cream helps [19]. Diaper rash is a variant with the same underlying basis and seen in incontinent patients, in hospitals and long-term care.

Candida infections may also involve dentures and cause stomatitis. Vaginitis with a creamy discharge from candida can be treated with a topical antifungal cream or suppositories or a single oral dose of fluconazole 150 mg [19].

The Skin and Cancer

The incidence of skin cancer increases with age [9]. Cancer is the second most common cause of death in the older adults (following cardiac disease). Persistent chronic skin problems have the potential to lead to malignant change over time [33]. The most common skin cancer by far is basal cell carcinoma, with squamous cell carcinoma the next common. Malignant melanoma is the third most common skin cancer, but the most malignant [9]. The risk factor for skin cancer that can be best minimized is sunlight exposure. In addition to UV light, genetic mutations and host factors play a role. UV light causes direct and indirect DNA damage through photo-oxidation [34].

Skin markers of systemic malignancy may be a result of metastases or syndromes secondary to humoral processes (Table 4.4). Metastatic lesions result from local, lymphatic or blood stream spread; their origin may be breasts, stomach, lungs kid-

Table 4.4 Skin involvement and cancer in older adults

Metastatic skin lesions:
  Origin: breast, colon, lung, stomach, kidneys, bladder, uterus and others
Nonmetatstatic manifestations:
  Endocrine syndromes: Carcinoid syndrome, gynecomastia
  Dermatomyositis (suggests carcinoma, lymphoma, melanoma)
  Pruritus or itching (may suggest lymphoma, leukemia)
  Thrombophlebitis, superficial or deep (may indicate pancreatic cancer)
  Blistering diseases (may parallel a cancer)
  Erythema gyratum repens (suggestive of cancer)
  Icthyosis (lymphoma, myeloma, carcinoma)
  Acanthosis nigricans (cancers, especially adenocarcinomas)
  Exfoliative dermatitis(lymphoma, leukemia)
Other facts about skin cancer
  Most common skin cancer is basal cell carcinoma
  Most malignant skin cancer is malignant melanoma
  Most preventable risk factor: diminished exposure to sunlight
  Gardener's syndrome: osteomas , sebaceous cysts and association with intestinal polyps
  Peutz–Jeghers syndrome : freckles on the lips and oral mucosa associated with intestinal or stomach polyps

neys, colon and uterus. The presence of unexplained manifestations especially with a history of recent or past history of malignancy or a poor response to treatment may indicate the need to initiate testing to detect underlying cancer [35]. Several nonmetastatic manifestations also may suggest the presence of an underlying malignancy; they are briefly listed in Table 4.4 and have been well detailed in a review by Braverman [35].

The role of primary care providers is to inspect the skin regularly and seek consultation from the dermatologist for any lesions that raise suspicion for malignancy; preventive measures for skin cancer are best instituted in time, at a young age.

Medication Effects

Older individuals are susceptible to and frequently develop infections. Antibiotics are commonly used in this age group, especially to treat staphylococci and streptococci (and enterococci); clinicians need to be aware of resistance to antibiotics, which easily develops in the geriatric age group [36]. The use of topical corticosteroids should be limited to shorter periods of time in older people; used beyond this period, would require consideration for steroid replacement for adrenal suppressed state and prophylactic treatment for osteoporosis.

Adverse drug reactions (ADRs) can present with cutaneous eruptions; these iatrogenic disorders may mimic systemic illness [37]. Because older adults tend to be on numerous prescribed and "over the counter" medications and are subject to polypharmacy, the frequency of drug reactions tend to be higher in the geriatric population [37]. Further, ADRs are a leading cause of death in the United States [38]. The timing of reaction occurring in relation to drug use varies from minutes as in the case of urticaria to months or years as with drug induced lupus [37]. Some drugs, while abused, such as hypnotics (associated with falls) and others such as estrogens, (side effects include cancer and vascular disease), are rarely associated with skin reactions [37]. Drug eruptions may take several forms and beyond the scope of description here; they can involve the skin, mucous membrane and several organ

Table 4.5 Medications and skin reactions: considerations in older adults

Altered pharmacokinetics and pharmacodynamics occur with age
Adverse skin reactions hence tend to increase with age
Association with higher prevalence of polypharmacy in elderly
Skin reactions may take minutes, days, months or years to manifest
Nature of reactions are highly variable
A good medication history is a key to diagnosis
Temporal relationship to drug may not be evident
Skin reactions may not occur in parallel with systemic side effects
Manifestations may be mistaken for systemic disease or aging
Secondary infection can be superimposed on drug reaction
Include drug reactions in the differential diagnosis of skin disorders

systems. Unusual but serious reactions, such as anticoagulant induced skin necrosis and drug induced vasculitis should not escape diagnosis (Table 4.5).

In summary, the wide array of disease processes and drug effects that manifest through the skin are surely a good reason for an adequate dermatology examination by health providers. It appears reasonable for inspection of all dermatomes to be performed at least annually in primary care. The skin might well be the gateway to the entire body!

References

1. Dharmarajan TS, Ugalino JT. The physiology of aging. In Dharmarajan TS, Norman RA, eds. Clinical Geriatrics, 1st ed. Boca Raton, CRC Press/Parthenon Publishing, 2003, pp. 9–22.
2. Dharmarajan TS, Tota R. Appropriate use of medications in older adults. Fam Pract Recertif. 2000; 22: 29–38.
3. Thomas DR. Age related changes in wound healing. Drugs Aging 2001; 18(8): 607–20.
4. Gerstein AD, Phillips TJ, Rogers GS et al. Wound healing and aging. Dermatol. Clin. 1993; 11: 749.
5. Yaar M, Gilchrest BA. Skin aging: postulated mechanisms and consequent changes in structure and function. Clinics Geriatric Med. 2001; 17: 617–3.
6. Ryan T. The ageing of the blood supply and the lymphatic drainage of the skin. Micron. 2004; 35: 161–71.
7. Millard TP, Hawk JLM. Photodermatoses in the elderly. Clin. Geriatr Med. 2001; 17: 691–714.
8. Elias PM, Ghadially R. The aged epidermal permeability barrier. Clin. Geriatr. Med. 2002; 18: 107–15.
9. Theodosat A. Skin diseases of the lower extremities in the elderly. Dermatol. Clin. 2004; 22: 13–21.
10. Sumino H, Ichikawa S, Abe M et al. Effects of age, menopause and hormone replacement therapy on forearm elasticity in women. J. Am. Geriatr. Soc. 2004; 52: 945–9.
11. Ashcroft GS, Dodsworth J, Van Boxtel E et al. Estrogen accelerates cutaneous wound healing associated with an increase in TGB-B1 levels. Nat. Med. 1997; 3: 1209–15.
12. MacLaughlin J, Holick MF. Aging decreases capacity of human skin to produce vitamin D 3. J. Clin. Invest. 1985; 76: 1536–8.
13. Holick MF. Vitamin D deficiency. What a pain it is. Mayo Clin. Proc. 2003; 78: 1457–9.
14. Hordinsky M, Sawaya M, Roberts JL. Hair loss and hirsutism in the elderly. Clin. Geriatr. Med. 2002; 18: 121–33.
15. Sperling LC. Hair and systemic disease. Dermatol. Clin. 2001; 19: 711–26.
16. Bowman PH, Hogan DJ. Leg ulcers: a common problem with sometimes uncommon etiologies. Geriatrics 1999; 54: 43–53.
17. Paquettte D, Falanga V. Leg ulcers. Clin. Geriatr. Med. 2002; 18: 77–88.
18. Cohen PR, Scher RK. The nails in older individuals. In Scher RK, Daniel CR, eds. Nails: Therapy, Diagnosis, Surgery. Philadelphia: WB Saunders, 1990, p. 127–50.
19. Martin ES, Elewski BE. Cutaneous fungal infections in the elderly. Clin. Geriatr. Med. 2002; 18: 59–75.
20. Norman D. The effects of age-related skin changes on wound healing rates. J. Wound Care 2004; 13: 199–201.
21. Reed MJ. Wound repair in older patients; preventing problems and managing the healing. Interview by Marc E. Weksler. Geriatrics 1998; 53(5): 88–94.
22. Ashcroft GS, Ashworth JJ. Potential role of estrogen in wound healing. Am. J. Clin. Dermatol. 2003; 4: 737–43.

23. Wilson JA, Clark JJ. Obesity: impediment to wound healing. Crit. Care Nurs. Q. 2003; 26(2): 119–32.
24. Gosain A, DiPietro LA. Aging and wound healing. World J. Surg. 2004; 28: 321–6.
25. Schneider JB, Norman RA. Cutaneous manifestations of endocrine-metabolic disease and nutritional deficiency in the elderly. Dermatol. Clin. 2004; 22: 23–31.
26. Schwartz KM. Dermopathy of Graves' disease (pretibial myxedema): long-term outcome. J. Clin. Endocrinol. Metab. 2002; 87: 438-46.
27. Kokkat AJ, Dharmarajan TS, Pitchumoni CS. Nutrition in older adults. Pract. Gastroenterol. 2004; 28(6): 22–44.
28. Balducci L. Epidemiology of anemia in the elderly: information of diagnostic evaluation. J. Am. Geriatr. Soc. 2004; 51: S2–S9.
29. Lipschitz D. Medical and functional consequences of anemia in the elderly. J. Am. Geriatr. Soc. 2004; 51: S10–S13.
30. Dharmarajan TS, Adiga GU, Norkus EP. B12 deficiency: recognizing subtle symptoms in older adults. Geriatrics 2003; 58: 30–8.
31. Etter L, Myers SA. Pruritus in systemic disease: mechanisms and management. Dermatol. Clin. 2002; 20: 459–72.
32. Elgart ML. Skin infections and infestations in geriatric patients. Clin. Geriatr. Med. 2002; 18: 89–101.
33. Adam JE. Skin cancer: a review. Geriatr. Aging 2002; 5: 14–16.
34. Sachs DL, Marghoob AA, Halpern A. Skin cancer in the elderly. Clin. Geriatr. Med. 2001; 17: 715–38.
35. Braverman IM. Skin manifestations of internal malignancy. Clin. Geriatr. Med. 2002; 18: 1–19.
36. Hutchison LC, Norman RA. Antibiotics and resistance in dermatology; focus for treating the elderly. Dermatol. Ther. 2003; 16(3): 206–13.
37. Sullivan JR, Shear NH. Drug eruptions and other adverse drug effects in aged skin. Clin. Geriatr. Med. 2002; 18: 21–42.
38. Lazarou J, Pomperanz B, Corey P. Incidence of adverse drug reactions in hospitalized patients. JAMA 1998; 279: 1200–5.

Chapter 5

White and Red Lesions of the Oral Mucosa

**Marcia Ramos-e-Silva, Tania Cestari,
and Cristiane Benvenuto-Andrade**

Introduction

Aging of the oral cavity is accompanied by intrinsic corporal changes that may affect its resistance to pathogens, such as reduction of the salivary flow, thinning of the mucosa with reduction of blood flow, and difficulties with oral hygiene caused by deterioration of body movements. However, a significant part of the oral lesions found in the elderly is caused by lifetime environmental aggressions and social problems. Some authors sustain that age by itself does not reduce the defense mechanisms of the oral cavity in healthy individuals. The lesions would be secondary to systemic diseases, malnutrition, and use of medications or poorly adapted dental prostheses [1]. Another peculiarity of elderly patients is the adjustment to some treatment regimens due to the increased rate of adverse effects of drugs and their probable interaction with other medications already in use [2].

A great diversity of oral lesions can be found in the geriatric patients, with prevalence varying between 28 and 61%, depending on the population studied [3]. The most common oral lesions include dermatoses secondary to trauma, neoplasia, immunological and hematological disturbances, oral manifestations of systemic diseases, and those that evolve with oral or facial pain [3,4]. Individuals using dental prostheses have up to three times more chances to present oral lesions than the general population [3]. Old or defective prostheses may lead to chronic mucosal alterations favoring the action of carcinogens such as the components of tobacco [5,6].

Some morphological alterations of the mucosa deserve special attention for their greater proneness to malignant transformation [7]. Initially, only leukoplakia and erythroplakia were included in this group. Gradually, actinic cheilitis, oral lichen planus, keratosis from tobacco use, sub-mucosal oral fibrosis, oral lupus, and some hereditary dermatoses, as congenital dyskeratosis, were also included [5]. A study performed in Finland demonstrated that only 17% of patients presenting lesions of the mucosa complained about pain [8]. The absence of alert signals demonstrates the importance of routine examinations of the oral cavity for an early diagnosis and treatment of its diseases, particularly those that may become malignant.

Lesions that evolve with a whitish or reddish appearance, and require attention for their differential diagnosis in the elderly patient will be approached in this chapter.

R.A. Norman (ed.), *Diagnosis of Aging Skin Diseases,*
© Springer-Verlag London Limited 2008

White Lesions

The pink color usually found in the normal oral mucosa is caused by the translucence of the epithelium and the lamina at that region, allowing penetration of light and its reflection by hemoglobin in the underlying vessels. The white lesions derive from superficial alterations of the mucosa that lead to the reflection and dispersion of the incident light. Those alterations may be caused by microbial colonies, exudates, necrosis of the superficial layers, epithelial thickening, or superficial sub-epithelial fibrosis [9]. The most frequent white lesions in the elderly patient will be discussed here.

Leukoplakia

The definition of leukoplakia has been undergoing changes during time [5]. In the Conference of Uppsala in 1994 it was established that it would be the predominantly white lesion of the oral mucosa which could not be clinically or pathologically characterized as another specific entity [7]. Lesions labeled clinically as leukoplakia can receive a more exact diagnosis after the histopathological study. In a work published in 1997, 17.8% of the clinically diagnosed leukoplakias received a final diagnosis of epithelial dysplasia or carcinoma after the histological study [10].

Leukoplakias can be found in all age groups although more common in the old population, in which its prevalence can range from 0.35 to 18.6%, depending on the sample, but usually lying between 2.5 and 4% [3,5]. The probable explanation is that the causative agents act cumulatively or require a long period of exposure [5]. The highest rates occur in populations using betel nuts and chewable tobacco, mainly in the solid form, very common in India and Southeast Asia [3, 5, 11]. Smokers have a six times higher risk of developing leukoplakia than non-smokers, despite lesions of non-smokers having a greater probability to evolve into cancer [11]. A comparative topographical analysis between smokers and non-smokers demonstrated that in those using tobacco the lesions usually appear at the soft palate while in non-smokers they affected the tongue borders more commonly [11]. In general, considering the whole population, the most frequent location of leukoplakic lesions is the vestibular mucosa [5, 12].

Leukoplakic lesions (Fig. 5.1) receive several classifications: homogeneous, verrucous, nodular, punctiform, pilous, candidiasic, erythro-leukoplakic, mixed, among others. From the practical point of view, one can speak about homogeneous and non-homogeneous forms [5]. The first is a white, uniform, and flat lesion, and the second, despite predominantly white in color, may present reddish areas, either flat, nodular, or exophytic.

It is believed that about 5% of the leukoplakias may develop into malignant processes in a period of 5 years [5]. The non-homogeneous lesions, as the verrucous proliferative and the erythro-leukoplakic lesions, are the ones of greater malignant potential [13], however, epithelial dysplasia can also be present in homogeneous

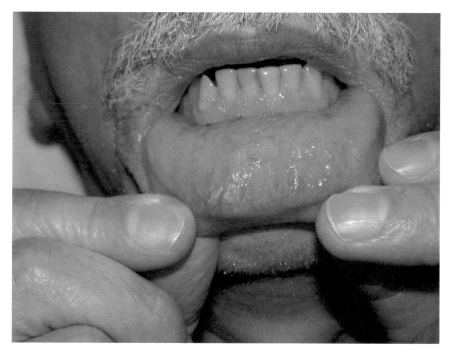

Fig. 5.1 Leukoplakia

lesions, signaling the possibility of a malignant transformation. In practice, the homogeneous form of the lesion or the absence of dysplasia are no warranty of benign evolution and all lesions should be followed [12].

Actinic Cheilitis

Cheilitis is the denomination given to non-specific inflammatory processes of the lips. Those with specific histology and eventual labial location, such as lichen planus, lupus erythematous, pemphigus, and syphilis, should be excluded from this designation [14]. Actinic cheilitis is an inflammatory and pre-malignant alteration of the lips, similar to the actinic keratosis of the skin. It is secondary to chronic exposure to ultraviolet radiation and affects mainly white males in the sixth or seventh decades of life [14, 15]. Its malignization ranges from 10 to 20% [15]. The lower frequency among blacks is usually explained by the protective effect of melanin, and in women by the use of lipstick, which would act as a protection [14]. Patients usually present other chronic cutaneous degenerative alterations in sun-exposed areas, such as actinic keratoses and/or skin cancer [14]. The lip may present a whitish aspect, with loss of both the uniform coloration of the semi-mucosa and the distinction of the border between the vermillion and the skin [14, 15] (Fig. 5.2). Atrophy, crusts, and erosions appear after continuous solar exposure, suggesting the

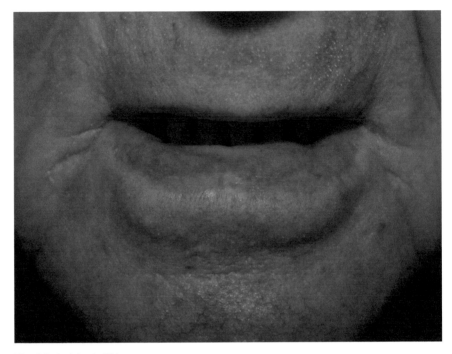

Fig. 5.2 Actinic cheilitis

occurrence of a malignant transformation [14]. The histopathology can demonstrate atrophic scaly epithelium, with increased keratin content and several degrees of dysplasia. Under the dysplastic area, there is a chronic inflammatory infiltrate composed by lymphocytes and some plasmocytes, in an elastotic dermis [15]. The biopsy for histological analysis of the lesion is essential to assure the early detection of malignant transformation [16]. Treatment can be made with ablative techniques, as vermilionectomy with cold knife or laser; with destructive techniques, as cryotherapy; or with the use of topical agents, as 5% fluoracil, and immunomodulators, as imiquimod [16, 17]. Lip sunscreens are indicated in prevention of recurrences [14].

Nicotinic Stomatitis

The expression "nicotinic stomatitis" designates alterations of the mucosa of the palate, secondary to the chronic exposure of smokers to tobacco and heat. The palate becomes whitish, wrinkled, and can present fissures [18] (Fig. 5.3). Small erythematous nodular areas can be observed, which represent inflamed glandular ducts. Malignant transformation is relatively rare, and histology shows reactive epithelial hyperplasia, with squamous metaplasia and chronic inflammation of the glandular ducts [9]. The clinical aspect is very similar to that of Darier's disease, an uncommon dominant autosomal dermatosis [19]. The treatment demands suspension of the irritating agent and observation [20].

Fig. 5.3 Nicotinic stomatitis

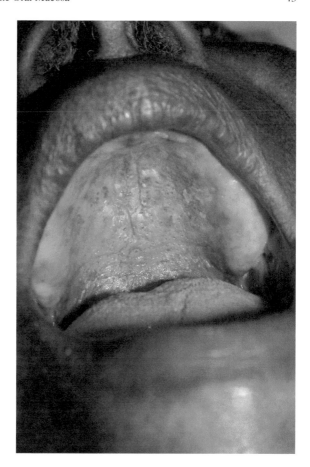

Oral Lichen Planus

Oral lichen planus (OLP) is a relevant differential diagnosis in red and white lesions of the oral mucosa for presenting clinical and histopathological similarity with several other mouth diseases [21]. It is an inflammatory dermatosis of unknown origin that affects 0.5–1% of the general population, apparently more common in women, with a proportion of 3:2 in relation to men. It is more precocious in males and does not present any familial pattern [3, 21–23]. The condition usually manifests in persons above 40, being very rare in children [23]. Any part of the oral mucosa can be affected, although the most usual locations are the buccal mucosa and the tongue [5, 23], with lesions in the palate being rare. In spite of the oral lesions being less common than the cutaneous ones, they cause greater discomfort and can generate pain and burning [23]. It is common for patients with OLP to present lesions in one or more extra-oral locations [21]. A study demonstrated vulvovaginal and cutaneous involvement in about 25 and 15% of affected women, respectively. Other locations are much less common [24].

The potential of those lesions for malignant transformation remains controversial, despite being much discussed, and ranges from less than 0.2 to 2.7% in the different studies [5, 25]. The clinical aspect can be extremely variable, with wheals, macules, striae, atrophic, eroded, or bullous areas [5]. The most classical form, with reticular pattern, presents bilateral arboriform striae of whitish coloration over an erythemato-violet area [23] (Figs. 5.4 and 5.5). The closest clinical form to oral cancer is the erosive type. The period of evolution and the location on the tongue were also described as indicative potential of a worsening prognosis [5].

Different from cutaneous lichen planus, the oral forms can have long evolution, reaching 25 years or more. The bullous, atrophic, and eroded variants are the most painful. Patients may refer burning in contact with irritating agents, such as

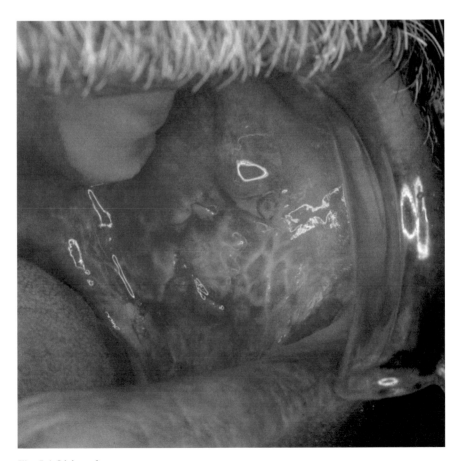

Fig. 5.4 Lichen planus

Fig. 5.5 Lichen planus

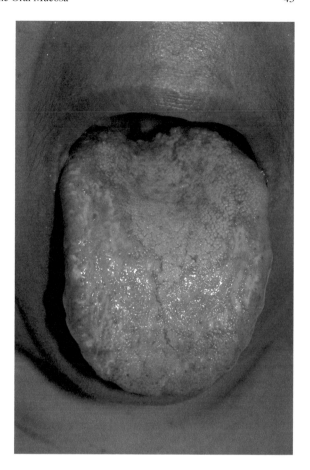

cigarettes and some foods [23]. The remaining forms are asymptomatic, usually found during routine examination [5, 23].

Although of unknown etiology, the current tendency is to consider lichen planus as an autoimmune disease, mediated by cells and unlocked by alteration in the antigens of the basal layer of the epidermis in genetically predisposed patients [23, 24]. The lymphocytic infiltrate and the amplified production of cytokines result in an increased expression of the intercellular-1 adhesion molecule (ICAM-1) and antigens of the histocompatibility complex, mainly of class II (MHC-II), by the keratinocytes [24]. Those events can lead to tissue destruction [24]. In histology, vacuolar degeneration and lysis of basal cells are observed, besides focal hyperparakeratosis, irregular acanthosis, and an amorphous eosinophilic band in the basal membrane [21]. Viruses, dental materials, and drugs can influence the triggering of the lesions. The influence of hepatitis C and HPV viruses is still controversial in the several published studies. The influence of amalgam, used in dental restorations, is also controversial, although there is regression of the lesions of OLP in some patients after removal of that material. The list of medications that can be related to the appearance of lesions is extensive and includes medications frequently used by the geriatric population: allopurinol, carbamazepine, diuretic thiazides, methyldopa, propranolol, salicylic acid, spironolactone, methacrylate, and non-steroid anti-inflammatories [23].

For diagnostic confirmation of OLP it is necessary to perform a biopsy for histopathological examination, preferentially of the reticular lesions [23]. The erythematous or erosive lesions frequently present with a diagnosis of unspecific mucositis [21]. Direct immunofluorescence is usually unspecific, showing deposits of IgM, IgG, IgA, C3, and fibrin in the Civatte corpuscles. That pattern can also be found in diseases like lupus erythematous and multiform erythema [23].

Treatment of OLP lesions is very variable, depending on the time of evolution and symptoms presented. As they are little symptomatic, they usually only require general care and attentive follow-up for the eventual appearance of a neoplasia. Before the beginning of any therapy, all medications identified as potential causes should be removed and traumas minimized. Odontologic follow-up and regular oral hygiene should be emphasized. In more serious cases, replacement of amalgam or gold restorations can be accomplished, since both metals have been implicated in the appearance of lesions [26].

The use of several systemic and oral medications has been indicated including: topical, oral, and intralesional corticosteroids, griseofulvin, cyclosporine, azathioprine, retinoids, dapsone, metronidazole, and levamisole. The choice of therapy should take into account the type of lesion, the symptoms, and the time of evolution of the picture. Good results were found in the most serious and difficult cases with photo-chemotherapy, surgical excision, or ablative laser, besides the use of adjuvant immunomodulators as levamisole and tacrolimus [26].

Oral Candidiasis

Oral candidiasis is the most common fungal infection in humans and is usually caused by the dimorphic fungus *Candida albicans*, although recurrent cases are often caused by more virulent types like *Candida glabrata* and *Candida tropicalis* [27, 28]. It is very common and insufficiently diagnosed in elderly patients, mainly in those using dental prostheses, affected by diabetes, and those immunocompromised [28]. In the elderly, decrease of salivation and of production of factors that promote the detachment of the fungus from the oral mucosa (as secretory IgA) and that inhibit their multiplication (lactoferrin and transferrin) contribute to colonization [29]. In non-insulin-dependent diabetes, the use of dentures and bad oral hygiene seem strongly associated to colonization by *Candida* [30]. Patients with non-insulin-dependent diabetes are also more predisposed to colonization by *Candida*, with larger significant prevalence of stomatitis related to dentures, especially when the diabetes is poorly controlled or associated to vitamin B deficiency [27,31]. Other risk factors for opportunistic infections by *Candida* are nutritional vitamin B12, folate, and iron deficiencies, besides psychotropic drugs and those that induce decrease of salivation [27]. Immunocompromised patients present a risk of hematogenic spreading or through the gastrointestinal tract, leading to significant increase of morbidity and mortality [28].

The infection by *Candida* has several possible clinical presentations as described below:

1. *Pseudo-membranous candidiasis.* It is characterized by whitish plaques of epithelial desquamated cells, fibrin, and hyphae. These plaques may occur in the labial or buccal mucosa, palate, tongue, periodontal, and oropharyngeal tissues (Fig. 5.6). Different from leukoplakias, these plaques are easily removable with the help of a spatula, exposing the underlying mucosa of erythematous aspect. The diagnosis is usually clinical, but can be accomplished by direct examination or culture for fungus [28].
2. *Acute atrophic candidiasis.* It is usually associated to burning sensation of the mouth or tongue. The tongue can acquire a lively red coloration, similar to that of vitamin B12 and folate deficiency. The diagnosis requires suspicion in cases of elderly patients using dentures, complaining about pain in the tongue, and who took antibiotics or corticosteroids [28].
3. *Chronic hyperplasic candidiasis.* It occurs in the buccal mucosa or at the borders of the tongue. It is associated to tobacco habits and resolves after its cessation.

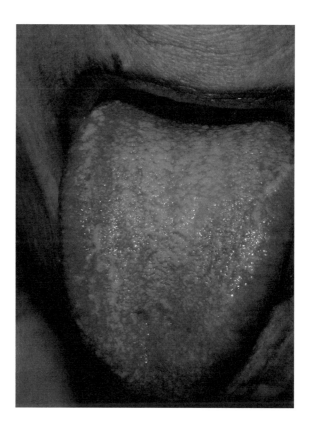

Fig. 5.6 Candidiasis

This form may become dysplastic, and some authors believe that *Candida* is only a secondary, instead of a causal, factor [28].

4. *Chronic atrophic candidiasis* (also known as denture-related stomatitis). This condition is described ahead in this chapter, under red lesions.

5. *Medium rhomboid glossitis.* This being an erythematous lesion, it is described ahead in this chapter.

6. *Angular cheilitis.* They are fissures of the angles of the mouth usually associated to oral infection by *Candida.* It can also be associated to the *Staphylococcus* and *Streptococcus* infection. Its appearance in the elderly is due to wrinkling and loss of skin elasticity of the face, creating a wet environment in the corner of the mouth that predisposes for those infections [32]. Other factors implicated in the appearance of angular cheilitis are anemia due to lack of iron and vitamin B12 deficiency.

Candidiases can be avoided in most cases with good oral hygiene. The dentures demand daily brushing for mechanical removal of the residues and cleaning with chlorhexidine. The combination with nystatin is not recommended because its simultaneous application with chlorhexidine results in deactivation of the two drugs [33]. Treatment can be made with topical, oral, or endovenous solutions of antifungal agents, according to the seriousness of the clinical picture [27]. Topical nystatin solutions and, with lesser frequency, amphotericin are recommended for the less complicated cases and in combination with systemic antifungals for the most extensive. They are not absorbed by the gastrointestinal tract and do not cause adverse systemic effects [28]. The remaining antifungals are related to the onset of nauseas and vomits.

The systemic treatment should be instituted in patients with intolerance or difficulty with the topical treatment, or in those with a high risk for development of systemic candidiasis. Due to the high saccharose contents in nystatin solutions, if the patient presents candidiasis complicated by diabetes or makes use of corticosteroids or immunosuppressors, oral medications may also be a good strategy. Although ketoconazole is as effective as itraconazole and fluconazole, it is not recommended in elderly patients due to risk of medication interactions and side effects. Itraconazole is suitable for immunocompromised patients that present a disease resistant to the treatment with fluconazole [28].

Red Lesions

The change of color of the oral mucosa from pink to red occurs when the blood pigment is seen more clearly due to congestion, hyperemia, hemorrhage, epithelial atrophy, acantholysis, or ulceration [9]. This aspect can be found in many oral alterations, but we will only approach here those of greater relevance in the geriatric patient.

Erythroplakia

Erythroplakia is an erythematous, velvet-like lesion, which does not differentiate clinically or pathologically from any specific entity. The prevalence is much smaller than for leukoplakias, usually below 0.1%. In several cases the erythroplakic areas connect with leukoplakic areas; this is the reason why some authors classify them as a type of leukoplakia called erythroleukoplakia [5]. Its clinical distinction from the atrophic-erosive forms of LPO is quite difficult, histopathology being very important in the differential diagnosis [10]. The anatomopathological examination demonstrates that more than 90% of cases have signs of dysplasia [5]. The probability of malignant transformation is 17 times greater than that of leukoplakias [20] and, for that reason, many authors suggest that they should be treated as true in situ carcinomas [5], being always excised and sent for histological study [20].

Prosthetic Stomatitis or Stomatitis Caused by Dentures and Papillary Hyperplasia of the Palate

Prosthetic stomatitis is the most prevalent oral disease among dental prostheses users [1]. In this condition, *Candida* infection development is favored by the use of dentures during the whole night, defective prostheses, xerostomia, as well as poor oral hygiene [27]. Not all prosthesis users develop this picture, more common in women, and still no individual hypersensitivity has been demonstrated to any type of material used in the manufacture of the prostheses [1, 20]. In general, erythema with little pain occurs in the contact area with the dentures, accompanied by angular stomatitis. The use of topical antifungals can be helpful, and, during the night, the prostheses should remain submerged in chlorhexidine solutions at 0.2% or sodium hypochlorite at 1% [20]. Cleaning with toothpaste usually used in natural teething is insufficient for the hygiene of prostheses [6].

Considering a variety of prosthetic stomatitis, papillary hyperplasia of the palate (PHP) is another relatively common condition found in dental prostheses users also known as papillomatosis of the palate, pseudo-papillomatosis, hypertrophic stomatitis, granulation of the palate, and pseudo-epitheliomatous hyperplasia of the palate. It is characterized by numerous small papillae with hyperplasia, no more than 2 mm in diameter, erythematous and edematous, with concentric disposition (Fig. 5.7). The lesions are, in general, asymptomatic, with greater incidence in the hard palate, especially in the areas in intimate contact with dental prostheses.

The conditions associated to PHP are countless, such as: use of dental prostheses during long periods during the day, bad dentures adaptation, an empty space between the prosthesis and the palate, poor oral hygiene, type of material involved in prostheses' manufacture and hygiene (it is five times more common in users of acrylic dentures than metallic ones), infection by fungi, traumas and systemic diseases, and the anemia from iron deficiency and other nutritional disorders [34,35]. Some authors believe that there is an important individual predisposing

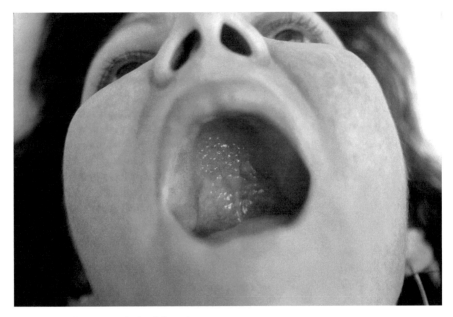

Fig. 5.7 Papillary hyperplasia of the palate

factor, given that not all the people that use prostheses and have poor oral hygiene present PHP [35].

The histopathological examination demonstrates hyperkeratosis with parakeratosis, exuberant papillomatosis, inflammatory infiltrate in the dermis, pseudoepitheliomatous hyperplasia with corneal pearls, koilocytes, mitosis figures, and hyperchromasia of the basal layer with cellular depolarization [35]. Occasional reports of malignant transformation associated to PHP justify the fact that some authors consider it a pre-malignant lesion, especially when there are focuses of dyskeratosis. However, the clinical evolution is usually benign, making that topic still controversial.

The diagnosis is made by anamnesis and physical examination using a good light source and a continuous air flow. An aspect of "wind blowing on wheat fields" is then observed. The differential diagnosis is made with nicotinic stomatitis, which does not occur in smokers with prosthesis, because the hyperplasia caused by the smoking habit protects the palate. Darier's disease can present a similar form, however, with smaller number of papillae, more keratinized and with more delicate projections [35]. When there is a clinical suspicion of squamous-cell carcinoma, the differentiation should be made through histopathology.

The most suitable treatments are: curettage, surgical excision, electrosurgery, laser, and cryosurgery. Topical medications have not shown satisfactory results [35]. The radical excision of the palate, including the adjacent periosteum, is acceptable only for small lesions, due to the risk of injury to important arteries, besides osteomyelitis and postoperative pain. The dental prosthesis and the oral hygiene should be reassessed, and the patient oriented to remove the dentures when sleeping.

Impressions of the Prosthesis and Dental Impressions

The suction of the mucosa against the teeth or against the prosthesis is the cause of these usually elevated impressions with the exact format of the causing agent. The diagnosis is made by history and physical examination, with great attention to the format and location of the lesions. Depending on the degree of aggression, some lesions can have tumorous aspect. They should be biopsied and differentiated from squamous-cell carcinoma [36].

Median Rhomboid Glossitis

The picture is characterized by depapillation with a rhomboid configuration in the central aspect of the dorsal area of the tongue, immediately above the terminal furrow [20] (Figure 5.8). It affects less than 1% of the adults and is asymptomatic [9]. Infection by *Candida* is common, and can be favored by the habit of smoking, use of dentures, and/or immunological deficiencies, as HIV infection [20,37]. Although histology can be very similar to that of a carcinoma, with pseudo-epitheliomatous

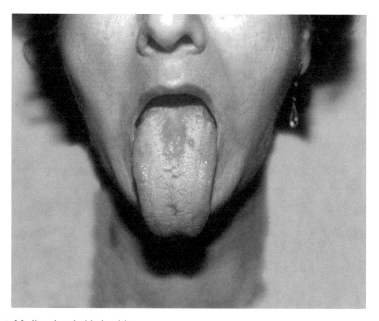

Fig. 5.8 Median rhomboid glossitis

epithelial hyperplasia, it is a benign disease [20]. Some cases, mainly in immuno-compromised patients are accompanied by candidiasis of the palate [9, 38]. The diagnosis is clinical; however, lesions with a nodular component may require biopsy to rule out malignancy [20]. The treatment consists of control of the symptoms and the irritating agents, and use of antifungals [38].

Purpura

Purpuric lesions usually occur by trauma, although the patient should be investigated to discard hematological conditions associated with bleeding, as leukemias. Petechiae in the palate are usually found in HIV-infected patients, while blood-filled vesicles are part of the clinical picture of localized oral purpura, pemphigoid, and, occasionally, amyloidosis [20].

Varicosities

Benign reddish-blue varicosities can be found in elderly patients, particularly in the ventral and lateral faces of the tongue [1] (Figure 5.9).

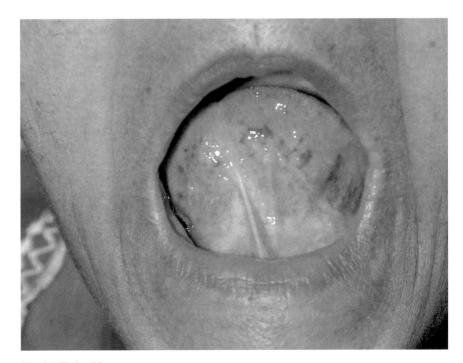

Fig. 5.9 Varicosities

Amelanotic Melanoma

Less than 2% of the melanomas are characterized by apparent absence of pigment. In the oral mucosa, however, this prevalence may reach up to two thirds [39]. The diagnosis is usually difficult and long delayed, worsening the prognosis [40]. About 50% of the patients present affected regional lymph nodes at the time of diagnosis, while 20% present disseminated lesions [41]. The presence of small-pigmented areas, which may be seen in a more meticulous examination of the lesions, can be useful to raise the suspicion index. If there is a suspicion of melanoma, the collected sample should be sent to routine histopathological examination and immunohistochemical analysis. The staining for S-100, HMB-45, and MART-1 are the most indicated and can help establish the diagnosis [39]. Treatment of oral melanoma is surgical. Bone involvement and presence of metastases point to a worst prognosis [9]. Some authors suggest the use of adjuvant chemotherapy, while the role of radiotherapy remains unclear [39].

Bullous Diseases

Although bullous diseases affect all age groups, elderly patients are more susceptible to the autoimmune and metabolic pictures, in particular pemphigoid (Figure 5.10), acquired bullous epidermolysis, and paraneoplastic pemphigus [42, 43]. Some

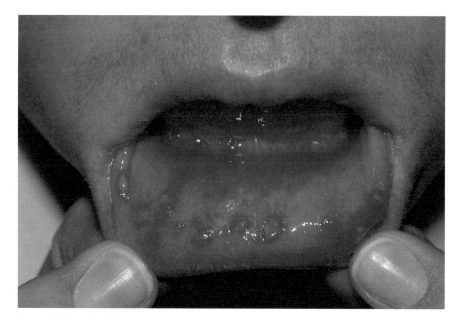

Fig. 5.10 Pemphigoid

patients do not present vesicles, only erythematosus or urticariform areas. When the diagnosis of bullous diseases is suspected, the specimen collected for direct immunofluorescence should include the adjacent normal skin. The accurate diagnosis is essential for the definition of the prognosis and therapeutics [42]. In the elderly, the prognostic is worse, with extensive vesiculation and slow healing, mainly in those with nutritional deficiencies. Secondary changes due to *Candida* infection are very common, delaying the diagnosis. The therapy for autoimmune bullous diseases includes immunosuppressive agents, such as systemic corticosteroids, mycophenolate mofetil, azathioprine, and cyclophosphamide [44]. Since elderly patients are more susceptible to drug-induced adverse effects, they should be kept under constant clinical and laboratorial evaluation.

Carcinoma

Most cases of oral cancer seem to evolve from an apparently normal epithelium, but in a percentage that varies from 30 to 50% they appear from pre-malignant lesions [5]. On the other hand, over 90% of the malignant lesions of the mucous oral membrane are squamous-cell or epidermoid carcinomas [45]. Several etiologic factors were already described: tobacco, alcohol, genetics, virus, radiations, occupational and nutritional exposure [5]. Most of them have a cumulative effect, causing large prevalence of oral cancer in the elderly [46]. About 95% of the cancers occur after the age of 40, with an average of diagnosis of 60 years [47]. Initially

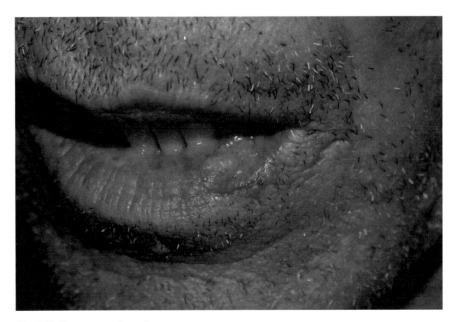

Fig. 5.11 Squamous-cell carcinoma

the oral carcinomas present as unspecific, asymptomatic, granular, neither ulcerated nor elevated lesions, with normal mucosal consistency, and absence of bleeding. They may vary from the erythematous to the whitish coloration (Figs. 5.11–5.14), hindering its diagnosis and worsening the prognosis [45,48]. When patients seek the doctor, they do it because of the presence of an ulcer or edema, although remaining asymptomatic [49]. Some characteristics should raise the suspicion of carcinomatous changes occurring in pre-malignant oral lesions: long duration, feminine sex, tongue or floor of the mouth location, tobacco use, non-homogeneous clinical aspect with erythematous or nodular areas, presence, and degree of dysplasia [50]. Factors suggesting the presence of a carcinoma include: erythroplakia, an ulcer with granular aspect, dilated blood vessels, hardening, a lesion attached to deeper tissues, and increased cervical lymph nodes (usually worsening the prognosis) [20]. These signs can occur very late in tumor progression, and only a high index of suspicion and routine revisions may increase the possibility of cancer detection in an early stage.

The biopsy of the suspicious lesions should include the red areas and tissue of normal appearance. Histopathological examination usually demonstrates epithelial

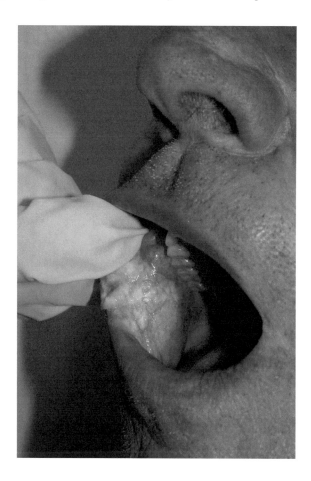

Fig. 5.12 Squamous-cell carcinoma

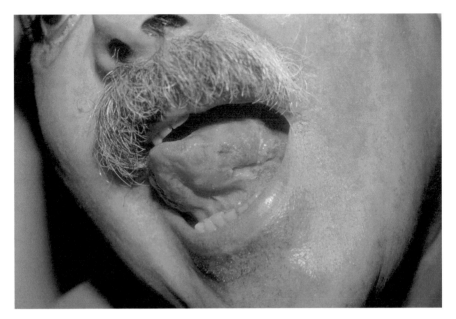

Fig. 5.13 Squamous-cell carcinoma

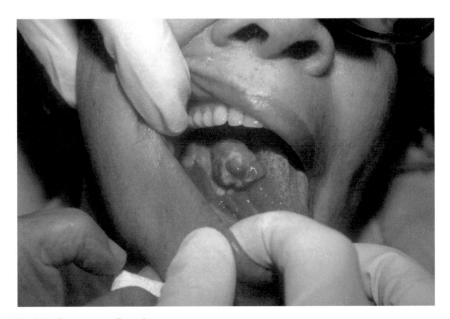

Fig. 5.14 Squamous-cell carcinoma

dysplasia invading the basal membrane. In more differentiated lesions there are concentric rings of keratin, called nests. The tumor infiltrates locally, and its metastases are primarily lymphatic. Treatment may range from local resection to debilitating surgeries, complemented with radiotherapy and/or chemotherapy [20].

Stomatodynia

Stomatodynia, also known as burning mouth syndrome or glossodynia (if only affecting the tongue), is more common in women over the age of 40 [20,51]. Patients refer a burning sensation in the tongue, which gets better on ingestion of foods. This sensation can also affect the lips, gingiva, and the palate [20]. Examination may reveal underlying causes like xerostomia, diabetes mellitus, some nutritional deficiency leading to infection by *Candida*, or, in lesser frequency, contact dermatitis and pressure urticaria [20]. In general, however, the examination of the oral cavity is normal, and most authors suggest that the discovery of some underlying cause for the burning sensation should exclude stomatodynia. Then this diagnosis should be reserved for patients without any other apparent cause for their symptoms [51]. The doctor should also be aware of possible symptoms caused by patient's anxiety for fearing an oral cancer or a sexually transmissible disease secondary to oral relations [20]. Psychological alterations, including anxiety and depression, are involved in up to 50% of cases in which no physical problems are found [51]. The differential diagnosis includes all inflammatory conditions of the oral mucosa, although these are frequently worsened by ingestion of foods and drinks [20].

Treatment is usually unsatisfactory and depends on the underlying cause [51]. Some patients request antidepressants and psychiatric support for a period that can vary from 3 to 18 months [20]. Some women in the menopause benefit from hormonal replacement [52]. In the apparently idiopathic cases treatment is little effective, but the symptoms remain mild [20], being necessary to explain that the disease does not have an organic cause nor relation to cancer [51]. Excellent results have been obtained with the use of pimozide, 1–2 mg a day, with total remission of the symptoms in almost all patients [51]. That medication, however, should be used with precaution due to its extra-pyramidal side effects, as rigidity, agitation, and akathisia.

Conclusion

Diseases of the oral mucosa, although very frequent in the elderly due to age-related physiological changes, dental prostheses use, and medications, are usually neglected during the clinical evaluation of those patients. Lesions of this epithelium are of interest not only to dermatologists, but also to dentists, otorhinolaryngologists, and head and neck surgeons.

The elderly patient needs orientation to get adapted to the modifications imposed on his/her organism, and the office visit can be the appropriate moment for this care. It is also important to emphasize the need for routine examination of the oral cavity, as well as the precocious clinical diagnosis, histopathological confirmation, and treatment of diseases as oral squamous-cell carcinoma, precancerous lesions, and other malignant tumors. This allows a better prognosis in relation to survival, mutilations, and cosmetic results after treatment.

References

1. Jainkittivong A, Aneksuk V, Langlais R. Oral mucosal conditions in elderly dental patients. Oral Dis. 2002; 8: 218–23.
2. Graham-Brown R. The ages of man and their dermatoses. In: Champion R, Burton J, Burns D, Breathnach S, eds. Rook/Wilkinson/Ebling Textbook of Dermatology, 6th ed. Oxford: Blackwell Science, 1998, pp. 3259–87.
3. Espinoza I, Rojas R, Aranda W, Gamonal J. Prevalence of oral mucosal lesions in elderly people in Santiago, Chile. J. Oral Pathol. Med. 2003; 32: 571–5.
4. Fantasia J. Diagnosis and treatment of common oral lesions found in the elderly. Dent. Clin. North Am. 1997; 41: 877–90.
5. Mallo Perez L, Rodriguez Baciero G, Lafuente Urdinguio P. Oral precancerous lesions in the elderly with special reference to the Spanish situation. RCOE 2002; 7: 153–62.
6. Coelho C, Sousa Y, Dare A. Denture-related oral mucosal lesions in a Brazilian school of dentistry. J. Oral Rehabil. 2004; 31: 135–9.
7. Axéll T, Pindborg J, Smith C, van der Waal I. Oral white lesions with special reference to precancerous and tobacco related lesions: conclusions of an international symposium held in Uppsala, Sweden, May 18–21 1994. J. Oral Pathol. Med. 1996; 25: 49–54.
8. Ekelund R. Oral mucosal disorders in institutionalized elderly people. Age Ageing 1988; 17: 193–8.
9. Ship JA, Phelan J, Kerr AR. Biology and pathology of the oral mucosa. In: Freedberg RM, Eisen AZ, Wolff K, Austen KF, Goldsmith LA, Katz SI, eds. Fitzpatrick's Dermatology in General Practice, 6th ed. New York: McGraw-Hill, 2003, pp. 1077–1090.
10. Onofre M, Sposto M, Navarro C, Motta M, Turatti E, Almeida R. Potentially malignant epithelial oral lesions: discrepancies between clinical and histological diagnosis. Oral Dis. 1997; 3: 148–52.
11. Schepman K, Bezemer P, van der Meij E, Smeele L, van der Waal I. Tobacco usage in relation to the anatomical site of oral leukoplakia. Oral Dis. 2001; 7: 25–7.
12. Schepman K, van der Meij E, Smeele L, van der Waal I. Malignant transformation of oral leukoplakia: a follow-up study of hospital-based population of 166 patients with oral leukoplakia from the Netherlands. Oral Oncol. 1998; 34: 270–5.
13. Batsakis J, Suarez P, el-Naggar A. Proliferative verrucous leukoplakia and its related lesions. Oral Oncol. 1999; 35: 354–9.
14. Rebello PF, Peninni S, Ramos-e-Silva M. Queilites. J. Bras. Med. 2000; 78: 104–10.
15. Santos J dos, Sousa S de, Nunes F, Sotto M, de Araujo V. Altered cytokeratin expression in actinic cheilitis. J. Cutan. Pathol. 2003; 30: 237–41.
16. Nieto MS, Albiol JG, Escoda CG. Surgical management of actinic cheilitis. Med. Oral 2001; 6: 205–17.
17. Smith K, Germain M, Yeager J, Skelton H. Topical 5% imiquimod for the therapy of actinic cheilitis. J. Am. Acad. Dermatol. 2002; 47: 497–501.
18. Rossie K, Guggenheimer J. Thermally induced nicotine stomatitis—a case report. Oral Surg. Oral Med. Oral Pathol. 1990; 70: 597–9.
19. Macleod R, Munro C. The incidence and distribution of oral lesions in patients with Darier's disease. Br. Dent. J. 1991; 171: 133–6.

20. Scully C. The oral cavity. In: Champion R, Burton J, Burns D, Breathnach S, eds. Rook/Wilkinson/Ebling Textbook of Dermatology, 6th ed. Oxford: Blackwell Science, 1998, pp. 3047–124.
21. Eisen D. The clinical features, malignant potential and systemic associations of oral lichen planus: a study of 723 patients. J. Am. Acad. Dermatol. 2002; 46: 207–4.
22. Bouquot J, Gorlin R. Leukoplakia, lichen planus and other oral keratoses in 23,616 white Americans over the age of 35 years. Oral Surg. Oral Med. Oral Pathol. 1986; 61: 373–81.
23. Jacques C, Pereira A, Cabral M, Cardoso A, Ramos-e-Silva M. Oral lichen planus part I: epidemiology, clinics, etiology, immunopathogeny and diagnosis. Skinmed 2003; 2: 342–349.
24. Eisen D. The evaluation of cutaneous, genital, scalp, nail, esophageal, and ocular involvement in patients with oral lichen planus. Oral Surg. Oral Med. Oral Pathol. Oral Radiol. Endod. 1999; 88: 431–6.
25. Holmstrup P. The controversy of a premalignant potential of oral lichen planus is over. Oral surg. Oral Med. Oral Pathol. Oral Radiol. Endod 1992; 73: 704–6.
26. Pereira A, Jacques C, Cabral M, Cardoso A, Ramos-e-Silva M. Oral lichen planus part II: therapy and malignant transformation. Skinmed 2004; 3: 19–22.
27. Dar-Odeh N, Shehabi AA. Oral candidosis in patients with removable dentures. Mycoses 2003; 46: 187–91.
28. Akpan A, Morgan R. Oral candidiasis. Postgrad. Med. J. 2002; 78: 455–9.
29. Kamagata-Kiyoura Y, Abe S, Yamaguchi H, Nitta T. Reduced activity of *Candida* detachment factors in the saliva of the elderly. J. Infect. Chemother. 2004; 10: 59–61.
30. Guggenheimer J, Moore P, Rossie K, et al. Insulin-dependent diabetes mellitus and oral soft tissue pathologies: II. Prevalence and characteristics of *Candida* and Candidal lesions. Oral Surg. Oral Med. Oral Pathol. Oral Radiol. Endod. 2000; 89: 570–6.
31. Dorocka-Babkowska B, Budtz-Joergensen E, Wolch S. Non-insulin-dependent diabetes mellitus as a risk factor for denture stomatitis. J. Oral Pathol. Oral Med. 1996; 25: 411–5.
32. Shay K, Truhlar M, Renner R. Oropharyngeal candidosis in the older patient. J. Am. Geriatr. Soc. 1997; 45: 863–70.
33. Barkvoll P, Attramadal A. Effect of nystatin and chlorhexidine digluconate on *Candida albicans*. Oral Surg. Oral Med. Oral Pathol. 1989; 67: 279–81.
34. Bhaskar SN, Beasley JD, Cutright DE. Inflammatory papillary hyperplasia of the oral mucosa: report of 341 cases. J. Am. Dent. Assoc. 1970; 81: 949—52.
35. Gavazzoni MF, Ramos-e-Silva M. Hiperplasia papilar do palato. Ann. Bras. Dermatol. 1994; 69: 28–31.
36. Ramos-e-Silva M, Fernandes N. Afecções das mucosas e semi-mucosas. J. Bras. Med. 2001; 80: 50–66.
37. van der Waal I. *Candida albicans* in median rhomboid glossitis: a post-mortem study. Int. J. Oral Maxillofac. Surg. 1986; 15: 322–5.
38. Holmstrup P, Besserman M. Clinical, therapeutic and pathogenic aspects of chronic oral multifocal candidiasis. Oral Surg. 1984; 56: 388–95.
39. Notani K, Shindoh M, Yamazaki Y, et al. Amelanotic malignant melanomas of the oral mucosa. Br. J. Oral Maxillofac. Surg. 2002; 40: 195–200.
40. Nandapalan V, Roland N, Helliwell T, Williams E, Hamilton J, Jones A. Mucosal melanoma of the head and neck. Clin. Otolaryngol. Allied Sci. 1998; 23: 107–16.
41. Rogers R, Gibson L. Mucosal, genital, and unusual clinical variants of melanoma. Mayo Clin. Proc. 1997; 72: 362–6.
42. Axt M, Wever S, Baier G, et al. Cicatricial pemphigoid: a therapeutic problem. Hautarzt 1995; 46: 620–7.
43. Rettore FC, Cardoso ICL, Sodré CT, Ramos-e-Silva M. Penfigóide cicatricial: relato de caso. Ann. Bras. Dermatol. 1995; 70: 339–42.
44. Vincent SD, Lilly GE, Baker KA. Clinical, historic, and therapeutic features of cicatricial pemphigoid. A literature review and open therapeutic trial with corticosteroids. Oral Surg. Oral Med. Oral Pathol. 1993; 76: 453–9.

45. Ramos-e-Silva M, Spitz LK, Magalhães TC, Corrêa AC, Aquino AM, Maceira JP. Carcinoma espinocelular da cavidade oral—4 casos. J. Bras. Med. 2003; 84: 83–5.
46. McIntyre G, Oliver R. Update on precancerous lesions. Dent. Update 1999; 26: 382–6.
47. Silverman S. Precancerous lesions and oral cancer in the elderly. Clin. Geriatr. Med. 1992; 8: 529–41.
48. Mashberg A, Feldman LJ. Clinical criteria for identifying early oral and oropharyngeal carcinoma: erythroplasia revisited. Am. J. Surg. 1988; 156: 273–5.
49. Amsel Z, Strawitz JG, Engstrom PF. The dentist as a referral source of first episode head and neck cancer patients. J. Am. Dent. Assoc. 1983; 106: 195–197.
50. Napier S, Cowan C, Gregg T, Stevenson M, Lamey P, Toner P. Potentially malignant oral lesions in Northern Ireland: size (extent) matters. Oral Dis. 2003; 9: 129–37.
51. Souza PRM, De Villa D, Carneiro SCS, Ramos-e-Silva M. Stomatodynia or burning mouth syndrome. Acta Dermatovenerol. Croat. 2003; 11: 231–235.
52. Wardrop RW, Hailes J, Burger H, Reade PC. Oral discomfort at menopause. Oral Surg. Oral Med. Oral Pathol. 1989; 67: 535–40.

Chapter 6

Nail and Hair Disorders in the Elderly

Marcia Ramos-e-Silva, Claudio de Moura–Castro Jacques, and Sueli Coelho Carneiro

Introduction

In the United States, people over 65 years of age represent almost 13% of the population, while in Brazil this is around 6% [1, 2].

The aging of the skin and its appendages is a complex phenomenon comprising genetic, endocrinological, immune and environmental factors added to free radicals generation. There is reduction of the number of keratinocytes, fibroblasts, and of the vascular network, particularly around hair bulbs and glands, resulting in decrease in hair and nail growth [3, 4]. The number of hair follicles, the rate of growth and diameter of hair, all are affected by age. The rate of growth of nails declines, the nail plate becomes thick and lunula size decrease [5–8].

Achten [9] and others [10–12] noted that the nail unit was comparable in some respects to a hair follicle. The hair bulb is similar to the intermediate nail matrix and the cortex to the nail plate. The hair bulb was considered analogous to the intermediate nail matrix and the cortex to the nail plate. The nail unit could be seen as an unfolded form of the hair follicle, producing a hair with no cortex, just hard cuticle. Diseases influence nail growth as seen in many statistical studies; and the nail analysis can be compared to a blood test in evaluating the general health of an individual [13].

Nail

The human nail has mechanical and social functions, and the most important of which are fine manipulation, scratching, physical protection of the extremity and a vehicle for cosmetics and aesthetic manipulation.

The nail unit components are [13]:

- lateral nail folds: cutaneous folded structure;
- proximal nail fold: cutaneous folded structure with proximal border of the nail;
- cuticle: the horny layer adherent to the dorsal nail plate;
- nail matrix: divided into three parts, the dorsal, the intermediate and the ventral matrix;

R.A. Norman (ed.), *Diagnosis of Aging Skin Diseases,*
© Springer-Verlag London Limited 2008

- lunula: the convex margin of matrix, seen through the nail;
- nail bed: the vascular bed;
- hyponychium: the cutaneous margin underlying the free nail, bordered distally by the groove; and
- distal groove: this is a cutaneous ridge demarcating the border between subungual structures and the finger pulp.

The nail shows colors that shine and seem to demonstrate the changes of the vascular nail bed and the organic tissue and system health.

The nail plate covers the nail bed and intermediate matrix. It is a keratinized structure, curved in both longitudinal and transversal axes. The upper surface of the nail plate is smooth and may have a variable number of longitudinal ridges that change with age.

Onychodystrophies most frequently observed are brittle and opaque nails, longitudinal striations, onychauxis, onychoclavus, onychogryphosis, splinter hemorrhages, subungual hematomas, and subungual exostosis. Some old age nail changes may be attributed to arteriosclerosis, even without evidence of obliteration of the vessel [13].

The care and adornment of the nail through variations in color, contour, and surface are considered of critical importance. Cleanliness does not achieve aesthetic satisfaction, and many products and procedures are on sale to fulfill the sources of attractiveness. The appearance of the nail is the best adornment of the hands of men and women. Attractive fingertips improve confidence and self-image [5, 8, 14].

Nail disorders, such as changes in color, contour, growth, surface, thickness, and histology, occur in the nail unit as the time goes by, and are common in the aged group. The onychodystrophies may represent changes associated with aging and related to systemic diseases and their treatments or altered local biomechanics [15].

Infections

Onychomycosis refers to involvement of the nail bed and undersurface of the nail plate by fungal organisms. It is common in the elderly, more often in males than females, and may involve both toenails and finger nails. It is divided in distal subungual onychomycosis (Fig. 6.1), proximal subungual onychomycosis, white superficial onychomycosis (Fig. 6.2), and Candida onychomycosis [16, 17]. Distal subungual onychomycosis is the most common dermatophytic infection, and is often caused by *Trichophyton rubrum*, characterized clinically by subungual hyperkeratosis. *Trichophyton mentagrophytes* is usually the causative organism of the proximal subungual onychomycosis. Saprophytic organisms, as *Scopulariopsis brevicaulis*, *Hendersonula toruloidea*, and *Scytalidium hyalinum*, may behave as nail pathogens in the elderly. It is well known that the elderly may have other multisystem diseases, which do not permit optimal foot and nail care, such as poor vision and mobility, and arthritis of the hands and other joints [18]. Only about 50% of all abnormal-appearing nails are due to onychomycosis, therefore, the clinical impression of onychomycosis should be confirmed, whenever possible [17].

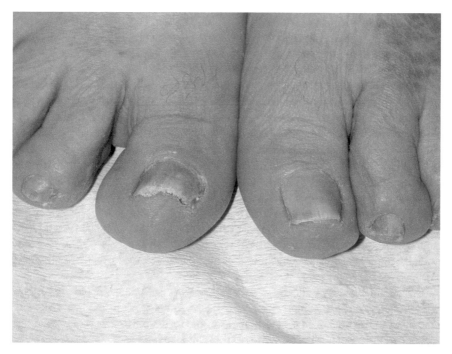

Fig. 6.1 Distal subungual onychomycosis

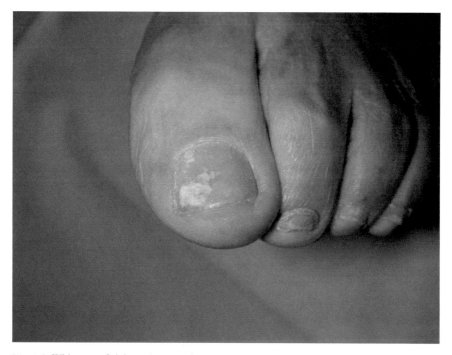

Fig. 6.2 White superficial onychomycosis

A direct mycological examination and a culture should be performed and confirm the diagnosis of onychomycosis before therapy is begun [15, 19].

Many treatments are available for onychomycosis. Topical therapy has low toxicity, prolonged duration and partial improvement [15, 17]. Systemic therapy has interactions with other systemic drugs, some adverse side effects and less treatment duration. Special care must be taken with the elderly due to the frequent interaction of the oral antifungal therapy, since they usually take many other medications.

Acute paronychial infections most commonly involve just one nail (Fig. 6.3). They are frequently caused by *Staphylococcus aureus* and treatment require opening of the abscess and oral antibiotics. Involvement of several nails will be considered as subacute or chronic paronychia secondary to chronic dermatitis, psoriasis vulgaris or Reiter's disease. Chronic paronychial infections are usually caused by Candida species or Gram-negative bacteria with a loss of the cuticle and appearance of the multiple transverse ridges. Treatment is often prolonged and a topical fungal lotion or cream should be applied two or three times a day. *Pseudomonas aeruginosa* may colonize nail plates that are onycholytic. Local therapy with antiseptic or antibiotic is effective [20].

Subungual hyperkeratotic debris may harbor *Sarcoptes scabiei* in elderly patients with ordinary or crusted (Norwegian) scabies. A cause of persistent infestations or epidemics of this condition in elderly patients and in nursing homes is the subungual location of the mite. It is necessary to cut the nails short and brush the fingertips with a scabicide when treating elderly patients for scabies [21].

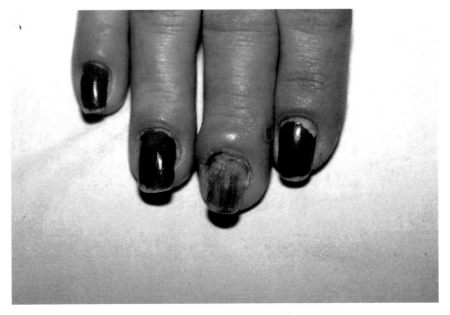

Fig. 6.3 Acute paronychial infection by *Candida* sp. and *Pseudomonas aeruginosa*

Elderly patients who are receiving immunosuppressive therapy may present peri-ungual warts caused by human papillomavirus, which may require aggressive treatment modalities [22, 23].

Trauma

Chronic trauma to the nail can result from faulty biomechanics, like digiti flexi, hallux rigidus, hallus valgus, overlapping, underlapping, and rotated toes. The onychodystrophies secondary to faulty biomechanism are onychauxis, onychoclavus, onychocryptosis, onychogryphosis, subungual exostosis, subungueal hematoma, and subungueal hyperkeratosis [24, 25]. The incompatibility between foot and shoe also result in trauma to the toe nails and subsequent onychodystrophy. Abnormal growth of the toenails secondary to pressure from the shoes may manifest as onychauxis and onychogryphosis. Subungual hematoma and subsequent onycholysis of the nail may occur [15].

The treatment of onychodystrophy should be directed to the underlying bony abnormality, to the foot care and appropriated shoes.

Brittle Nails

This disorder is common in elderly people and is characterized by excessive longitudinal ridging, horizontal layering (lamellar separation) of the distal nail plate, roughness (trachyonychia) of the nail plate surface, and/or irregularity of the distal edge of the nail plate [15, 26]. The origin of the brittle nail is varied, and can be endogenous or exogenous disease. In the elderly the problem may be secondary to dehydrating agents.

The treatment involves the elimination of precipitating habits, agents or systemic disorders and to dehydrate the nail plate, cuticle and surrounding nail folds with a moisturizer under occlusion at bedtime.

Onychauxis

Onychauxis or pachyonychia is a localized hypertrophy of the nail plate. It is characterized by hyperkeratotic, discolored nails and loss of translucency of the nail plate, subungual hyperkeratosis and debris. It is associated with aging, as with several disorders more common in the geriatric population. Local complications include distal onycholysis, increased susceptibility to acquiring onychomycosis, and pain. As a result of constant pressure of the hyperkeratotic nail on the underlying and surrounding tissues, subungual ulceration and hemorrhage may occur [15]. The treatment involves periodic partial or total debridement of the thickened nail plate by electric drills, chemical avulsion (urea paste 40%), surgically remotion [27, 28].

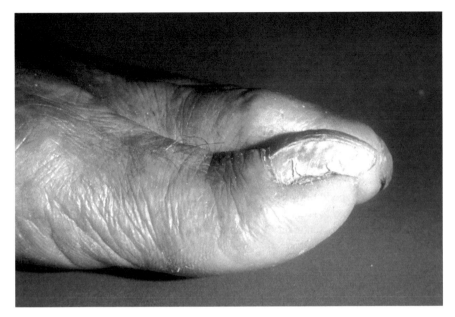

Fig. 6.4 Onychogryphosis

Onychogryphosis

It is a common exaggerated enlargement involving the great toe nails in elderly persons that permits the nail to continue to grow without treatment. The treatment consists of nail avulsion with or without ablation of the nail matrix. Chemical nail destruction or surgical avulsion may be used to remove the nail plate [29] (Fig. 6.4).

Onychophosis

It is common in the elderly patients and results from repeated minor trauma to the nail plate, involving the first and fifth toes with localized or diffuse hyperkeratotic tissue that develops on the lateral or proximal nailfolds. The treatment consists of debriding the hyperkeratotic tissue with keratolytics. Emollients and wearing comfortable shoes may prevent the development of onychophosis [15].

Onychoclavus

It is a subungual heloma or a subungual corn. This represents a hyperkeratotic process in the nail area that is caused by either anatomic abnormalities or mechanical changes in foot function. It is most commonly located under the distal nail margin and results from repeated minor trauma with accompanying localized pressure on the distal nail bed and hyponychium. The subungual corn occurs beneath the great toe nail and appears as a dark spot under the nail plate. The treatment consists of removal of the lesion and prevention of recurrence by modification of the footwear and protective pads [15].

Onychocryptosis

This condition results when part of the nail plate pierces the lateral nailfold and it is characterized by inflammation with or without granulation tissue, tenderness at rest, and pain on ambulation or with pressure to the digit [15] (Fig. 6.5). Improper cutting of the nails and external pressure secondary to poorly fitting footwear, long toes, hereditary nail abnormalities, poor foot hygiene, and prominence of the nailfolds are among the common causes of onychocryptosis [30].

In the elderly patient with decreased sensation of their feet or toes secondary to an underlying systemic disease, such as diabetes mellitus, peripheral vascular disease or arteriosclerosis, onychocryptosis can be a devastating problem with significant morbidity. A conservative treatment involves the elevation of the lateral border of the nail and local care consisting of topical antibiotics. When the onychocryptosis is more severe surgical approaches for complete or partial avulsion of the ingrown nail may be necessary. In order to correct the severe nail overcurvature orthonyx technique may be used with a series of adjustments of stainless steel wire nail brace

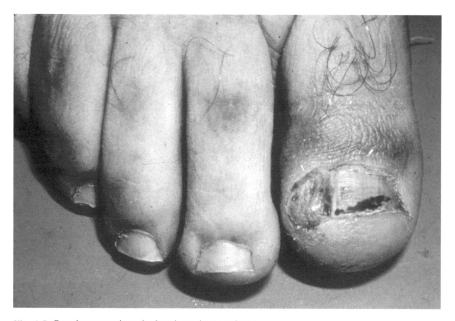

Fig. 6.5 Onychocryptosis and telangiectasic granuloma

that maintains constant tension of the nail plate. Liquid nitrogen spray cryotherapy may provide initial treatment of patients with onychocryptosis [31].

Subungual Hematomas

Trauma to the fingernail or toenail is the most frequent cause of hematoma. The others are anticoagulant therapy, amyloidosis, bullous pemphigoid and diabetes mellitus [28] (Fig. 6.6).***

Subungual Exostosis

It is a benign, tender, bony proliferation acquired during the fourth through sixth decades of life probably related to faulty pedal biomechanics [32].

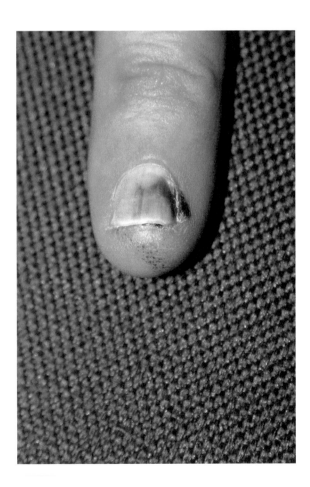

Fig. 6.6 Subungual hematoma

Onychotilomania

Some persons maybe subject to dysmorphic symptoms and may have manifestations of obsessive–compulsive pathology, like neurotic excoriations and repetitive scratching of the nail plate. These patients, commonly female who frequently have depressive tendencies, are unable to control the activity [14].

Hair

At birth there are approximately 1,000,000 hair follicles on the scalp of men and women and no new hair follicles are formed after fetal life [33]. There is a decrease in follicle density as one ages, from more than 1000 follicles/cm^2 in the newborn until less 500 in the elderly [33, 34].

Hair changes related to aging include diffuse hair loss and graying, among other problems [35–37].

Gray Hair

They are the result of a progressive and, sometimes, total loss of melanocytes by the hair bulb [38]. The hair is thinner and sparse, but it is not weaker than pigmented hair. Thin hair may become a severe problem. The beginning of graying process does differ among racial groups. In whites, graying initiates more or less 10 years earlier than in blacks; whereas in the Japanese, graying is reported to occur midway between the blacks and whites. The graying process initiates at the temples in men and in the 2 in. around the hairline in women; it spread to the vertex and slowly involves the entire scalp. Body hair grays later [39].

A permanent does give the hair more body and hair coloring corrects the graying [39]. It is advisable that these procedures be done by a professional hair dresser (Fig. 6.7).

Hair Loss

Hair loss in men and women may be idiopathic, associated with aging, related to a genetic predisposition, caused by drugs or associated with hormonal or metabolic abnormality (Fig. 6.7). The patients must be submitted to a meticulous review of the family and personal histories, diet and medication and hair care habits, and, last but not least, the clinical examination. The count of the hair shedding daily is necessary to establish a shedding pattern or thinning. Laboratory tests can be performed to look for chronic diseases like diabetes, renal or hepatic pathology, diminished albumin or iron storage.

Fig. 6.7 Gray hair and hair loss

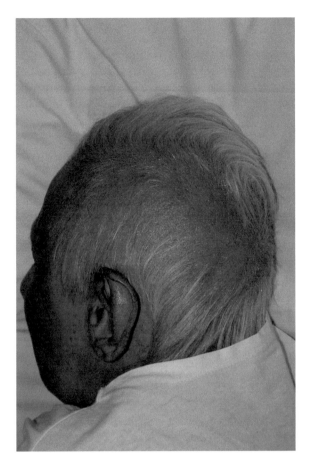

Telogen Effluvium

Telogen effluvium occurs when anagen hair follicles are cycled simultaneously into the telogen phase with increasing hair shedding daily. Several mechanisms are implicated and five functional types have been described recently. Women 30 to 60 years old are affected and complain of continuous scalp-hair loss over a long time [40].

Therapy for telogen effluvium is not specific. Finding and treating the underlying cause should be the solution. Topical minoxidil (2–5%) may be recommended.

Senescent Alopecia

Senescent alopecia is the name for the hair thinning that does not become apparent until after 50 years of age [41]. The phenomenon results from a reduction in follicle size and alterations in hair cycling [41, 42]. Not everyone is affected in the same.

There are many differences between individuals. Hair density and rate of hair growth in the axilla, pubic region and on the extremities typically decrease with aging [42].

Alopecia Areata

Alopecia areata is an autoimmune T-cell-mediate disease, which is directed against hair follicle antigens. Twelve percent of patients are over 50 years old [42]. It is characterized by patches of nonscarring hair loss that can affect any hair-bearing region. Alopecia areata commonly attacks pigmented hair fibers, sparing white and gray hairs [43].

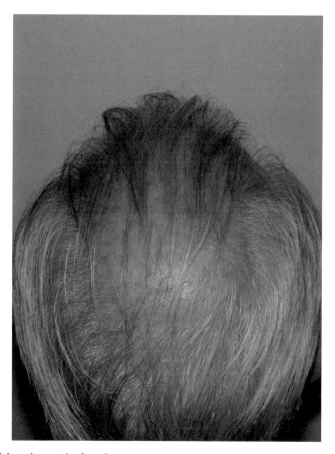

Fig. 6.8 Male androgenetic alopecia

Androgenetic Alopecia

Androgenic alopecia is more prevalent in the elderly. Some male pattern baldness affects well over one half of the adult male population. Genetic, endocrine, and aging factors are interdependent. Although the inherited predisposition, male pattern alopecia will not result if androgens are not present. Androgens are not able to induce baldness in individuals without genetic predisposition to baldness. Aging acts promoting the hair loss as the year goes by [44, 45].Norwood [45] shows that male pattern baldness is a progressive condition that accompanied advanced age, and is much more common than generally believed (Fig. 6.8).

The patterns of hair loss in women are not easily recognized although it is currently defined and be present as late as the sixth decade of life (Fig. 6.9). In women,

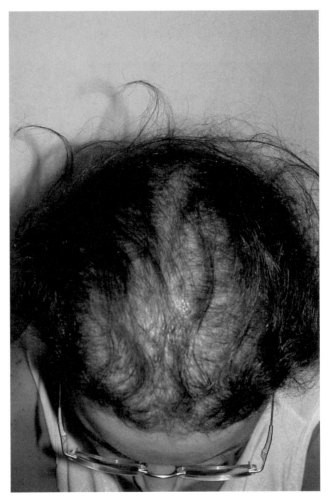

Fig. 6.9 Female androgenetic alopecia

androgenetic alopecia androgen dependence and hereditary nature are not as obvious as they are in affected men. The incidence of frontoparietal loss increases from 13% in premenopausal women to 37% in postmenopausal women [46,47].

Vierhapper et al. demonstrate that the majority of balding young men present normal production rates of testosterone (T) and a marked rise in the production rates of dihidrotestosterone (DHT), and consequently with a shift of the ration between the production rates of T and DHT. The findings in early-onset female-pattern hair loss are quite the opposite.The majority of these women are characterized by subnormal to low-normal production rates of DHT, but an increase in the production rate of T [48,49].

There are few drugs, minoxidil and antiandrogenic agents, as spironolactone, cimetidine and cyproterone acetate, for hair loss. When this treatment does not satisfy, good results have been achieved with surgical hair transplant [35,36].Cosmetic therapy is particularly beneficial for depressed patients and, in low periods, cosmetics provide readily accessible psychological boost [50].

Hirsutism

The term 'hirsutism' is defined by the presence, in women, of terminal and vellus hairs in a male pattern. It is related to an increase in androgen level or to an end-organ response to androgens [51]. It may be idiopathic, reflect a familial trait, become prominent with aging, or be associated with adrenal or ovarian disease. The most common ovarian cause is polycystic ovarian syndrome, whereas the most common adrenal cause is congenital adrenal hyperplasia [42].

Conclusion

Both men and women may experience severe alteration in hair and nails in the aging process, and these structures are important agents of variation in self-image and self-esteem of the elderly. It is necessary to provide conditions to improve the aspect of these skin appendages so that this elderly population, that is growing in number, can feel safe and satisfied.

Physicians, especially dermatologists, must be acquainted with these problems in the elderly and must know how to treat them. We must also be familiarized with the cosmetic procedures available to disguise them, when complete treatment is unavailable.

References

1. Administration on Aging. Statistics on the Aging Population. Profiles of older Americans: 2004. http://www.aoa.gov/prof/Statistics/profile/profiles.asp.
2. Instituto Brasileiro de Geografia e Estatística. IBGE. Censo demográfico 2000. http://www1.ibge.gov.br/home/estatistica/populacao/censo2000/tabelabrasil111.shtm.

3. Cerimele D, Celleno L, Serri F. Physiological changes in ageing skin. Br. J. Dermatol. 1990; 122: 13–20.
4. Cestari TF, Trope BM. The mature adult. In: Parish LC, Brenner S, Ramos-e-Silva M, eds. Women's Dermatology: From Infancy to Maturity. Lancaster: Parthenon, 2001, pp. 72–80.
5. Kurban RS, Bhawan J. Histologic changes in skin associated with aging. J. Dermatol. Surg. Oncol. 1990; 16: 908–14.
6. Bean W. Nail growth: 30 years of observation. Arch. Intern. Med. 1974; 134: 497–502.
7. Baran R, Dawber RPR. The ageing nail. In: Fry L, ed. Skin Problems in the Elderly. Edinburgh: Churchill Livingstone, 1985, pp. 315–30.
8. Baran R, Dawber RPR. The nail in old age. In: Baran R, Dawber RPR, eds. Diseases of the Nails and Their Management. Oxford: Blackwell, 1994, 116–20.
9. Achten G. Normale histologic und histochemie des nagels. In: Jadassohn J, ed. Handbuch der Haut-und Geschlechtskrankheiten. 1V. Berlin: Springer-Verlag, 1968, pp. 339–76.
10. Lynch MH, O'Guin WM, Hardy C et al. Acid and basic hair/nail ('hard') keratins: their co-localization in upper cortical and cuticle cells and the human hair follicle and their relationship to soft keratins. J. Cell Biol. 1986; 103: 2593–606.
11. Shono S, Mataga N, Toda K. The two dimensional peptide mappings of the nail low-sulfur S-carboxyl-methyl keratins. J. Dermatol. 1987; 14: 419–26.
12. Kitahara T, Ogawa H. Cultured nail keratinocytes express hard keratins characteristics of nail and hair. Arch. Dermatol. Res. 1992; l: 253–6.
13. Dawber RPR, De Berker D, Baran R. Science of the nail apparatus. In: Baran R, Dawber RPR, eds. Diseases of the Nails and Their Management. Oxford: Blackwell, 1994, pp. 1–34.
14. Koblenzer CS. Psychologic aspects of aging and the skin. Clin. Dermatol. 1996; 14: 171–7.
15. Cohen PR, Scher RK. Geriatric nail disorders: diagnosis and treatment. J. Am. Acad. Dermatol. 1992; 26: 521–31.
16. Zaias N. Onychomycosis. Arch. Dermatol. 1972; 105: 263–74.
17. Gupta AK. Onychomycosis in the elderly. Drugs Aging 2000; 16(6): 397–407.
18. Hay RJ. Infections affecting the nails. In: Samman PD, Fenton DA, eds. The Nail in Disease. London: William Heinemann, 1986, 27–50.
19. Gupta AK, Jain HC, Lynde CW, Watteel GN, Summerbell RC. Prevalence and epidemiology of unsuspected onychomycosis in patients visiting dermatologists' offices in Ontario, Canada—a multicenter survey of 2001 patients. Int. J. Dermatol. 1997; 36(10): 783–7.
20. Haley L, Daniel CR III. Fungal infections. In: Scher RK, Daniel CR III, eds. Nails: Therapy, Diagnosis, Surgery. Philadelphia: WB Saunders, 1990, pp. 106–19.
21. Scher RK. Subungual scabies. Am. J. Dermatopathol. 1983; 5: 187–9.
22. Shumer SM, O'Keef EJ. Bleomycin in the treatment of recalcitrant warts. J. Am. Acad. Dermatol. 1983; 9: 91–6.
23. Gibson JR, Harvey SG. Interferon in the treatment of persistent viral warts. Dermatologica 1984; 169: 47–8.
24. Wernick J, Gibbs RC. Pedal biomechanics and toenail disease. In: Scher RK, Daniel CR III, eds. Nail Therapy, Diagnosis, Surgery. Philadelphia: WB Saunders, 1990, 244–9.
25. Riccitelli ML. Foot problems of the aged and infirmed. J. Am. Geriatr. Soc. 1966; 14: 1058–66.
26. Lubach D, Cohrs W, Wurzinger R. Incidence of brittle nails. Dermatologica 1986; 172: 144–7.
27. South DA, Farber EM. Urea ointment in the nonsurgical avulsion of nail dystrophies—a reappraisal. Cutis 1980; 25: 609–12.
28. Helfand AE. Nail and hyperkeratotic problems in the elderly foot. Am. Fam. Physician 1989; 39: 101–10.
29. Buselmeier TJ. Combination urea and salicylic acid ointment nail avulsion in nondystrophic nails: a follow-up observation. Cutis 1980; 25: 397–405.
30. Lloyd-Davies RW, Brill GC. The aetiology and out-patient management of ingrowing toenails. Br. J. Surg. 1963; 50: 592–7.
31. Sonnex TS, Dawber RPR. Treatment of ingrowing toenails with liquid nitrogen spray cryotherapy. Br. Med. J. 1985; 291: 173–5.

32. Oliveira AS, Picoto AS, Verde SF, Martins O. Subungual exostosis: treatment as an office procedure. J. Dermatol. Surg. Oncol. 1980; 6(7): 555–8.
33. Dawber RPR. Aetiology and pathophysiology of hair loss. Dermatologica 1987; 175(Suppl. 2): 23–28.
34. Spindler JR, Data JL. Female androgenetic alopecia: a review. Dermatol. Nurs. 1992; 4(2): 93–9.
35. Fenske NA, Albers SE. Cosmetic modalities for aging skin: what to tell patients. Geriatrics 1990; 45: 59–67.
36. Fenske NA, Lober CW. Structural and functional changes of normal aging skin. J. Am. Acad. Dermatol. 1986; 15: 571–85.
37. Montagna W, Carlisle K. Structural changes in ageing skin. Br. J. Dermatol. 1990; 122: 61–70.
38. Dalziel KL. Aspects of cutaneous ageing. Clin. Exp. Dermatol. 1991; 16: 315–23.
39. O'Donoghue MN. Cosmetics for the elderly. Dermatol. Clin. 1991; 9: 29–34.
40. Whiting DA. Chronic telogen effluvium. Dermatol. Clin. 1996; 14: 723–31.
41. Kligman AM. The comparative histopathology of male-pattern baldness and senescent baldness. Dermatol. Clin. 1988; 6: 108–18.
42. Hordinsky M, Sawaya M, Roberts JL. Hair loss and hirsutism in the elderly. Clin. Geriatr. Med. 2002; 18(1): 121–33.
43. Hordinsky M. Alopecia areata: pathophysiology and latest developments. J. Cut. Med. Surg. 1999; 3: S28–30.
44. Hamilton JB. Male hormone stimulation is prerequisite and an incitant in common baldness. Am. J. Anat. 1942; 71: 451–80.
45. Norwood OT. Male pattern baldness: classification and incidence. Southern Med. J. 1975; 68(11): 1359–65.
46. Olsen EA. Androgenetic alopecia. In: Disorders of Hair Growth: Diagnosis and Treatment. New York: McGraw-Hill, 1994, pp. 257–83.
47. Olsen EA. Female pattern hair loss. J. Am. Acad. Dermatol. 2001; 45(3): S70–80.
48. Vierhapper H, Maier H, Nowotny P, Waldhausl. Production rates of testosterone and of dihydrotestosterone in female pattern hair loss. Metabolism 2003; 52(7): 927–29.
49. Vierhapper H, Nowotny P, Maier H et al. Production rates of dihydrotestosterone in healthy men and women and in men with male pattern baldness: determination by stable isotope/dilution and mass spectrometry. J. Clin. Endocrinol. Metab. 2000; 86: 5762–4.
50. Kligman AM, Graham JA. The psychology of appearance in the elderly. Dermatol. Clin. 1986; 4(3): 501–7.
51. Camacho-Martinez F. Hypertrichosis and hirsutism. In: Bolognia JL, Jorizzo JL, Rapini RP, eds. Dermatology. London: Mosby 2003: 1051–9.

Chapter 7

Rosacea in the Elderly

Ronald Marks

Introduction and Definition

Rosacea is a common disorder that can only be defined in clinical terms as there are no diagnostic tests or reliable laboratory markers. It is a chronic disorder of the convexities of facial skin characterised by persistent erythema and telangiectasia that is punctuated by episodes of intensification of the erythema, swelling and the appearance of papules and less often pustules.

Rosacea is a disease with an impressive history. It was described by Shakespeare and before that by Chaucer in rumbustious and jovial (and alcoholic) characters. Unfortunately it was not clearly distinguished from acne vulgaris by medical writers until the latter half of the 20th century. This probably explains how the prefix acne became attached to the term rosacea to describe the disorder. In fact any popular disorder of facial skin was described as "acne." Rosacea should no longer receive a qualifying "acne" prefix as acne and rosacea share only the face as a site of involvement and a tendency to develop papular lesions.

Epidemiology

Rosacea mostly affects fair skinned, blue-eyed individuals and is endemic in North West Europe. It is especially prevalent in Celtic types from Ireland, Wales and Scotland as well as those derived from Celts but who live in the United States and elsewhere. It is very much less common in darker complexioned individuals on the Mediterranean littoral. It is quite uncommon in Asian people although is seen in lighter skinned individuals from the Indian sub-continent as well as the Chinese and Japanese. It is rare in black skinned people. The age of onset is enormously variable but it is essentially a disorder of mature adults and is certainly not uncommon in the seventh and eighth decades. One characteristic needs to be mentioned in this context and this is the persistence of the condition. At least two studies have demonstrated that patients who have once had an attack are liable to experience further attacks some years hence [1, 2].

R.A. Norman (ed.), *Diagnosis of Aging Skin Diseases,*
© Springer-Verlag London Limited 2008

Rosacea is no respecter of social class and does not seem to have a predilection for any particular profession or trade.

Clinical Features

The cardinal feature of rosacea is a persistent redness of the convexities of the skin of the face, i.e. the cheeks, chin front of nose and forehead (Fig. 7.1). Alongside the erythema there is telangiectasia which is more marked in patients who have had the disease over a long period. The cheeks do not feel warm to the touch and the redness is due to "pooling" rather than increased blood flow. The pooling is due to loss of dermal fibrous connective tissue support to the vasculature (see under "Pathology" and "Aetiopathogenesis"). At this stage patients also complain of frequent blushing or flushing.

In some patients the reddened areas are slightly thickened and oedematous. This is especially noticeable over the forehead. Apart from the erythema, telangiectasia and slight swelling which are persistent, the condition is subject to episodic inflammation with the appearance of papules and sometimes pustules (Fig. 7.2). These must not be confused with acne. Papules in acne tend to be tender and irregular in shape whereas in rosacea the papules are usually hemispherical and non-tender.

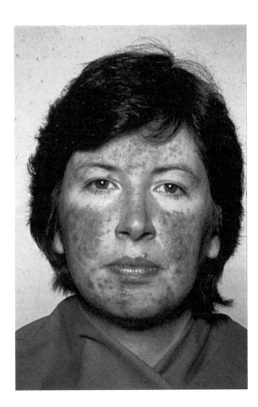

Fig. 7.1 Typical distribution of rosacea

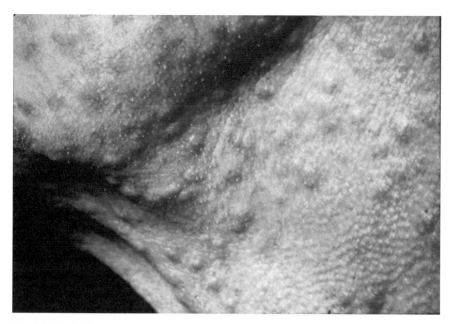

Fig. 7.2 Papules in rosacea

Accompanying the papules there is some increase in the erythema and the degree of swelling during the acute episode. Untreated the acute episode subsides although a few papules continue to appear.

Rosacea is usually confined to the face although the front and sides of the neck is uncommonly also involved. Very rarely a few papules develop on the limbs [3]. This extrafacial or disseminated variety should only be diagnosed if the papules look like rosacea papules and occur during the course of typical facial rosacea.

Complications of Rosacea

The eye is often affected in rosacea. In most patients the ocular involvement takes the form of a conjunctivitis and/or a stye or a chalazion. The complaint of "dry eyes" is curiously common and when tested a surprising number of patients give a positive Schirmer test.

Some of the complications of rosacea are very much more common in men. This is certainly true of one ophthalmological complication—keratitis. Luckily rare, this disease is painful and threatening to the eyesight. Although keratitis is much more common in men other quite common ocular complications of rosacea occur equally in both sexes. Blepharoconjunctivitis and keratoconjunctivitis sicca are both extremely common and quite troublesome.

Lymphoedema is a quite rare complication and much more commonly seen in men. It is usually confined to one side of the face (Fig. 7.3) and is annoyingly

Fig. 7.3 Lymphoedema in rosacea

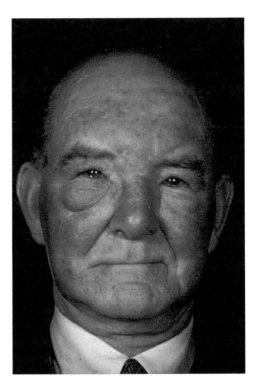

Fig. 7.4 Rhinophyma. Note dilated follicular orifices and "irregular craggy surface"

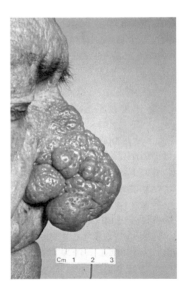

persistent. It resists all treatment although some cosmetic help has been claimed by surgical debulking [4].

Rhinophyma is usually listed as a complication of rosacea although the writer's experience is that this curious nasal disorder may occur in isolation, with minimal rosacea, or the condition may even with acne. Traditionally rhinophyma is associated with alcohol excess but careful studies [5] have shown that this is not the case. Once again it is much more often seen in men although it is occasionally seen in a mild form in women. The nose is usually a dull red or mauve and the skin surface often has numerous telangiectatic vessels over the surface. The whole structure is swollen—usually irregularly so and in the worst cases the clinical results are grotesque (Fig. 7.4). Rhinophyma is for the most part confined to the nose but patients have been described where the "phymatous" enlargement affects other parts of the face—such as the ear lobes or the chin.

Differential Diagnosis

Any disorder in which redness of the skin of the cheeks is part of the clinical picture may be mistaken for rosacea. Weathering in healthy Celtic types is often accompanied by redness of the cheeks which may be mistaken for rosacea. Indeed this may indeed be the first stage of rosacea (see later). The disorders that cause most problems are those in which the underlying disorder is systemic lupus such as systemic erythematosus, dermatomyositis and polycythaemia rubra vera as they tend to cause symmetrical signs with erythema without any major change in the skin surface. In general these diseases can be distinguished by the presence of physical signs and symptoms outside of the facial skin as well as there being characteristic laboratory findings. Where there is any doubt at all it is worthwhile arranging for haematological tests, ANF and anti-DNA antibody blood tests and muscle enzyme studies.

Acne causes considerable confusion in the inexperienced. Acne is a disease characterised by the presence of comedones and seborrhoea—which is not a feature of rosacea [6]. Rosacea is confined to the face whereas in acne lesions usually also occur over the back, shoulders and chest. Acne causes scarring, rosacea does not. Cystic lesions may develop in acne but never do in rosacea. Finally, acne is a disease of the "teenager" and young adult whereas rosacea occurs characteristically in the middle aged and elderly.

Other common skin disorders that may sometimes cause difficulty include seborrhoeic dermatitis and perioral dermatitis. The former of these is mainly a disease of skin flexures rather than convexities and, being a dermatitis, is also marked by scaling. Perioral dermatitis is very much more frequently seen in young (15–25) females. It develops around the mouth and in the nasolabial folds—which rosacea avoids. Furthermore perioral dermatitis is characterised by very small papules and papulopustules without the background of erythema typical of rosacea.

The photodermatoses may occasionally cause confusion although the occurrence of rash on other light exposed areas (e.g. back of hands) usually distinguishes these from rosacea. Also telangiectasia and papules are seen in rosacea alone.

Pathology of Rosacea

When there is redness and telangiectasia clinically but no inflammatory papules the predominant histological change is in the dermis. Large irregular vascular channels are present throughout the upper dermis which is often strikingly oedematous. In addition the fibrous component of the dermis is itself abnormal in two ways. Firstly there is marked solar elastotic degenerative change—more than one would have expected in an individual of a similar age, skin colour and life style but without rosacea and from a similar site on the face [7]. Secondly the dermal fibres appear less well organised into bundles than expected and are thinner and less intensely staining than normal (Fig. 7.5). This dermal dystrophy is evident in the background even when there is marked inflammation.

If a papule is biopsied the above dermal changes are present but swamped by the presence of a variably heavy monoclear inflammatory cell infiltrate consisting of lymphocytes and histiocytes arranged perivascularly. In a small proportion of samples perhaps 10% giant cells are found in the inflammatory foci without any specific arrangement. The inflammation does not appear focussed on follicular structures but is consistently arranged around the walls of small blood vessels. If pustules are sampled, a similar histological picture emerges but in this case follicles are involved by collections of polymorphonuclear neutrophils in the superficial parts of the follicle. Close inspection will often show that these follicles are infested with the mite *Demodex folliculorum*, which for some reason are much more numerous in rosacea than in control skin.

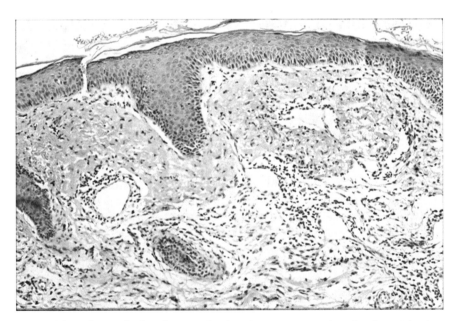

Fig. 7.5 Photomicrograph of erythemato telangiectatic rosacea—note dermal oedema, telangiectasia and dermal disorganisation (haematoxylin and eosin × 45)

In rhinophyma the same background dermal changes are present and in addition there is sebaceous gland hypertrophy and massive dilation of the follicular structures. Inflammation and fibroplasia are also present.

Aetiopathogenesis

The cause of rosacea is not known. Hopeless hypotheses and mysterious myths [8] have abounded in the past half-century and agencies as diverse as psychological abnormality, gastrointestinal disease, dietary indiscretion and skin infections (and/or infestations) have been blamed. Recently infection with *Helicobacter pylori* has been investigated but is now thought an unlikely contender in the aetiological stakes. The role of *Demodex folliculorum* is still hotly debated. In this writer's view it may play some subsidiary (but not primary) [9] role.

A striking clinical feature of rosacea is the distribution of the rash on the light exposed areas on the skin of the face—in fact the disorder occurs in a similar distribution to that of the photodermatoses. As mentioned above there is marked solar elastosis in the dermis of patients with rosacea as well as a dermal dystrophy. The pronounced telangiectasia histologically may well result from this lack of dermal integrity as a result of loss of perivascular support. The redness and oedema may also result from this basic structural problem. How the inflammation would result in this scheme is less certain but it is possible that the dilated vessels, which will contain pooled stagnant blood, will have hypoxic endothelium allowing potentially inflammatory molecules to permeate from the blood into the dermis. Whatever else is clear the detail of the aetiopathogensis is not, and much more research is needed in this area.

Management

Broadly speaking the management can be thought of under three headings. The first are *simple measures* applicable to all patients. These include sympathy and reassurance directed to information concerning the excellent response to treatment and ways of improving the appearance, for example, using green-tinted cosmetics. Advice concerning sun avoidance and/or protection should also be given. In addition simple emollients will assist by reducing the burning sensation that some patients experience. Avoidance of flushing/blushing by cutting back on hot and spicy foods is of doubtful value but a few patients may benefit.

Topical treatments. This is the second category of measures that may be employed. Topical metronidazole was the first topical treatment to be found of value in papular rosacea; 0.75% metronidazole gel assists some 60–70% patients over a 6–8 week period [10]. It stings but does not cause any other significant side effects. More recently azelaic acid preparations (15 or 20%) have been found effective in rosacea [11] though how either those or metronidazole preparations work is utterly mysterious. Azelaic acid preparations not only reduce the inflammation but also appear to reduce the erythema.

Systemic treatments. The most effective remedy that we have for treatment of papular rosacea is the tetracycline group of antibiotics [12]. The great majority of patients are considerably improved by administration of these drugs in full dosage. Improvement usually begins some 2–3 weeks after starting treatment and continues for several weeks. After subsidence of the disease reduction in dosage may be attempted but restarting the original dose may be needed if new lesions appear. It is often the case that the drug has to be continued for 6 months before it can be stopped without a recurrence of the lesions. Other antibiotics can be used—notably erythromycin or clarithromycin—and seem as effective. Metronidazole [13] was the first antibiotic to be described as effective for rosacea but is not now often used. Isotretinion has been suggested by some but has not been effective in my hands.

Phototherapy. Either high intensity pulsed light or pulsed dye laser therapy has been shown to effectively reduce the erythema when used over a period of 3–6 weeks.

Conclusion

All patients with rosacea can be helped. At times in some patients the disorder is more stubborn than in others but there are no patients who at the end of 2–3 months are not substantially improved.

References

1. Marks R, Irvine C. Prognosis and prognostic factors in rosacea. In Marks R, Plewig G, eds. Acne and Related Disorders, Proceedings of an International Symposium Cardiff. Martin Dunitz, 1989, pp. 331–3.
2. Knight AK, Vickers CFH. A follow up of tetracycline treated rosacea. Br. J. Dermatol. 1975; 93: 577–80.
3. Marks R, Wilson Jones E. Disseminated rosacea. Br. J. Dermatol. 1969; 81: 16–28.
4. Bernardin FP, Kersten RC, Khouri LM, Kulwin M, Mutasim DF. Chronic eyelid lymphedema and acne rosacea. Report of two cases. Ophthalmology 2000; 12: 2220–3.
5. Marks R. Concepts in the pathogenesis of rosacea. Br. J Dermatol. 1968; 80: 170–7.
6. Marks R, Lever L. Diagnostic discrimination between acne and rosacea. In Marks R, Plewig G, eds. Acne and Related Disorders Proceedings of an International Symposium Cardiff. Martin Dunitz, 1989, pp. 317–20.
7. Marks R, Harcourt Webster JN. Histopathology of rosacea. Arch. Dermatol. 1969; 100: 683–91.
8. Marks R. Rosacea: hopeless hypotheses, marvellous myths and dermal disorganization. In Marks R, Plewig G, eds. Acne and Related Disorders Proceedings of an International Symposium Cardiff. Martin Dunitz, 1989, pp. 293–9.
9. Zülal E, Orhan O. The significance of *Demodex folliculorum* density in rosacea. Int. J. Dermatol. 1998; 37: 421–5.
10. Neilson GP. Treatment of rosacea with 1% metronidazole cream: a double-blind study. Br. J. Dermatol. 1983; 108: 327–32.

11. Maddin S. A comparison of topical azelaic acid 20% cream and topical metronidazole 0.75% cream in the treatment of patients with papulopustular rosacea. J. Am. Acad. Dermatol. 1999; 40: 961–5.
12. Marks R, Ellis J. Comparative effectiveness of tetracycline and ampicillin in rosacea. Lancet 1971; ii: 1049–52.
13. Pye RJ, Burton JL. Treatment of rosacea by metronidazole. Lancet 1976; i: 1211–2.

Chapter 8

Variations in Aging in Ethnic Skin and Hair: Corrective and Cosmetic Treatment

Margaret I. Aguwa and Marcy Street

Introduction

The changing racial and ethnic demographic of patients coming into both the primary care and dermatological settings requires medical practitioners to move beyond the "one size fits all" when it comes to providing corrective and cosmetic treatment of the skin and hair for these individuals. By all accounts, the complexion of the United States is rapidly changing, and so are the needs of our present and future patient base.

It is predicted that by the year 2050, people of color, including Hispanics, Asians and Pacific Islanders, Native Americans and individuals of African decent, will be in the majority in the United States. In view of the ongoing discussion of racial and ethnic disparities in health care, it is important to address the needs of these groups of patients, in terms of screenings, diagnoses and treatments of a whole host of conditions, including dermatological problems, which may or may not manifest themselves in the traditional ways. Not only will the ethnicity of our patients undergo a metamorphosis, but so will the age base of our patients. We are clearly in a time of the aging of America and must be well versed on how the skin of diverse populations ages, and how it reacts to treatment during the aging process.

Medical professionals must be informed and alerted to the ever- changing needs of an aging racial and ethnic population and be prepared to meet their very specific needs. Variability exists in the way the racial or ethnic skin functions and reacts to preventative, corrective and cosmetic treatment.

One of the difficulties is that there has been little study of and limited medical literature produced and available to the practitioner on the differences in dermatological care, disorder diagnosis and treatment among the various people of color (African-American, African, Hispanic, Asian and Native American) and how it should differ from that of their fair skin counterparts of European origin. Thus the unique care, diagnosis and treatment of individuals with skin of color, through the ages and stages of their lives, are often neglected.

As we begin to more effectively address these needs we must not only utilize the limited documented knowledge base, but also push for more research, clinical studies and information on effective practices that help enlighten our general and specialty practices when it comes to the screening, diagnosis and treatment of racial and ethnic skin and hair.

R.A. Norman (ed.), *Diagnosis of Aging Skin Diseases,*
© Springer-Verlag London Limited 2008

Biological Differences in Skin and Hair

The primary external racial or ethnic difference that characterizes the biological difference in skin and hair is color. The significant biological difference between people of color and their Caucasian counterparts is the amount of cutaneous pigment or melanin in the skin. Skin reactions to chemical and environmental changes manifest themselves in a host of ways, especially as patients advance in age. For example, sun exposure has a greater effect on the aging process over time of fairer skinned individuals, with less melanin, than with people of color. The medical professional needs to be aware of hypertrophic scarring, keloids, hyperpigmentation and melasma that occur more typically in patients with more cutaneous pigment in their skin.

Data support the evidence that there is no appreciable difference in the number of melanocytes between people of different races or ethnicities. Yet there may be individual variances in the number of melanocytes from one person to another, and in concentrations in different parts of the body, such as arms and legs.

The racial and ethnic differences occur due to variations in size, number and aggregation of the melanosomes within the melanocyte and the keratinocyte. As an example, a dark-skinned black patient may have non-aggregated, large melanosomes, whereas a light-skinned black patient may have both large and smaller aggregated melanosomes. Another significant racial and ethnic difference is found in the thickness of the epidermis. Darker skins not only tend to have thicker skin layers, but also experience epidermal thinning as part of the aging process. This is significant because evidence suggests these racial differences in the thickness of the skin can effect transcutaneous penetration of chemicals and drugs.

Researchers have raised questions regarding what these differences in skin could mean when examining the effects of aging, the environment and the care of skin of color. A few researchers have not only defined skin of color but also presented some medical inquiry into why it is less likely to burn, yet readily tans, resulting in a lower proportion of persons of color with skin cancer and other pigmentation disorders, who remain poorly diagnosed and managed when suffering from other skin-related illnesses.

Biological Differences Between Patients of Color and Other Skin Types

- Increased melanin content, melanosomal dispersion
- Multinucleated and larger fibroblasts in black persons compared with their white counterparts
- Curved hair follicle/spiral hair type in black persons compared with white persons
- Fewer elastic fibers anchoring hair follicles to dermis in black persons

Therapeutic Differences Between Patients of Color and Other Skin Types

- Lower rates of skin cancer in people of color
- Higher mortality rate from skin cancer due to late diagnoses and less aggressive surgical, chemotherapeutic and other treatment modalities
- Less pronounced photo-aging
- Higher rates of pigmentation disorders due to biologic predisposition and more pigment reactions to over-the-counter and prescription medications
- More pronounced keloid formation among black patients than other racial and ethnic groups
- More pseudofolliculitis in blacks who shave with razors
- More scalp and hair disorders among black patients who practice hair braiding and/or use strong chemicals on the hair
- Increased incidents of tension alopecia in black patients, due to pulling of the fragile hair shaft and application of strong chemicals used in straightening and coloring the hair.

Ethnicity and Aging

While increased melanin does protect some ethnic and racial groups from some of the damage of ultra violet (UV) rays, the medical practitioner should not assume that

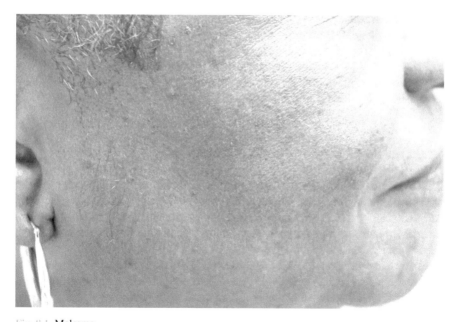

Fig. 8.1 Melasma

pigmented skin never suffers the effects of environmental exposures. People of color can experience photodamage, skin atrophy, loss of collagen and elastin damage as well as hyper and hypopigmentation as they age (Fig. 8.1).

In addition to the damage that the sun can cause, the long-term effects of poor lifestyle choices, such as alcohol and tobacco use, lack of sleep, poor hydration, lack of proper nutrition and family history, are important in addressing the skin of minority populations. These factors can intensify specific physical signs of aging like accelerating the development of fine and coarse skin wrinkling, irregular mottled pigmentation and skin laxity. These factors not only negatively affect the skin and hair, but can also trigger chronic health conditions such as diabetes, hypertension, various cancers, as well as renal, hepatic and cardiac diseases.

Family Practitioner and Dermatologist as a Team

Since the majority of patients enter the healthcare system through their primary care physician, it is therefore important for these physicians to have a strong knowledge base of dermatological problems and to establish and maintain a good relationship with a dermatologist. Clinic visits present good opportunities to dialogue with the patient about skin and hair concerns. The skin and hair can often indicate the presence of disorders within the thyroid, connective tissue and the immune and hormonal systems. The individual's skin and hair may also manifest the effects of emotional stress and exposure to environmental toxins. It is therefore important for all physicians to be aware that clinical symptoms may present differently in patients of African descent.

These visits with the family practice physician should be viewed as valuable opportunities to perform visual screening of the skin for suspicious lesions and moles that may indicate precancerous or malignant conditions. Subsequently, a dermatologist or a skin cancer specialist should conduct thorough full body skin examinations for those patients with higher risk factors or suspicious lesions.

Understanding the Role Culture Plays

Biology is not the only factor that determines skin and hair differences between racial and ethnic groups. Grooming practices of a particular group affect the skin, hair and scalp and can potentially impact the development of certain related diseases. Medical practitioners who treat diverse populations should understand the need to perform a comprehensive evaluation that includes taking an appropriate history of products used on the skin, hair and scalp in addition to the grooming practices such as frequency of hair washing, types of hair styles like braiding, perming, flat ironing and texturing, twisting and dred-locking.

These questions become important when evaluating patients that present with a rash, hyperpigmentation, contact dermatitis or hair and scalp complaints, since these

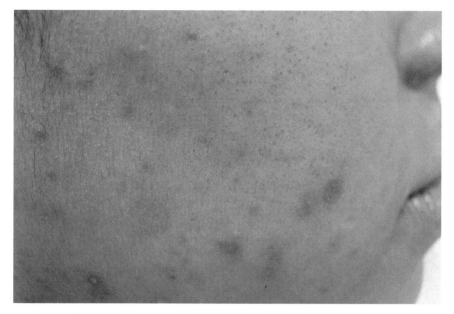

Fig. 8.2 Scarification of acne

practices and products could trigger such reactions. Dermatologists who often see ethnic patients with severe hairline and forehead acne and rashes know that these eruptions can be due to the use of oil-based skin, hair and scalp products.

In treating the ethnic patient, the physician should consider the skin's melanin response to certain topical medications in order to minimize hypo or hyperpigmentation. A patient's skin color, use of chemicals, cultural and grooming practices and response to treatment regimens ought to be considered when evaluating and developing a medical or cosmetic treatment plan (Fig. 8.2).

Skin Cancers and Moles

Although the incidence of skin cancers is less common in ethnic minority populations, it is still essential that darker skin shades be protected from prolonged exposure to the ultraviolet rays of the sun by the use of sunscreens, limiting sun exposure during the peak hours and wearing protective clothing. Medical literature indicates that the lesser the pigmentation, the greater the risk of melanoma on sun-exposed skin. While fairer skinned Caucasians are more susceptible to melanomas than Hispanics, Asians and Blacks, all patients should be screened regularly for a variety of skin cancers.

Therefore a thorough skin evaluation should not be neglected in people of color and considered routine. This includes examining the scalp, face, neck, trunk, limbs, hands, feet, genitalia, oral mucosa and nail beds (Fig. 8.3).

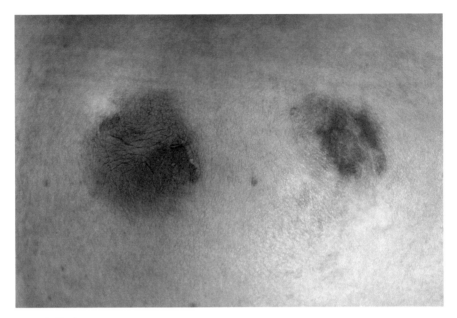

Fig. 8.3 Nevi

According to a study in the *American Journal of Dermatology*, patients of color—especially black patients—are being diagnosed with skin cancers at Stages III and IV, when the cancer has already metastasized to other parts of the body. The most positive outcomes for patients of color come from early detection, diagnosis and appropriate treatment.

Melanomas and other skin cancers in white patients are usually found in areas that are sun-exposed. Practitioners doing routine screenings in ethnic skin must go beyond "the usual suspect" sites, since many lesions are often found in unusual sites on the body such as the mucous membranes in the mouth, nasal passages, genitals, the palms of the hands, soles of the feet and toe web spaces. Incidentally, as people of African decent age, the incidence of skin cancer located under the nail bed rises significantly.

The practitioner should be aware that the two most frequently occurring carcinomas in African-Americans are squamous cell carcinoma (SCC) and basal cell carcinoma (BCC). SCC accounts for 67% of all skin tumors and is most often located on legs, rather than in the exposed skin. These SCCs may develop in an old burn or vaccination site or on chronically irritated skin. Black males over 50 years of age have twice the incidence of SCC than black females. So, total body screening is essential. BCC often occurs on the head and neck regions. While African-American women have an incidence rate of BBC that is similar, this cancer acts more aggressively in the African-Americans than in Caucasians. Patient education is key!

In addition to regular skin screening for suspicious growths in the clinical setting, practitioners should educate ethnic patients on their risks for skin cancers, including the ABCDE of melanomas (*A* asymmetry, *B* irregular borders, *C* variegated color, *D* diameter greater than 6 mm or a pencil head eraser, *E* sudden elevation). The patients also become more aware of what to look for if they are shown photographs of suspicious lesions in brochures. These handouts are essential in patient education as they depict examples of red, scaly or pearly lesions. Keep in mind that the hue of the lesion on ethnic skin may be different and appear brown to violaceous or purple. Educating the patient on how precancers and skin cancer appear helps create an awareness of the importance of early diagnosis and treatment of skin cancers.

Treatment of Skin Cancers

When planning the best treatment plan for each patient, the physician should consider the type of skin cancer, its location and size and the person's general health and medical history. A variety of treatment modalities are available for managing skin cancers. These treatments may involve the use of topical agents, oral medications, surgical procedures, radiation treatment and chemotherapy or a combination of these.

In treating skin cancer, a physician/dermatologist should be aggressive in removing the cancer and destroying cancerous cells through a host of surgical procedures, including simple excision and the very specialized Mohs micrographic procedure. Mohs surgery permits immediate and complete microscopic examination of the excised cancerous tissue and allows for all the roots and extensions of the cancer to be removed in the one surgical procedure. Of all the skin cancer surgical procedures, it has been recognized as the leading treatment with the highest reported cure rate.

Mohs surgery is reserved for skin cancers that have recurred following a previous treatment or that are at a high risk for recurrence or that involve deeper structures of the skin. Mohs surgery is often used in areas such as the face, especially on the nose, eyelids, lips and hairline. Also cancers on the ears, hands, feet and genitals benefit from using the Mohs technique as it is important to preserve as much normal skin tissue as possible for cosmetic or functional purposes. Regardless of the surgical procedure type, the main goal of treatment is the same for the ethnic patient as it is for the Caucasian patient—to remove or destroy cancer completely, leaving as small a scar as possible.

Racial and Ethnic Differences in Hair and Scalp

The ethnic differences in hair are probably more pronounced that the phenotypic characteristics of skin color. There are four basic hair types: straight, wavy, helical and spiral—which is the primary type for the majority of blacks. There are few differences between the thickness of the cuticle, the shape, size or scale of the hair and the cortical cells between white and black subjects. The existing literature does suggest that the total hair density of blacks may be lower than their white counterparts.

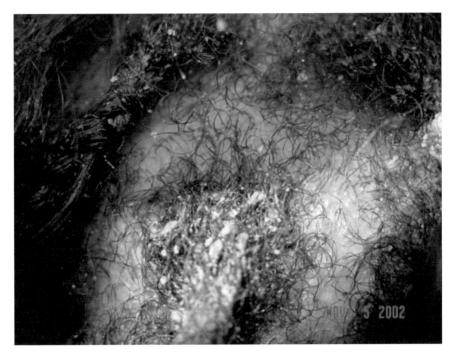

Fig. 8.4 Traction alopecia

Research also suggests that blacks have fewer elastic fibers that anchor the hair follicles to the dermis. This should be kept in mind when a patient presents with certain types of alopecia, such as traction alopecia or follicular degeneration syndrome. Patients of African decent may present with a higher incidence of certain types of alopecia that may be genetic. Physicians may also find that the harsh chemicals that are often used on the fragile hair of the black patient can also lead to severe hair breakage, sometimes down to the scalp level. The products a patient uses to groom the hair are not the only thing that affects breakage and loss, but the tools used can cause damage, and even scalp burns (if heated styling tools, such as hot combs, flat or curling irons, are used).

There is often a higher incidence of contact dermatitis among black men and women than among other users of hair dye. It is suggested that the darker shades of dyes have a more irritating effect on the scalp over time (Fig. 8.4).

Black Men and Hair Loss

Although there is a trend among some black men to shave their heads for cosmetic reasons, alopecia can be devastating for some black men. Medical literature on hair loss in black and Hispanic men is sparse. There is some evidence that white males begin to lose their hair at younger ages than other ethnic patients, but by the age of 35 one-third of all men experience some degree of baldness. Based on the overwhelming amount of hair restoration advertising and programs, this is clearly a matter of widespread and serious concern for a large segment of our society.

There are a variety of products, mostly topical, on the market for hair regrowth. Minoxidil, trade-named Rogaine, is the main hair loss treatment on the US market, formerly offered by prescription only, but now the lower strengths are sold over the counter. It is the most widely used agent for hair restoration. This agent works best if use starts within the first 5 years of hair thinning. Rogaine has also been reported to have some positive effects on women.

Other procedures used for hair restoration involve surgical treatment. One is hair transplantation performed by a practitioner who has specialized training in the procedure. Hair transplantation involves taking donor hair follicles from unaffected scalp and placing them in the areas of hair loss. This transplanted hair has many advantages, including a good color, texture match and degree of curliness. Hair follicles taken from the donor site generally last a lifetime, in areas where they are transplanted. Also, once the scalp is healed, the hair is expected to grow, and a patient can use any type of hair product, including perms and relaxers. Side effects for the procedure can include scar or keloid formation and scalp irritation. Appropriate patient evaluation is essential before this procedure can be performed.

Hairlifting is a cosmetic surgery procedure where an area of bald scalp is removed and the entire hair-bearing scalp is lifted and stretched upward and forward into the areas of hair loss. Depending on the degree of hair loss and the scalp's flexibility, the desired coverage may be achieved in one to several sessions. The procedure is often combined with hair transplantation to reconstruct a natural looking frontal hairline. In a similar procedure, scalp reduction or excision, the bald area is cut out and the remaining hair-bearing scalp is pulled together and stitched. Similar surgical complications may occur which include keloids, scars and irritation.

Cosmetic Procedures

It has been suggested that ethnic patients are less likely candidates for cosmetic procedures. Although pigmented skin shows signs of aging later than fairer skinned patients, many cosmetic procedures can have a positive effect in keeping a patient's skin looking more youthful longer.

Cosmetic procedures in ethnic skin should be mild. Chemical peels have long been an accepted practice for the improvement of the appearance of fine lines and wrinkles that develop with aging of white skin. Yet physicians should proceed with great caution when performing these procedures on ethnic skin. The skin's melanocytes may over- or underproduce in response to the inflammation of harsh topical creams or chemical peels, resulting in hypopigmentation or hyperpigmentation. Deeper peels may even produce keloids.

Patients of color are increasingly interested in anti-aging products they can use at home that will prevent damage and improve the appearance of fine lines, rough and dry skin and irregular pigment.

What Works

There are more and more cosmetic advances to slow down the appearance of aging that work well in ethnic skin. These include microdermabrasion, tissue tightening with radiofrequency, fillers such as collagen, hyaluronic acid, botulinum toxin injections and salicylic acid chemical peels. Take home treatment advice may include establishing a good cleansing and moisturizing routine and the use of mild topical retinoids and antioxidants. Improper use of the products or procedures can lead to a myriad of other skin problems including acne blemishes, dry flaky skin and hypo or hyperpigmentation.

Dermatologists who take care of people of color have been using microdermabrasion on pigmented skin with success in reducing the effects of wrinkles and acne scars without creating additional damage. They have also used laser treatments for hair removal successfully. The 1064 NdYAG or 810 diode lasers have worked well.

Cosmetic Treatment for Keloids

As patients age, the keloids they have lived with for years may become a source of discomfort and concern. Corticosteroid (Kenalog 10–40 mg/cc) injections to the site of the keloid may reduce the size, pain and itching often associated with keloids. Also excisional surgery may be effective even though the keloid may reoccur or enlarge. Subsequent Kenalog injections into the surgical site may be necessary for up to 1 year or more to minimize the chance of recurrence (Fig. 8.5).

Non-cancerous Skin Lesions

Patients of color, both male and female, are more likely to develop raised, dark, painless lesions, as they age, called papulousa nigra. They appear as flat or raised, even colored papules on the face, neck and trunk and are usually asymptotic. Patients may want them removed, especially if they are on the face or in areas that rub against their clothing. Skin tags may also appear as raised pedunculated tan to brown raised papules on the face, neck and inframmary areas. They may be irritated by jewelry or clothing. Seborrheic keratoses are warty, verrucous papules and plaques that may develop on the face, neck trunk or limbs. They represent an overgrowth of the top layer of the skin and may be irritated by sweat and clothing and are cosmetically unsightly (Fig. 8.6).

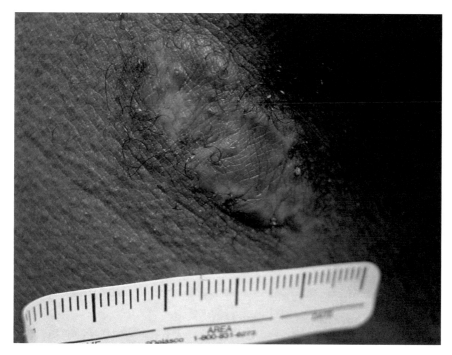

Fig. 8.5 Keloid formation

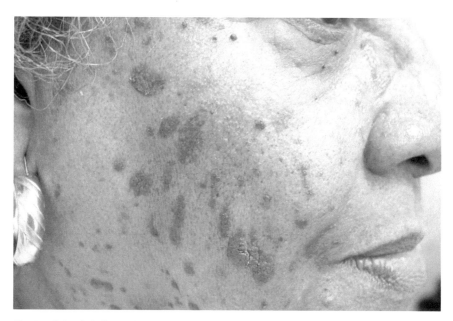

Fig. 8.6 Seborrheic keratosis

Summary

The key to successful treatment, both corrective and cosmetic in ethnic patients, is to first understand that race and ethnicity do impact the skin. As with all patients, how we provide appropriate, preventative, corrective and cosmetic treatment is an essential of good clinical management. As our patient base becomes more diverse, so must our ability to treat these patients in their aging processes.

References

1. Projections of the resident population by race, Hispanic origin and nativity: middle series, 2006 to 2010. Populations Projections Program, Population Division, U.S. Census Bureau, Washington, DC, 2001.
2. Berardesca E, Maibach H. Racial differences in skin pathophysiology. J. Am. Acad. Dermatol. 1996; 34(4): 667–72.
3. Halder R, Nootheti PK. J. Am. Acad. Dermatol. 2003; 48(6).
4. McDonald CJ. Structure and function of the skin: are there differences between black and white skin? Dermatol. Clin. 1988; 6(3).
5. Berardesca E, Maibach H. Ethnic skin: overview of structure and function. J. Am. Acad. Dermatol. 2003; 48(6).
6. Jackson B. J. Am. Acad. Dermatol. 2003; 48(6).
7. McMichael AJ. Scalp and hair disease in the black patient. In Johnson BL Jr, Moi RL, White GM, eds. Ethnic Skin: Medical and Surgical. St. Louis: Mosby, 1998.
8. Montagna W, Carlisle K. The architecture of black and white facial skin. J. Am. Acad. Dermatol. 1991; 24(6).
9. Taylor SC. Epidemiology of skin diseases in ethnic populations. Dermatol. Clin. 2003; 21(4).
10. Richards GM, Oresajo CO, Halder RM. Structure and function of ethnic skin and hair. Dermatol. Clin. 2003; 21(4).

Chapter 9

Skin Cancer in Elderly Patients

Charles Dewberry

The dermatologist that engages in health care for the elderly is far and away the physician that is expected to be the frontrunner for detection and treatment of skin cancers. It is much like the other inherent medical sub-specialty expectations. The OB-GYN performs c-sections; cavities are the responsibility of the dentist; the cardiac surgeon performs the triple bypass; and the geriatric dermatologist assumes the responsibility of integumental neoplasms. Family practitioners, general practitioners, nurses, assistants, and other healthcare workers in the field of geriatric medicine and nursing home management are all involved. Often, it is these healthcare providers that alert the dermatologist about suspicious lesions.

A sizable demographic percentage of many dermatologists' patient populations are geriatric patients. The geriatric population is afflicted with a great many dermatology concerns, due to not only the normal aging process but the additional stressors acquired from environmental causes. The long-term effects of exterior causes such as UV radiation, chemical irritants, temperature, humidity, dryness, pathogens, and so on are compounded for those who have had to endure longer. This cumulative damage profoundly affects the health of the elderly. They simply have accumulated more of everything, including quantitative decay, which might be a good definition of "aging" of humans as biologic organisms [1].

The future dermatology practice will increase in the number of geriatric patients. Not only is the geriatric population one of the fastest growing segments of our society but also the baby boomer generation is now at the geriatric doorstep. The age group of 50- to 65-year-olds represents a significant fraction of the total population [2].

The popularity of the public to engage in purposeful exposure to get that "tan" look will probably affect the baby boomers just as the geriatric population had higher amounts of "occupational" exposure. The generation of yesterday may have spent more time working out of doors than today's workforce. The availability of ultraviolet protection and the education of patients about ultraviolet protection have only come into vogue in the last decade or so. Using demographic reasoning we can expect an exponential increase in the growth rate of cutaneous malignancies presenting in the ever-increasing pool of geriatric patients.

Even considering the trend in recent years to use sun block and tint auto windows as preventative medicine is extremely important, it is retrospect, especially

R.A. Norman (ed.), *Diagnosis of Aging Skin Diseases,*
© Springer-Verlag London Limited 2008

when neoplasms are concerned. Genetic mutations that eventually lead to neoplastic lesions happen by either spontaneous event or mutagenic induction from extrinsic factors. Larger amounts of time and heavier chronic exposure only serve to increase their incidence [1].

Sound clinical advice includes recommending to a patient to make a habit of avoiding peak sunlight hours, wearing appropriate clothing, and applying barrier creams. However, it has not been demonstrated that following this advice will cause any regression or remission in cutaneous tumors.

And how does all this cumulative decay add up? Often to skin cancer, whether it is a primary lesion or metastasis of an internal malignancy.

Recognizing that skin cancers are going to present more often, and that we are relied upon to manage them collectively, is only part of the equation. We must also accept the responsibility of treatment. The geriatric patient is living longer today than the same patient of yesterday and the quality of life is higher. It is therefore more important today than ever to diagnose and treat the elderly. Our geriatric patient is much more likely to be impacted by untreated tumors because they are likely to live long enough to allow for the growth and development and eventual morbidity of cancer.

It is not unusual to field questions from patients and their family members about why we should bother with treatment. This thought process stems from both a fear that the treatment could be worse than the disease and that the patient is too old to benefit from treatment of any cancers. Neither line of reasoning is sound. The patient may not live long enough before any such lesion becomes mortally significant but may encounter more than casual morbidity. Neoplastic lesions are, by their very physiologic make-up, pockets of poorly healing tissue. At the very least, the cost that simple wound care and dressing changes, which are chronic in nature, could incur can at least be limited to a week or two following curative surgery. Consider also the eventual spread of any neoplasm into the surrounding tissue. Vascular invasion can lead to bleeding, and nerve invasion can lead to loss of function. Bone invasion compounds the already serious issue of brittle bones and instability.

The psychological impact on the patient is also very real and tangible. Our geriatric patients deserve the best attempts to keep them disease free and maximize quality of life.

The available treatment options offer a variety of avenues to choose from. Draconic and heroic measures need not be employed, especially if lesions are diagnosed early. Chemotherapy and radiation therapy can be effective in some instances, but not particularly well tolerated. Conservative surgical measures are often very well tolerated. Local anesthesia allows for surgical intervention using methods done in the office setting or even at bedside. ED&C, cryotherapy, wide excision, and Mohs micrographic surgery can be utilized for almost every patient [3]. Topical agents such as 5-fluorouracil, blistering agents, escharic agents, and even some immune modulators designed for warts can also be utilized. The expected efficacy may not always approach 100% but the tolerability and ease of application can be attractive.

The geriatric patient is also concerned about the cosmetic implications of any treatment. Surgical repair considerations as well as collateral damage from destruction-oriented procedures are very important aspects as well.

The geriatric patient is at a higher risk of developing cutaneous neoplasms and will benefit from prompt diagnosis and treatment. Quality of life for patients is the real target.

Skin cancer comes in a variety of types, divided by the tissue of origin (see Table 9.1).

After a diagnosis has been made, preferably by proven biopsy, appropriate treatment options can be entertained. Treatment of several types of skin cancer can be reasonably well achieved using one or more of several special topical creams and other compounds. These are divided into two different groups, either an "escharic" or an "immunologic" treatment. The escharic compounds are designed to cause destruction of the tissue. They are applied topically to the intended site and a little beyond, and through chemical means the tissue is cauterized and the diseased tissue sloughed off as the intended gain. Salicylic acid, podophylin, other acids, and several more concoctions and colloquial remedies are cheap and available. They can also be applied to any lesion with success. Effectiveness is maximized with appropriate follow-up and retreating as necessary. Two weeks for follow-up is a reasonable time frame to start with, and allows for adequate time to assess efficacy. The immunologic class differs only in the way the treatment compound interacts with the tissue. These interfere with molecular pathways and are tumor cell specific. 5-fluorouracil, Aldara (imiqumod), Condylox, and other receptor-specific treatment creams are available but are sometimes more expensive than the escharic type. Furthermore, only a few types of lesions can be treated. Squamous cell in situ, bowenoid, actinic keratosis, superficial basal cell carcinoma, and possibly morpheaform type, are the only real candidates. Unfortunately, with the exception of 5-FU for SCC in situ, the effectiveness has been encouraging but supported by only level-four and level-five evidence.

Despite the limitations that can be encountered when using one of the topical treatments they can still be attractive options for some patients. Often in geriatric medicine we must provide treatment for patients who are not good surgical candidates. Apart from being elderly with medical reasons, sometimes it can be a matter of transportation, follow-up, and other psychosocial issues as well. It is also important that a decision might be made to stop the treatment regimen. The decision to do so is made clinically, with psychosocial issues taken into account. The lesion can present as clinically clear and be so diagnosed, or a biopsy can be done after appropriate healing time to definitively ascertain clearance of cancerous tissue.

The next treatment options are considered mechanical destruction. The physician causes destruction of the diseased tissue by a variety of means. Liquid nitrogen cryotherapy has been utilized with some anecdotal effectiveness, especially in superficial tumor growth. Thai et al. has reported the exceptional usefulness of cryosurgery. The astute clinician can nearly perform "cold soft excision" of a myriad type of lesions using skillful and judicious use of liquid nitrogen. Electric

Table 9.1 Types of skin cancer

Epidermis [4]	Hyperplastic	Keratoacanthoma Pseudoepitheliomatous Hyperplasia		
	Atypical proliferation	Actinic keratosis	Hypertrophic Acantholytic Lichenoid	
	Squamous cell carcinoma	In situ Invasive	Well differentiated Poorly differentiated Bowen's Erythroplasia of D'Queryat Epithelioma of Jadassohn	
	Basal cell carcinoma	Superficial Nodular	Sclerosing Morpheaform Multifocal Basosquamous	
Melanocytic	Lentigo maligna Malignant melanoma	Lentigo maligna melanoma Superficial spreading melanoma Acral letiginous melanoma Nodular melanoma		
Reticular dermis neoplasias	Neurilemmoma	Shwanoma	Metastatic carcinomas	Dermatofibrosarcoma
	Desmoid tumor	Fibrosarcoma	Epithelioid cell sarcoma	Protuberans
	Granular cell tumor	Pyogenic granuloma	Angiokeratoma	Fibroxanthosarcoma
	Glomus tumor	Kaposi's sarcoma	Leiomyoma	Lymphangioma circumscriptum Hemangiopericytoma
Neoplasia of panniculus	Liposarcoma			
Pilosebacious tissue	Sebaceous adenoma	Nevus sebaceous	Sebaceous carcinoma	
	Sebaceous epithelioma	Trichofolliculoma	Pilar tumor	
	Trichilemmoma	Trichoepithelioma Eccrine spiradenoma	Pilomatrixoma Eccrine poroma	
Sweat gland tumors	Syringoma Clear cell hidradenoma	Cutaneous mixed tumor	Syringocystadenoma	
	Hydradenoma papilliferum	Cylindroma		

desiccation and curettage has been a standby for many years. In the hands of a skillful physician this can be quite successful. Lasers have allowed for even more skillful application in the place where hyfrecators and Boveys have been used. Using local anesthesia, the procedure cauterizes and nearly vaporizes the tissue. Effectiveness relies solely on whether or not all the cancerous cells are desiccated. This is determined by the operator and, with expertise, can have a high curative rate. Postoperative wound care is very important, as healing will be by secondary intention.

Radiation has been used for many years with a great degree of success and is still a viable option. Radiation therapy is generally not utilized for strictly cutaneous lesions, but still very appropriate in the field of internal malignancies. Also, it is to be noted that some radiation treatments can cause squamous cell atypia some years post op, and radiation burns are not uncommon [5].

Surgical excision is the final option and very often an excellent choice. The high curative rates and high tolerability make surgical possibilities very attractive [3]. Extra consideration should be given to not only the patients' candidacy for surgery but the pharmacological aspects as well as both prescription and OTC products [6]. A wide excision with appropriate margins and a good surgical eye such as what is needed for electric desiccation and curettage is one of two methods. Mohs's micrographic surgery is the other. Mapping of concentrically excised tissue that is intra-operatively examined under magnification to dictate surgical removal is the gold standard. This procedure enjoys the highest curative rate and facilitates healing by primary intention. It also imparts a level of tissue sparing that is attractive to both patient and practitioner. The procedure employs local anesthesia and can be done outpatient, but not at bedside. Specific equipment, trained staff and technicians, and appropriately trained physicians can be a little hard to come by, especially in the nursing home, but recent interest has prompted mobile units to be assembled and services to be provided on site [7].

Putting all of this together in a meaningful way that benefits the patient is the real goal. In order for the diagnosis to be made, the lesion has to be located and biopsied first. Start with the initial approach to the patient. Often, the chief complaint will be the lesion itself. If not, take the opportunity to fully examine the patient. Pay attention to the expected areas of increased sun exposure like the forearms, face, auricular helices, shoulders, and back. It is important to remember that skin cancer can arise anywhere in the integumental system and examination of all areas including nails, mucosa, and plantar surfaces should be done [8]. If the patient has a history of skin cancer excision or treatment, be sure to carefully examine that site for possible recurrence also. Organ transplant recipients represent a subpopulation with a higher incident of skin cancers [9].

The ability to find a cancerous or otherwise suspicious lesion is not a difficult skill to achieve. A good plan would be considering a biopsy for any lesion that presents suspiciously. Suspicious clinical findings that may indicate neoplastic lesions include ulceration, pearly bordered, keratotic, spontaneously bleeding, etc. The key is that all neoplastic lesions are made up of atypical cells and as such, normal appendegeal cells such as hair follicles and pores are significantly reduced or altogether absent. Depending on the cell type of origin, the clinical findings of different types of skin cancer can be appreciated. Squamous cell cancer begins with the squamous layer and atypical proliferation presents as erythematous scaly plaques with cloudy semi-translucent thickening of underlying tissue in later stages. Basal cell cancer presents as a proliferation of basal cells. These are cuboidal and form a pearly mass with erythema and ulceration in later stages. Melanocyte-proliferative lesions present as pigmented macule with thickening, erythema, and ulceration in later stages.

Special consideration should be given to neoplasms of melanocyte origin [8]. The insidious nature and significant morbidity and mortality associated with melanomas increases the need for early detection and intervention. Unfortunately, pigmented macules and papules are found in abundance in the geriatric population and clearly they cannot all be biopsied. The popular anachronism ABCD has been employed to help distinguish clinical significance: reviewing with A = asymmetry, B = borders, C = colors, D = diameter. If the suspected lesion displays any characteristic of being malignant, do not waste the opportunity to biopsy and secure a diagnosis [8, 10].

On the subject of biopsy, there are a few judicious points to remember: take the extra effort to ensure hemostasis after the tissue sample is collected. If the lesion appears superficial, consider increasing the size of the tissue collected during the biopsy to increase your chance of removing the entire lesion. Use the larger diameter of a punch knife or excision margins and even a well-guided dermatology flex blade. This can be very beneficial to both the patient and the medical professional in a variety of common scenarios.

Review of current literature brings several issues to the forefront and reveals some pertinent pearls. Ailken et al. [11] reports that although skin examinations, both self and clinical, have increased in the 65-year-old and younger population, they have decreased in the elderly population. Rosso and Budroni [12] conclude that the prevalence of NMSC and melanoma have both increased 5–7% with a slightly larger increase for males over females. With respect to melanoma itself and the recent trendy belief that mortality rates have stabilized in the last decade, Swetter et al. [13] produced results from a study that showed that incidence and mortality have continued to rise in the elderly population, especially in male patients. Mortality was also considered by Nolan et al. and a report published reviewing lethal nonmelanoma skin cancers. They reported that of the lethal cases the average age of diagnosis was 79 years and 68 years for immune-compromised patients. A median age of survival after diagnosis was 17 months! SCC was identified in 70% of the cases [13]. Consideration of all that is geriatric medicine and geriatric dermatology and the need for more frequent and thorough examinations of elderly patients are outlined and described by Landow [16] and should be considered.

The role of the dermatologist that provides care to the geriatric patient assumes the care for the integumental system. The ability to affectively diagnose and treat cancerous lesions with special care given to the needs of the geriatric patient might be considered as indispensable. Accept the responsibility of skin cancers and perform biopsies with empathy and care. Treat cancerous lesions with the same empathy and care and aggressively search for them with thorough and frequent examinations.

References

1. Korting GW. Geriatric Dermatology. Philadelphia: WB Saunders, 1980, pp. 113–6.
2. Extermann M. Cancer in the older patient: a geriatric approach. Ann. Long-Term Care 2002; 10(1): 49–54.
3. Alam M, Norman RA, Goldberg LH. Germatologic surgery in geriatric patients: psychosocial considerations and perioperative decision-making. Dermatol. Surg. 2003; 28: 1043–50.
4. Hood AF, Kwan TH, Burnes DC, Mihm MC. Primer of Dermatopathology. Boston: Little Brown, 1984.
5. Futrell JW, Myers GH. The burn scar as an immunologically privileged site. Surg. Forum No. 25. 1972:124–31.
6. Collins CC, Dufresne RG. Dietary supplements in setting of Mohs surgery. Dermatol. Surg. 2002; 28(6): 447–52.
7. Brio D. Choosing the right modality to treat non-melanoma skin cancer. Skin Aging 1999; 7(6): 40–51.
8. Brenner S, Tamir E. Early detection of melanoma: the best strategy for a favorable prognosis. Clin. Dermatol. 2002; 20(3): 203–9.
9. Orengo I, Brown T, Rosen T. Cutaneous neoplasia in organ transplant recipients. Client Prob. Dermatol. 1999; 11(4): 127–60.
10. Miller SD, Elston D. How best to approach a suspicious pigmented lesion? Consulant 2002; 42(4): 449–0.
11. Ailken JK, Janda M, Lowe JB. Prevalence of whole body skin examination in a population high risk for skin cancer. Cancer Causes Control 2004; 15(5): 453–63.
12. Rosso S, Budroni M. SkinCancers! Melanoma, NMSC, and Kaposis sarcoma. Epidemiol. Prev. 2004; 28(2 Suppl): 57–63.
13. Nolan RC, Chan MT, Heenan PJ. A review of lethal nonmelanoma skin cancers. J. Am. Acad. Dermatol. 2005; 52(1): 101–8.
14. Swetter SM, Geller AC, Kirkwood JM. Melanoma in the older person. Oncology 2004; 18(9): 1187–96.
15. Thai KE, Fergin P, Freeman M. A prospective study in the use of cryosurgery for the treatment of AK's. Int. J. Dermatol. 2004; 43(9): 687–92.
16. Landow K. Skin cancer screening guidelines for older patients? Postgrad. Med. 2003; 116(5): 57.

Chapter 10

Differential Diagnosis of Autoimmune Bullous Diseases in the Elderly

Diya F. Mutasim

Overview

The primary lesion in bullous diseases is a vesicle (0.1–1 cm) or bulla (> 1 cm). Although these diseases affect patients in all age groups, the elderly are particularly susceptible. Bullous diseases may be divided into five subgroups based on the etiology and pathogenesis of blister formation: autoimmune, allergic, mechanical, metabolic and infectious (Table 10.1). The following review is limited to autoimmune bullous diseases.

The high incidence of bullous diseases in the elderly may result from several factors. The experimental induction of blisters is easier in the elderly than in younger individuals [1], probably because of loss of structure and function of adhesion molecules that normally maintain the integrity of cell–cell and cell–matrix adhesion [2]. The normal rete ridge pattern of the dermal–epidermal junction is gradually lost during aging. This results in a diminution in the surface area and thus the strength of dermal–epidermal adhesion, which results in easy blistering. In addition, the incidence of immune dysregulation increases with age. This results in a higher incidence of autoantibody production and several autoimmune diseases including autoimmune bullous diseases [3].

The autoimmune bullous diseases result from an immune response to molecular components of desmosomes or the basement membrane zone [4]. The various types of pemphigus are associated with antibodies to desmosomal proteins [5–12]. There is strong direct experimental evidence that antibodies in pemphigus vulgaris and pemphigus foliaceus cause acantholysis and blister formation by directly interfering with desmosomal function [5, 6, 13]. On the other hand, all the subepidermal autoimmune bullous diseases except dermatitis herpetiformis result from antibodies against one or more components of the basement membrane zone [14, 15]. In general, subepidermal vesicles result from activation of complement by the bound antibody molecules, followed by the influx of a cellular inflammatory infiltrate that may be neutrophil-rich or eosinophil-rich [16, 17]. Table 10.2 shows the target molecules for the various autoimmune bullous disorders.

R.A. Norman (ed.), *Diagnosis of Aging Skin Diseases,*
© Springer-Verlag London Limited 2008

Table 10.1 Classification of bullous diseases

Autoimmune
  Pemphigus
  Pemphigoid
  Epidermolysis bullosa acquisita
  Dermatitis herpetiformis
  Linear IgA disease
Mechanical
  Epidermolysis bullosa simplex
  Junctional epidermolysis bullosa
  Dystrophic epidermolysis bullosa
Metabolic
  Porphyria (and pseudoporphyria)
  Diabetic bullae
  Bullous amyloidosis
Allergic
  Toxic epidermal epidermolysis
  Bullous erythema multiforme
  Stevens–Johnson syndrome
  Bullous acute allergic contact dermatitis
Infectious
  Bullous impetigo
  Staphylococcal scalded skin syndrome
  Bullous herpes virus infections

Table 10.2 Molecular classification of bullous diseases

Bullous disease	Targeted molecule
Pemphigus vulgaris	Desmoglein III (and Desmoglein I)
Pemphigus foliaceous	Desmoglein I
Paraneoplastic pemphigus	Desmoplakin I, Desmoplakin II, BP 230, Envoplakin, Periplakin, Desmoglein III
IgA pemphigus	Desmocollin I
Bullous pemphigoid	BP 180, BP 230 (hemidesmosome and lamina lucida)
Herpes gestationis	BP 180, BP 230 (hemidesmosome and lamina lucida)
Mucous membrane pemphigoid	BP 180, laminin 5 (hemidesmosome and lamina lucida)
Epidermolysis bullosa acquisita	Type VII collagen (anchoring fibrils)
Linear IgA dermatosis (adults and children)	LAD antigen (BP 180) (hemidesmosome and lamina lucida), occasionally type VII collagen

Diagnosis

The accurate diagnosis of autoimmune bullous diseases requires evaluation of clinical findings, histopathology, direct immunofluorescence and indirect immunofluorescence [18]. The diagnostic specificity of the clinical findings varies among bullous diseases [19-27]. There is clinical overlap among various groups of bullous diseases. For example, linear IgA disease [28, 29] may mimic bullous pemphigoid and dermatitis herpetiformis. IgA pemphigus [30] mimics pemphigus foliaceous, pemphigus herpetiformis and subcorneal pustular dermatosis. Paraneoplastic pemphigus [31] may mimic pemphigus vulgaris and Stevens–Johnson syndrome. Inflammatory epidermolysis bullosa acquisita may be indistinguishable from bullous pemphigoid [32]. The non-inflammatory mechanobullous form of epidermolysis bullosa acquisita [33-39] may be indistinguishable from porphyria cutanea tarda and pseudoporphyria. Mucous membrane pemphigoid [40] is clinically indistinguishable from anti-epiligrin disease, mucosal epidermolysis bullosa acquisita, mucosal linear IgA disease and occasionally mucosal lichen planus. Bullous systemic lupus erythematosus [41–43] may be indistinguishable from epidermolysis bullosa acquisita [33–39], linear IgA disease [44, 45] and bullous pemphigoid.

The specimen for histological examination should include an early, intact vesicle with adjacent skin. The shave technique is preferred. Ruptured or old vesicles reveal secondary changes of epithelial regeneration, secondary inflammation or secondary infection. These changes may mask the primary diagnostic findings. The specimen for direct immunofluorescence should include normal-appearing skin immediately adjacent to a lesion (perilesional skin). If the patient presents with erythematous or urticarial plaques, the specimen for direct immunofluorescence should include normal-appearing skin adjacent to such a lesion. For indirect immunofluorescence, blood, serum or blister fluid should be submitted. Immunofluorescence tests are usually performed in specialized immunopathology laboratories and are best interpreted by a dermatopathologist or immunodermatologist with special expertise in the area of bullous diseases.

An accurate diagnosis is essential for predicting the course and prognosis of bullous diseases, and for choosing therapy. The accuracy in making a diagnosis of an autoimmune bullous disease increases as more findings are available. For example, epidermolysis bullous acquisita may have clinical and histological overlap with bullous pemphigoid and linear IgA disease. These three diseases, however, may be differentiated on the basis of direct and indirect immunofluorescence findings. Similarly, paraneoplastic pemphigus may have similar clinical and histological features to pemphigus vulgaris and other mucocutaneous diseases, especially erythema multiforme. Immunological studies help to differentiate paraneoplastic pemphigus from other diseases. An accurate diagnosis of paraneoplastic pemphigus is essential for appropriate workup and treatment.

Prognosis

The prognosis of bullous diseases in the elderly is generally worse than in younger individuals. Extensive blistering leads to extensive erosions that heal slowly, especially in patients with nutritional deficiencies or systemic disease. Slow healing of extensive erosions predisposes to loss of fluids and electrolytes as well as secondary bacterial infection and sepsis. In addition, superficial erosions may progress to ulcers because of increased local pressure in immobile and bedridden patients. Finally, temperature regulation may be compromised following the loss of large areas of epidermis. Over the past several decades, mortality from the bullous disease has decreased significantly. Presently, the common causes of death are complications secondary to the therapeutic agents used [46].

Differential Diagnosis of Subepidermal Bullous Diseases

The subepidermal diseases that affect the elderly are bullous pemphigoid, mucous membrane pemphigoid, epidermolysis bullosa acquisita, linear IgA disease and dermatitis herpetiformis.

Clinical Differential Diagnosis

The clinical findings of the non-inflammatory, classical type of epidermolysis bullosa acquisita are characteristic. Vesicles and bullae are induced by minor trauma over the dorsum of the hands as well as other trauma prone sites. In patients who present primarily with involvement of the hands and forearms, differentiation from porphyria cutanea tarda and pseudoporphyria is not possible. The classical presentation of dermatitis herpetiformis (pruritic papulovesicles over the lower back, buttocks, elbows and knees) is also characteristic. The classical presentation of bullous pemphigoid is also characteristic (tense bullae over flexural areas) (Figs. 10.1 and 10.2). Differentiation between atypical presentations of bullous

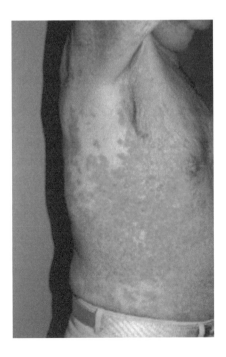

Fig. 10.1 Bullous pemphigoid. Note tense vesicles and bullae on erythematous base

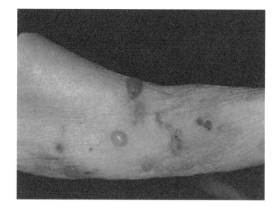

Fig. 10.2 Bullous pemphigoid. Tense, intact and ruptured bullae on erythematous plaque

pemphigoid, inflammatory epidermolysis bullosa acquisita (Fig. 10.3) and linear IgA disease is difficult.

Histologic Differential Diagnosis

A subepidermal vesicle may be non-inflammatory (or pauci-inflammatory), associated with a neutrophil-rich infiltrate or associated with an eosinophil-rich infiltrate [18]. Non-inflammatory and pauci-inflammatory vesicles are characteristic of epidermolysis bullosa acquisita, porphyria, pseudoporphyria and rarely bullous pemphigoid. Subepidermal vesicles with an eosinophil-rich infiltrate are characteristic of bullous pemphigoid. Subepidermal vesicles with neutrophil-rich infiltrate are characteristic of dermatitis herpetiformis, linear IgA disease, inflammatory epidermolysis bullosa acquisita, bullous systemic lupus erythematosus and, extremely rarely, bullous pemphigoid [18]. The histological findings in mucous membrane pemphigoid are non-specific and may reveal neutrophils, eosinophils or both.

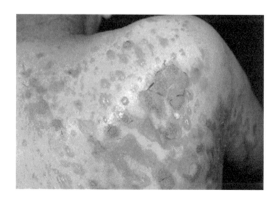

Fig. 10.3 Inflammatory epidermolysis bullosa acquisita. Note inflammatory bullae and erosions

Direct Immunofluorescence Differential Diagnosis

Granular deposition of IgA and C3 along the basement membrane and the tips of dermal papillae is characteristic of dermatitis herpetiformis. Continuous linear deposition of IgA along the basement membrane with or without deposition of C3 is characteristic of linear IgA disease. Deposition of IgG and C3 in a linear pattern along the basement membrane is characteristic of both bullous pemphigoid and epidermolysis bullosa acquisita (all types). The intensity of deposition of IgG compared to C3 may be helpful in differentiating between bullous pemphigoid and epidermolysis bullosa acquisita. C3 deposition tends to be more intense than IgG deposition in bullous pemphigoid (Fig. 10.4) while the opposite is true in epidermolysis bullosa acquisita. Differentiation between bullous pemphigoid and epidermolysis bullosa acquisita with almost complete certainty may be obtained by direct immunofluorescence using the salt-split technique. The biopsy specimen is incubated in 1 M sodium chloride that results in a dermal–epidermal cleft. Direct immunofluorescence is then performed. Based on the sites of bullous pemphigoid and epidermolysis bullosa acquisita antigens (hemidesmosomes/lamina lucida vs. anchoring fibrils), deposition in epidermolysis bullosa acquisita is limited to the dermal site of the cleft while deposition in bullous pemphigoid is either limited to the epidermal side or both epidermal and dermal sides of the cleft.

Indirect Immunofluorescence Differential Diagnosis

Indirect immunofluorescence using salt-split normal human skin may be helpful in differentiating between bullous pemphigoid and epidermolysis bullosa acquisita. Normal human skin is incubated in 1 M sodium chloride that results in a subepidermal cleft through the lamina lucida allowing epidermolysis bullosa acquisita antigen to be solely on the dermal side, and bullous pemphigoid antigens primarily on the epidermal side and to a lesser degree on the dermal side of the cleft. Indirect immunofluorescence in epidermolysis bullosa acquisita is positive in 50% of the cases and is limited to the dermal side. Immunofluorescence in bullous pemphigoid

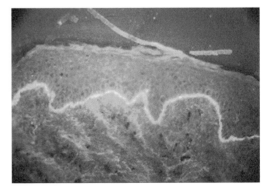

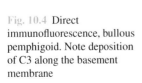

Fig. 10.4 Direct immunofluorescence, bullous pemphigoid. Note deposition of C3 along the basement membrane

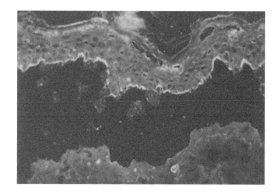

Fig. 10.5 Indirect immunofluorescence using human salt-split skin. Note deposition of IgG limited to the epidermal side of the cleft

is positive in approximately 90% of cases and is commonly limited to the epidermal side (Fig. 10.5) and occasionally to the epidermal and dermal sides [47]. Table 10.3 summarizes the approach to the differential diagnosis of subepidermal bullous diseases based on histology, direct immunofluorescence and indirect immunofluorescence.

Table 10.3 Algorithm for the Diagnosis of subepidermal autoimmune bullous disease

Histopathology	Direct immunoflu-orescence	Indirect immunofluo-rescence	Diagnosis
Subepidermal non-inflammatory	IgG, C3 ± IgM, IgA at BMZ	(1) Dermal side of SSS	EBA
		(2) Epidermal side of SSS	BP
Subepidermal with eosinophil-rich infiltrate	C3, IgG at BMZ	Epidermal side of SSS	BP, HG, mucosal pemphigoid
Subepidermal with neutrophil-rich infiltrate	(1) Granular IgA in dermal papillae and BMZ	Negative on epithelium (+anti-endomysial antibodies)	DH
	(2) Linear IgA ± C3, BMZ	IgA at BMZ	LAD
	(3) IgG, IgM, C3, IgA, fibrinogen	(1) Dermal side of SSS	EBA, rare anti-epiligrin disease
		(2) Dermal side of SSS and positive lupus serology	Bullous SLE

Abbreviations: BMZ, basement membrane zone; BP, bullous pemphigoid; DH, dermatitis herpetiformis; EBA, epidermolysis bullosa acquisita; HG, herpes gestationis; LAD, linear IgA disease; SLE, systemic lupus erythematosus; SSS, salt-split skin; ±, with or without.

Differential Diagnosis of Intraepidermal Bullous Diseases

There are four main types of pemphigus: pemphigus vulgaris, pemphigus foliaceous (superficial pemphigus), paraneoplastic pemphigus and IgA pemphigus.

Clinical Differential Diagnosis

Mucosal involvement is consistently present in paraneoplastic pemphigus (Fig. 10.6) and pemphigus vulgaris (Fig. 10.7). The initial presentation of most patients with pemphigus vulgaris is with oral lesions that are slowly followed by skin lesions (Fig. 10.8). Mucosal involvement does not occur in patients with pemphigus foliaceous or IgA pemphigus. Scalp involvement is common in both pemphigus vulgaris and pemphigus foliaceous. The skin lesions of paraneoplastic pemphigus are highly polymorphous and may mimic those of erythema multiforme, Stevens–Johnson syndrome, lichen planus, lichen planus pemphigoides and other bullous diseases. The vesicles in pemphigus foliaceous are superficial and collapse rapidly, resulting in an appearance that makes suspicion for a bullous disorder rather low

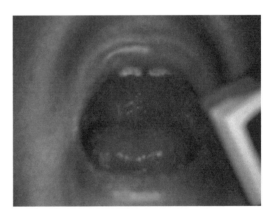

Fig. 10.6 Paraneoplastic pemphigus. Note erosions on the palate

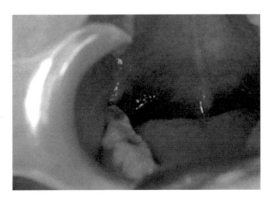

Fig. 10.7 Pemphigus vulgaris. Note erosions over the posterior buccal mucosa

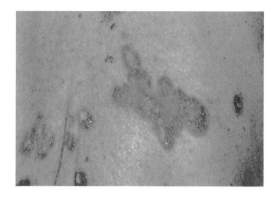

Fig. 10.8 Pemphigus vulgaris. Note crusted erosions over the back

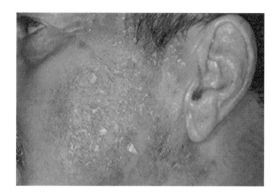

Fig. 10.9 Pemphigus foliaceus. Note erythematous patches with shallow erosions and fine crusting

(Figs. 10.9 and 10.10). The distribution of pemphigus foliaceous, however, is rather characteristic involving primarily the upper trunk, face and scalp and, to a lesser degree, the rest of the skin surface. The primary lesion of IgA pemphigus may be similar to that of pemphigus foliaceous as well as subcorneal pustular dermatosis (Fig. 10.11). There are no diagnostic histological findings for IgA pemphigus. A high index of suspicion is required in order to perform appropriate immunofluorescence studies.

Histologic Differential Diagnosis

Histological examination is helpful in this group of disorders. The primary finding in pemphigus vulgaris is a suprabasal acantholytic cleft that extends only to the lower spinous layers. There is a variable inflammatory infiltrate. The main findings in paraneoplastic pemphigus are suprabasal acantholytic cleft that is usually admixed with interface vacuolization and dyskeratosis. Pemphigus foliaceous reveals subcorneal or intragranular acantholytic cleft. The primary lesion of IgA pemphigus may reveal an intraepidermal neutrophilic pustule or a subcorneal acantholytic cleft with neutrophils.

Fig. 10.10 Pemphigus foliaceus. Note extensive eruption of erythematous patches with shallow, finely crusted erosions

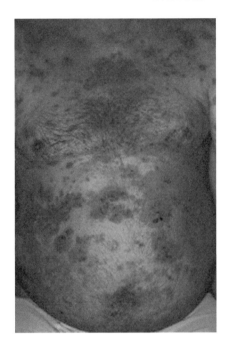

Fig. 10.11 IgA pemphigus. Note erythematous vesicopustules

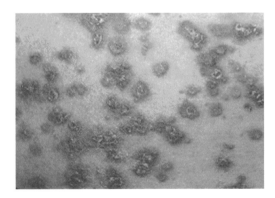

Immunofluorescence Differential Diagnosis

Direct immunofluorescence in IgA pemphigus reveals IgA with or without C3 around epidermal cells. IgG and C3 deposition around epidermal cells is characteristic of pemphigus vulgaris, pemphigus foliaceous and paraneoplastic pemphigus. Additionally, paraneoplastic pemphigus reveals frequent deposition of C3 along the basement membrane. Table 10.4 summarizes the approach to the diagnosis of intraepidermal bullous diseases.

While the combination of clinical, histological and direct immunofluorescence findings is diagnostic of pemphigus vulgaris, pemphigus foliaceous and IgA pem-

Table 10.4 Algorithm for the diagnosis of intraepidermal bullous disease

Histopathology	Direct immunofluorescence	Indirect immunofluorescence	Diagnosis
Suprabasal	(1) IgG ± C3 at ICS	IgG at ICS, monkey esophagus	PV > PNP
	(2) IgG ± C3 at ICS + BMZ	IgG at ICS, rat bladder	PNP
Subcorneal	(1) IgA at ICS	IgA at ICS	IgA pemphigus
	(2) IgG ± C3 at ICS	IgG at ICS	PF
	(3) IgG ± C3 at ICS, Ig ± C3 at BMZ	IgG at ICS, + ANA	PE

Abbreviations: BMZ, basement membrane zone; PE, pemphigus erythematosus; PF, pemphigus foliaceous; PNP, paraneoplastic pemphigus; PV, pemphigus vulgaris; >, more likely than.

phigus, the specific diagnosis of paraneoplastic pemphigus requires further laboratory evaluation. Unlike IgG antibodies in pemphigus vulgaris and pemphigus foliaceous, which recognize and bind to stratified squamous epithelium only, IgG antibodies in paraneoplastic pemphigus recognize other proteins in desmosomes of other epithelia. Indirect immunofluorescence using rat urinary bladder is highly sensitive and specific for paraneoplastic pemphigus antibodies. There is approximately 20% incidence of false positivity (by pemphigus vulgaris antibodies) and false negativity. In cases in which the diagnosis of paraneoplastic pemphigus is highly suspected, immunoprecipitation of the patient's serum using a skin extract is extremely helpful and positive in approximately 100% of patients. Confirming the diagnosis of paraneoplastic pemphigus is essential for initiating a systemic workup for associated neoplasm.

Differential Diagnosis of Predominantly Mucosal Bullous/Erosive Disease

The following discussion will be limited to the two mucous membranes that are most frequently involved with a bullous disease, namely, oral and ocular mucosa. Involvement of other mucous membranes lined by stratified squamous epithelium is frequently accompanied by involvement of the oral or ocular mucosa.

Differential Diagnosis of Ocular Disease

Chronic conjunctival inflammation and scarring is a characteristic feature of cicatricial (or mucous membrane) pemphigoid (Fig. 10.12). Involvement of the eyes may occasionally be accompanied by involvement of the oral mucosa. Rarely, few scattered skin lesions may be seen on the upper trunk and arms [26]. In contradistinction, ocular involvement in pemphigus is usually accompanied by extensive involvement

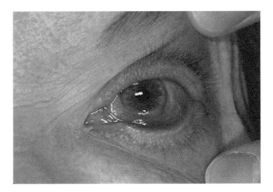

Fig. 10.12 Mucous membrane pemphigoid. Note conjunctival erythema and mild early scarring

of skin and other mucous membranes, especially the oral mucosa. Involvement of the ocular mucosa with pemphigus is usually mild and transient and consists of conjunctival injection. Ocular involvement in paraneoplastic pemphigus, however, may be severe and result in cicatrization [26].

Histological evaluation of a biopsy specimen from inflamed conjunctiva is usually of little benefit in differentiating among the above disorders. Immunofluorescence examination, however, may be helpful (refer to sections on "Direct Immunofluorescence Differential Diagnosis," "Indirect Immunofluorescence Differential Diagnosis" and "Immunofluorescence Differential Diagnosis"). In general, if there is extraocular involvement, biopsy specimens should be obtained from the skin or oral mucosa.

Differential Diagnosis of Oral Disease

Oral blisters and erosions are characteristic of pemphigus vulgaris and mucous membrane pemphigoid (Fig. 10.13). They may occasionally be a manifestation of erosive lichen planus, mucosal epidermolysis bullosa acquisita and mucosal linear IgA disease. Pain tends to favor pemphigus vulgaris and lichen planus. There are no characteristic morphologic features that are diagnostic of a specific disease. The presence of whitish, striated patches with erosions favors lichen planus. Involvement of the posterior buccal mucosa may favor pemphigus vulgaris and involvement of the gingiva may favor mucous membrane pemphigoid.

The specific diagnosis is based on histological and immunofluorescence evaluation. A biopsy specimen may be obtained from a vesicle. Vesicles, however, tend to rupture rapidly. Alternatively, a biopsy for histological examination may be obtained from the inflamed margin of an erosion. The presence of suprabasal acantholysis is characteristic of pemphigus vulgaris while a subepithelial cleft is characteristic of mucous membrane pemphigoid. A band-like lymphocytic infiltrate with or without a subepithelial cleft is characteristic of lichen planus. Epidermolysis bullosa acquisita and linear IgA disease are not distinguishable from pemphigoid.

Fig. 10.13 Mucous
membrane pemphigoid. Note
vesicles of the palate

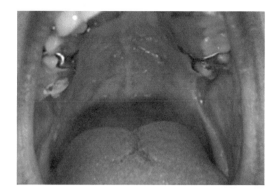

Direct immunofluorescence is essential in the differentiation among the various mucosal disorders. Deposition of IgG and C3 around epithelial cells is characteristic of pemphigus. Linear deposition of IgG and C3 along the basement membrane is characteristic of pemphigoid and epidermolysis bullosa acquisita. Linear deposition of IgA with or without C3 along the basement membrane is characteristic of linear IgA disease. Deposition of fibrinogen along the basement membrane with or without cytoid bodies is characteristic of lichen planus.

Indirect immunofluorescence may also be helpful. The majority of patients with active oral pemphigus vulgaris have circulating antibodies. Approximately 20–30% of patients with mucous membrane pemphigoid, linear IgA disease and epidermolysis bullosa acquisita have circulating antibodies. There are no specific circulating antibodies in patients with lichen planus.

References

1. Grove GL, Duncan S, Kligman AM. Effect of aging on the blistering of human skin with ammonium hydroxide. Br. J. Dermatol. 1982; 107: 383–400.
2. Montagna W, Carlisle K. Structural changes in aging human skin. J. Invest. Dermatol. 1979; 73: 47–53.
3. Dubey DP, Yunis EJ. Aging and nutritional effects on immune functions in humans. In Stites DP, Terr AI, eds. Basic and Clinical Immunology, 7th ed. Norwalk, CT: Appleton and Lange, 1991, pp. 190–3.
4. Burgeson RE, Christiano AM. The dermal–epidermal junction. Curr. Opin. Cell Biol. 1998; 9: 651–8.
5. Roscoe JT, Diaz L, Sampaio SA, Castro RM, Labib RS, Takahashi Y, et al. Brazilian pemphigus foliaceus autoantibodies are pathogenic to BALB/c mice by passive transfer. J. Invest. Dermatol. 1985; 85: 538–41.
6. Anhalt GJ, Labib RS, Voorhees JJ, Beals TF, Diaz LA. Induction of pemphigus in neonatal mice by passive transfer of IgG from patients with the disease. N. Engl. J. Med. 1982; 306: 1189–96.
7. Amagai M, Klaus-Kovtun V, Stanley JR. Autoantibodies against a novel epithelial cadherin in pemphigus vulgaris, a disease of cell adhesion. Cell 1991; 67: 869–77.
8. Beutner EH, Jordon RE. Demonstration of skin antibodies in sera of pemphigus vulgaris patients by indirect immunofluorescent staining. Proc. Soc. Exp. Biol. Med. 1964; 117: 505–10.

9. Rappersberger K, Roos N, Stanley JR. Immunomorphological and biochemical identification of the pemphigus foliaceus autoantigen within desmosomes. J. Invest. Dermatol. 1992; 99: 323–30.

10. Karpati S, Amagai M, Prussick R, Cehrs K, Stanley JR. Pemphigus vulgaris antigen, a desmoglein type of cadherin, is localized within keratinocyte desmosomes. J. Cell Biol. 1993; 122: 409–15.

11. Stanley JR. Cell adhesion molecules as targets of autoantibodies in pemphigus and pemphigoid, bullous diseases due to defective epidermal cell adhesion. Adv. Immunol. 1993; 53: 291–325.

12. Eyre RW, Stanley JR. Identification of pemphigus vulgaris antigen extracted from normal human epidermis and comparison with pemphigus foliaceus antigen. J. Clin. Invest. 1988; 81: 807–12.

13. Hu CH, Michel B, Schlitz JR. Epidermal acantholysis induced in vitro by pemphigus autoantibody. Am. J. Pathol. 1978; 90: 345–51.

14. Diaz LA, Giudice GJ. End of the century overview of skin blisters. Arch. Dermatol. 2000; 136: 106–12.

15. Stanley JR. Pemphigus and pemphigoid as paradigms of organ-specific, autoantibody-mediated diseases. J. Clin. Invest. 1989; 83: 1443–8.

16. Liu Z, Giudice GJ, Zhou X, Swartz SJ, Troy JL, Fairley JA, et al. A major role for neutrophils in experimental bullous pemphigoid. J. Clin. Invest. 1997; 100: 1256–63.

17. Liu Z, Diaz LA, Troy JL, Taylor AF, Emery DJ, Fairley JA, et al. A passive transfer model of the organ-specific autoimmune disease, bullous pemphigoid, using antibodies generated against the hemidesmosomal antigen, BP 180. J. Clin. Invest. 1993; 92: 2480–8.

18. Mutasim DF, Diaz LA. The relevance of immunohistochemical techniques in the differentiation of subepidermal bullous diseases. Am. J. Dermatopathol. 1991; 13: 77–83.

19. Bilic M, Mutasim DF. Bullous pemphigoid. xPharm On-Line Pharmacology Reference and Database. Amsterdam: Elsevier Science, 2004.

20. Hawayek LH, Mutasim DF. Paraneoplastic pemphigus. xPharm On-Line Pharmacology Reference and Database. Amsterdam: Elsevier Science, 2004.

21. Hawayek LH, Mutasim DF. Pemphigus folieaceus. xPharm On-Line Pharmacology Reference and Database. Amsterdam: Elsevier Science, 2004.

22. Hawayek LH, Mutasim DF. Pemphigus vulgaris. xPharm On-Line Pharmacology Reference and Database. Amsterdam: Elsevier Science, 2004.

23. Pipitone MA, Mutasim DF. Epidermolysis bullosa acquisita. xPharm On-Line Pharmacology Reference and Database. Amsterdam: Elsevier Science, 2004.

24. Sluzevich JC, Mutasim DF. Intraepithelial IgA bullous disease. xPharm On-Line Pharmacology Reference and Database. Amsterdam: Elsevier Science, 2004.

25. Anhalt GJ, Mutasim DF. Bullous pemphigoid, cicatricial pemphigoid, and pemphigoid gestationis. In Jameson JL, ed. Principles of Molecular Medicine. Totowa, NJ: Humana Press, 1998, pp. 817–20.

26. Mutasim DF, Pelc NJ, Anhalt GJ. Cicatricial pemphigoid. Dermatol. Clin. 1993; 11: 499–510.

27. Mutasim DF, Pelc NJ, Anhalt GJ. Paraneoplastic pemphigus. Dermatol. Clin. 1993; 11: 473–81.

28. Bean SF. Linear IgA bullous dermatosis and chronic bullous dermatosis of childhood. In Jordon RE, ed. Immunologic Diseases of the Skin. Norwalk, CT: Appleton and Lange, 1991, pp. 347–51.

29. Chorzelski TP, Jablonska S. IgA linear dermatosis of childhood (chronic bullous disease of childhood). Br. J. Dermatol. 1979; 101: 535–42.

30. Beutner EH, Chorzelski TP, Wilson RM, Kumar V, Michel B, Helm F, et al. IgA pemphigus foliaceus. Report of two cases and a review of the literature. J. Am. Acad. Dermatol. 1989; 20: 89–97.

31. Anhalt GJ, Kim S, Stanley JR, Korman NJ, Jabs DA, Kory M, et al. Paraneoplastic pemphigus. An autoimmune mucocutaneous disease associated with neoplasia. N. Engl. J. Med. 1990; 323: 1729–35.

32. Gammon WR, Briggaman RA, Wheeler CE Jr. Epidermolysis bullosa acquisita presenting as an inflammatory bullous disease. J. Am. Acad. Dermatol. 1982; 7: 382–7.
33. Nieboer C, Boorsma DM, Woerdeman MJ, Kalsbeek GL. Epidermolysis bullosa acquisita: Immunofluorescence, electron microscopic and immunoelectron microscopic studies in four patients. Br. J. Dermatol. 1980; 102: 383–92.
34. Palestine RF, Kossard S, Dicken CH. Epidermolysis bullosa acquisita: a heterogeneous disease. J. Am. Acad. Dermatol. 1981; 5: 43–53.
35. Pass F, Dobson RL. Epidermolysis bullosa acquisita. Arch. Dermatol. 1965; 91: 219–23.
36. Provost TT, Maize JC, Ahmed AR, Strauss JS, Dobson RL. Unusual subepidermal bullous diseases with immunologic features of bullous pemphigoid. Arch. Dermatol. 1979; 115: 156–60.
37. Richter BJ, McNutt NS. The spectrum of epidermolysis bullosa acquisita. Arch. Dermatol. 1979; 115: 1325–8.
38. Roenigk HH Jr, Pearson RW. Epidermolysis bullosa acquisita. Arch. Dermatol. 1981; 117: 383.
39. Roenigk HH Jr, Ryan JG, Bergfield WF. Epidermolysis bullosa acquisita: report of three cases and review of all published cases. Arch. Dermatol. 1971; 103: 1–10.
40. Bean SF. Cicatricial pemphigoid. In Beutner EH, Chorzelski TP, Kumar V, eds. Immunopathology of the Skin, 3rd ed. New York: John Wiley, 1987, pp. 355–60.
41. Barton DD, Fine JD, Gammon WR, Sams WM Jr. Bullous systemic lupus erythematosus: an unusual clinical course and detectable circulating autoantibodies to the epidermolysis bullosa acquisita antigen. J. Am. Acad. Dermatol. 1986; 15: 369–73.
42. Briggaman RA, Gammon WR, Woodley DT. Epidermolysis bullosa acquisita. In Wojnarowska F, Briggaman RA, eds. Management of Blistering Diseases. New York: Raven Press, 1990, pp. 127–38.
43. Camisa C, Sharma HM. Vesiculobullous systemic lupus erythematosus. J. Am. Acad. Dermatol. 1983; 9: 924–33.
44. Chorzelski TP, Jablonska S, Beutner EH, Wilson BD. Linear IgA bullous dermatosis. In Beutner EH, Chorzelski TP, Kumar V, eds. Immunopathology of the Skin, 3rd ed. New York: John Wiley, 1987, pp. 407–20.
45. Leonard JN, Haffenden GP, Ring NP, Fry L. Linear IgA bullous dermatosis in adults—The St Mary's view. In Beutner EH, Chorzelski TP, Kumar V, eds. Immunopathology of the Skin, 3rd ed. New York: John Wiley, 1987, pp. 421–9.
46. Anhalt GJ, Nousari HC. Bullous diseases. In Rakel RE, Bope EJ, eds. Conn's Current Therapy. Philadelphia, PA: Saunders, 2003, pp. 918–25.
47. Mutasim DF, Adams BB. Immunofluorescence in dermatology. J. Am. Acad. Dermatol. 2001; 45: 803—22.

Chapter 11

Geriatric Fungal Infections

Sadia Saeed, Elizabeth Sagatys, Justin R. Wasserman, and Michael B. Morgan

Introduction

Fungal infections are one of the most prevalent dermatologic conditions affecting the geriatric population. Fungi originate from several environments. Anthropophilic fungi grow only on humans, zoophilic fungi grow on animals, and geophilic fungi live in the soil. Three groups cause cutaneous fungal infections: dermatophytes (*Trichophyton*, *Microsporum*, and *Epidermophyton*); yeasts, (*Malassezia* and *Candida*); and non-dermatophyte molds (*Scopulariopsis, Aspergillus,* and *Fusarium*).

Several factors contribute to increased prevalence of fungal infections in the elderly, including an age related decline in immune response, diabetes mellitus, peripheral vascular disease, malnutrition, vitamin deficiency, infections requiring the use of broad spectrum antibiotics, lymphoproliferative disorders, malignancies, chemotherapy, corticosteroid use, cutaneous trauma, and denture use. Immunosuppressive therapy is commonly used in the geriatric population for transplantation, inflammatory disorders, and autoimmune disorders. Warm, humid climates provide favorable conditions for fungal growth. Certain fungi, like *Candida albicans* is considered normal flora of the mouth, vagina, and gut. Disease usually occurs only when the *Candida* can grow beyond the capability of the host's immune defenses.

Superficial Mycoses

Dermatophytes are defined by their ability, under the majority of conditions, to live only off of dead keratin derived from the superficial stratum corneum of the skin, hair, and nails. Since mucosal surfaces contain no keratin layer dermatophytes cannot survive on these surfaces. In an immunosuppressed host, it is possible for the dermatophytes to undergo deep local invasion, or systemic dissemination. Dermatophytes are known to be responsible for the majority of infections of the scalp, face, trunk, extremities, groin, hands, feet, and nails.

R.A. Norman (ed.), *Diagnosis of Aging Skin Diseases,*
© Springer-Verlag London Limited 2008

Epidemiology

While the elderly population is susceptible to all of the superficial mycoses, there is an increased prevalence of tinea pedis, mucosal and cutaneous candidiasis, and onychomycosis in geriatric populations compared to other age groups [1].

Most superficial mycoses are caused by infection with specific organisms that have a predilection for different anatomical sites. Tinea capitis is commonly associated with *Trichophyton tonsurans* and *Microsporum canis*. Infections of the oral mucosa are almost exclusively caused by *Candida albicans*. The pathogen most commonly associated with tinea versicolor is *Malassezia globosa* [2] and *Malassezia furfur*. Tinea corporis has been linked to *Trichophyton rubrum, Trichophyton tonsurans, Trichophyton mentagrophytes,* and *Microsporum canis*. Tinea cruris will commonly isolate *Trichopyton rubrum* and *Epidermophyton floccosum*, while other intertriginous site infections are associated with *Candida albicans*. Genital infections such as balanitis and vulvovaginitis usually occur due to overgrowth of *Candida albicans*. Tinea manuum as well as tinea pedis are primarily caused by infection with *Trichophyton rubrum*. Tinea pedis will often isolate other species such as *Trichophyton mentagrophytes and Epidermophyton floccosum*. Tinea pedis is the most common of the dermatophyte infections [1]. The prevalence of onychomycosis increases directly with age and is nearly 20% in patients greater than 60 [3]. In 90% of the cases of onychomycosis *Trichophyton rubrum* and *Trichophyton mentagrophytes* are the cause, however, 8% are cause by non-dermatophyte molds such as *Aspergillus* and *Fusarium,* and 2% are caused by *Candida albicans* [3].

Etiology and Pathogenesis

Zoophilic and geophilic dermatophytes typically engender a more pronounced inflammatory response than anthropophilic pathogens [4].

Tinea pedis is usually transmitted by walking barefoot in areas with infectious desquamated scales, or in bathing and swimming facilities. Favorable environments for fungal growth include moist warm areas such as between the toes. Tinea pedis serves as a primary source of infection, which can then be spread to the nails, hands, and groin.

Clinical Manifestations

Tinea capitis is a dermatophyte infection of the hair shaft that presents as

- Black-dot type consists of patches of alopecia with broken hair shafts.
- Gray-patch type is scaly and pruritic. Oral candidiasis has three distinct forms.
- Thrush appears as loose white plaques on any mucosal surface that are easily removed by rubbing with an instrument.

- Atrophic candidiasis acutely has painful erythema of the oral mucosa with atrophy of dorsal papillae of the tongue. Chronically it appears as well circumscribed erythematous lesions in areas covered by dentures.
- Angular chelitis appears with erythema, maceration, crusting, and fissures at the commisures.

Tinea versicolor presents as small 1–2 cm macules or patches that may be pink, hypopigmented, or hyperpigmented. A fine scale may be present.

Tinea corporis and tinea cruris appear as ring-like erythematous plaques with scaling at the periphery (Fig. 11.1).

Tinea pedis has three forms.

- Interdigital presents as dry scale between the toes.
- Moccasin type involves the sole and sides of the foot with hyperkeratotic scale.
- Vesicobullous is usually located in the arch and appears as a vesicle flattened into a reddish brown macule.

Candidal intertrigo presents as pustules on an erythematous base, which become confluent into eroded patches with small pustules at the periphery (Fig. 11.2).

Onychomycosis presents in three forms:

- Distal–lateral subungual: distal subungual hyperkeratosis and onycholysis
- Superficial white: chalky white plaque on the dorsal surface of the nail
- Proximal subungual: white discoloration at the proximal nail plate.

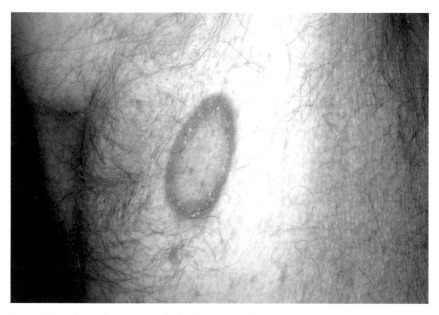

Fig. 11.1 Annular, scaly patches typical of tinea corporis

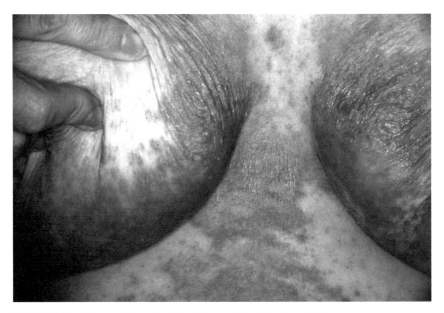

Fig. 11.2 Intertriginous scaly and erythematous rash typical of candidiasis

Diagnosis and Pathology

Diagnosis of superficial fungal infections is primarily accomplished by direct microscopy of KOH-treated scraping from the lesion. Care should be taken to obtain scrapings from the leading edge of cutaneous infections and the undersurface of presumed nail infections. Properly done sensitivity can be as high as 83–96% [5,6]. Dermatophyte infections appear as branching hyphae of uniform width with irregularly spaced septa. *Candidal* infections will appear as pseudohyphae, which branch only at septa, and spores (Fig. 11.3). *Malassezia* species will appear as short filamentous hyphae and spores have the typical "spaghetti and meatballs" appearance. If scrapings are insufficient for diagnosis biopsy may provide further information.

Fungal cultures are indicated for Tinea capitis and Onychomycosis. Dermatophyte culture mediums include Dermatophyte Test Medium (DTM), Mycosel agar, and Sabouraud's dextrose agar. Fungal cultures have been shown to have low sensitivity averaging just 50% [7]. DTM has been shown to be rapid and effective, with a sensitivity of 77% as compared to laboratory cultures, and positive predictive value of 61% [8].

Skin biopsy offers the best overall sensitivity and specificity in the diagnosis of dermatophytes. An additional advantage is the ability to diagnose inflammatory or neoplastic entities that clinically simulate fungal infection. The H&E appearance is subtle consisting of delicate, clear filamentous strands, located in the stratum corneum (Fig. 11.4). The fungal elements may be highlighted with Periodic Acid Schiff (PAS) or Gomori Methanamine Silver (GMS) staining.

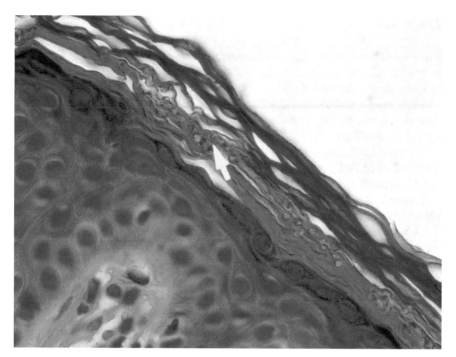

Fig. 11.3 Microscopic section showing dermatophyte hyphae located in the stratum corneum (*arrow*)

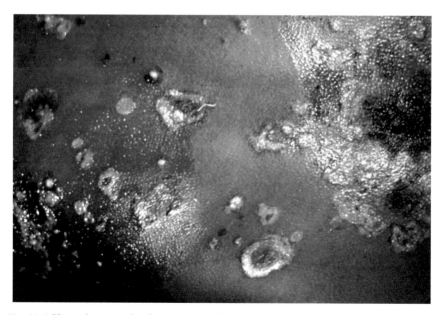

Fig. 11.4 Unusual presentation for cryptococcosis consisting of ulcers in HIV-positive patient

Treatment

Tinea versicolor can be treated with over the counter shampoos or ketoconazole creams/shampoos. One dose therapy for tinea versicolor with systemic azoles may be more practical in the elderly.

Tinea capitis can be treated with either griseofulvin or terbinafine and dosage depends on weight [9]. Duration of treatment with terbinafine depends on the pathogens identified [10, 11].

Candidal infections respond well to topical azoles. In some cases treatment alone is not sufficient. Patients with oral candidiasis should remove dentures at night. *Candidal* intertrigo must be kept dry with application of antifungal powders.

Tinea cruris, tinea pedis, and tinea corporis can be treated with topical azoles or 1% terbinafine cream twice daily for 2 to 4 weeks. Oral therapy may be necessary for elderly patients with poor eyesight or difficulty reaching their feet, terbinafine would be a first choice, but griseofulvin, fluconazole and itraconazole may also be used [12].

Unless the patient has pain or a limitation in mobility it may be okay not to treat onychomycosis. However, in diabetics, onychomycosis may be a route by which foot ulcers and gangrene develop. Terbinafine has been shown in several studies to be the best treatment for dermatophyte onychomycosis [13–15], while *Candidal* onychomycosis is best treated with itraconazole or fluconazole.

Many elderly patients are on multiple medications, it is important to choose treatment based on minimization of side effects and drug–drug interactions. Itraconazole is a CYP3A4 inhibitor and is well known to effect the plasma concentration of many drugs. When treating geriatric patients it is important to assess liver and renal function.

Subcutaneous and Deep Infections

Cryptococcosis

Epidemiology

The causative organism is *Cryptococcus* neoformans. Two subtypes have been identified, namely *Cryptococcus* neoformans var neoformans (responsible for virtually all cases seen in the United States) and *Cryptococcus* neoformans var gatti (mostly confined to the tropics). The source of microorganisms is bird (especially pigeon) and bat droppings, or soil contaminated with their guano.

Cell-mediated immunity plays an important protective role; most patients acquiring infection have impaired cellular immunity [16–18], are on chronic immunosuppressive therapy [19] or have chronic debilitating diseases. HIV infection has become an important risk factor, and cryptococcosis is one of the defining features in classifying patients with AIDS [20, 21].

Clinical Features

The route of entry is inhalation, with primary infection most commonly resulting in pulmonary granulomas. Hematologic spread to other organ systems, especially to the brain, can occur. Other affected sites include bones, prostate, and skin [22]. Cutaneous involvement occurs in approximately 10–15% of cases [22, 23], commonly involving the head and neck [24]. Cutaneous manifestations include formation of papules, plaques, pustules, ulcers (Fig. 11.5) and even cellulitis [25]. Ulcers may exude thin fluid containing yeasts. Nodules may sometimes be large enough to simulate keloids [26]. Lesions resembling herpes virus [27] or molluscum contagiosum [28] have also been reported. Primary cutaneous cryptococcosis is rare [24, 29, 30].

Histopathology

Tuberculoid granulomas are confined to the dermis and upper subcutaneous tissue, with chronic inflammation and multinucleated cells. Rare accompanying neutrophils may be identified. Organisms are found both free and within the giant cells. Microscopic reaction is generally limited [31, 32], with non-capsulated strains producing a greater granulomatous response. Unencapsulated forms are commoner in AIDS [22].

The epithelium displays reactive acanthosis, pseudo- epitheliomatous hyperplasia, and may be ulcerated.

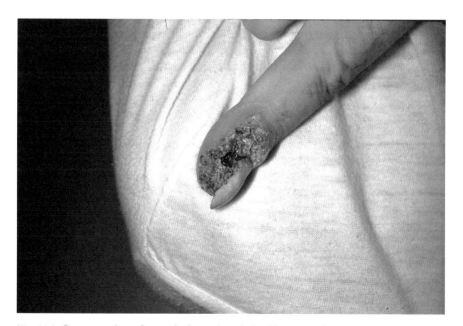

Fig. 11.5 Crusty papule on finger of primary inoculation blastomycosis

Diagnosis

Rapid tissue diagnosis is achieved with India Ink or Tzank smears. The cell wall is accentuated with PAS or methanamine silver stains. Mucicarmine staining also highlights the capsule helping to differentiate from other organisms, which are generally negative [18]. Combination stains with PAS-Alcian blue will contrast cell wall and capsule. Phagocytosed organisms however may not have a well-defined capsule. Fontana Masson demonstrates melanin and is helpful in strains lacking capsules [33]. The organisms are refractile under polarized light. *Cryptococcus neoformans* is a 3– 15 μm organism, showing narrow-based budding [18]. Rudimentary pseudohyphae are rarely present, causing a diagnositic dilemma with other yeast [34]. Morphologic clues favoring cryptococcosis include round shape, thick capsule, good growth on blood agar plates, inhibited in the presence of cyclohexamide. Indirect immunoflourescence staining is available [35], and definitive identification requires thorough biochemical staining.

Coccidiodomycosis

Epidemiology

The causative organism is *Coccidioides immitis*. Organisms are highly infectious [36] and endemic in Southwestern United States, Mexico, and South America [37, 38]. Mode of entry is usually inhalation, which generally results in an asymtomatic [39] or self-limited pulmonary infection [40]. Cutaneous, meningeal and muscle involvement may occur as a part of disseminated disease. Dissemination is seen in less than 1% of cases, mostly in the immunocompromised [40, 41], and is more commonly observed in Native Americans and Filipinos [40].

Primary infection is exceedingly rare, confined mostly to cases of occupational exposure, in farmers and laboratory workers [39].

Clinical Features

Signs and symptoms, if present, are confined to the lungs, and are more likely seen in immunosuppressed individuals [42]. Skin lesions are almost invariably secondary, sometimes accompanied with CNS, bone and joint involvement [39]. Lesions are often multiple, involving the face, especially the nasolabial fold [39]. Verrucous plaques, papules, nodules, pustules, subcutaneous abscesses with draining ulcers [43, 44] may be seen.

Histopathology

Non-caseating granulomas containing multinucleated giant cells are seen in the upper-mid dermis [43]. The histiocytes within granulomas may rarely contain endospores or microorganisms, 80–100 μm in diameter. Spherules are PAS positive [32] unlike the endospores, which can be visualized with Congo red stain [45].

Suppuration, with perivascular neutrophils, eosinophils and lymphocytes, may be seen in the early phase [32, 46]. The epidermis shows pseudo-epitheliomatous hyperplasia.

Diagnosis

Spherules may be seen on examination of the sputum or bronchioalveolar lavage [47]. Colonies of variable morphology appear on blood agar in approximately 1 week. The arthroconidia consist of distinct barrel shaped viable alternating with "empty" cells, which make them highly infective on inhalation. Serologic testing with complement fixation is helpful in determining the extent of disease and has prognostic implications [48].

Blastomycosis

Epidemiology

The causative organism is *Blastomyces dermatitidis.* It is found in bird droppings and rotting wood, commonly in North and South America, India, and Africa [49–51]. The disease is often sporadic, and for unclear reasons is commoner in men than in women.

Clinical Features

Disease may manifest in three forms. The commonest presentation is insidious, subclinical pulmonary involvement. Dissemination may occur to the bones, joints, CNS, prostate, testis, or skin [32]. Unlike with other fungal infections, the host is usually immunocompetent [52]. Primary cutaneous infection is rare. Skin lesions start as a gradually enlarging papule (Fig. 11.6), which ultimately results in a pus-filled ulcer with serpingious border. Healing results in a central, spreading scar.

Histopathology

Neutrophils infiltrate the dermis in early stage, later with the development of granulomas. Round yeast forms, 8–30 µm in diameter, with thick capsules may be identified in multinucleated giant cells or in the center of abscesses. PAS or Silver stains may be required to illustrate their presence. Histopathology is more subtle in primary cutaneous infections [32]. The epidermis characteristically displays pseudo-epitheliomatous hyperplasia [32].

Diagnosis

Organisms are easily found on tissue section. Calcofluor white may enhance visualization. *Blastomyces* is a dimorphic organism, which exists in a yeast form at 37°C

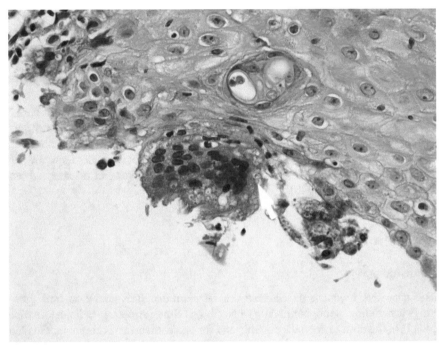

Fig. 11.6 Microscopic section showing multinucleated giant cell containing histoplasma spores (*arrow*)

and is mycelial at room temperature. It exhibits broad based budding. Relatively fast growing colonies are identified on culture. Exoantigen, serologic complement fixation and nucleic acid hybridization tests are available, and may be used as an adjunct to cultures.

Histoplasmosis

Epidemiology

The organism exists in soil and rotten wood contaminated with poultry and bat droppings [53]. It is endemic in Africa (*Histoplasma duboisii*), Asia, and America (*Histoplasma capsulatum*). The organism is found along the Mississippi Valley where in some parts, a majority of the local population reacts positive to skin testing.

Clinical Features

The American form usually presents as a subclinical infection with positive skin test [54]. Primary involvement of the lungs requires a large innoculum, and is mostly self-limited. Chronic cavitary lesions (Buckshot calcifications) may develop, and are commoner in COPD patients [55]. Disseminated infection, spreading through the reticuloendothelial system to involve the splenic and hepatic lymph nodes [54], can occur in the elderly or immunocompromised [56]. This may be the presenting picture in patients with AIDS, who are also at a higher risk of fatal disseminated disease. Cutaneous involvement is present in a minority (5–10%) of cases [57]. Lesions are commonest on the face, arms and trunk [58]. Clinically, they may appear as papules, pustules, an eczematous rash, ulceration, cellulitis or panniculitis [58].

The African subtype generally presents as osteomyelitis with a single overlying skin and subcutaneous lesion [59].

Histopathology

The dermis and sometimes subcutaneous tissue will contain a caseating or non-caseating granulomatous reaction with lymphoplasmacytic and multinucleated giant cells. Numerous organisms are seen within multinucleated histiocytes (Fig. 11.7). The organisms are surrounded by an artifactual halo, giving the false impression of a capsule. Cutaneous nerve infiltration with parasites and dermal necrosis with only minimal inflammatory response may be seen in immunosuppresed patients [58].

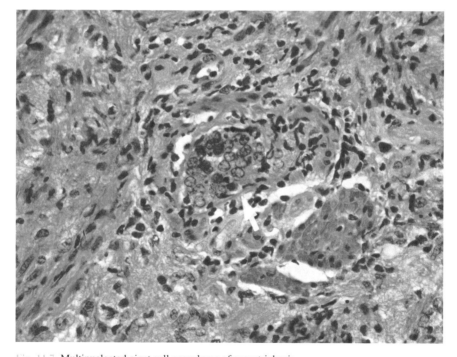

Fig. 11.7 Multinucleated giant cell granuloma of sporotrichosis

Diagnosis

Rapid presumptive diagnosis can be made by a stained wet preparation. Ovoid microorganisms with narrow-based budding [60] and maximal dimension of 3–5 μm: *H. capsulatum* and 7–15 μm: *H. duboisii* are also easily identified on H&E tissue sections. Special staining with PAS may be necessary to find organisms in old, healed granulomas. *H. capsulatum* is a misnomer; the organism lacks a capsule. Blood culture on blood agar plates is carried out in suspected disseminated cases. The organism is dimorphic and exists as yeast at body temperature and mycelium at room temperature. Nucleic acid hybridization may be used for final confirmation. Skin testing is no longer performed, as it cannot differentiate old from recent infections.

Sporotrichosis

Epidemiology

The causative organism is *Sporothrix schenckii*. Organisms thrive in rotting vegetable and wood [61]. Direct inoculation into open wounds or traumatically through splinters is the common mode of infection. The disease is more prevalent in males, mostly as an occupational exposure. Rarely, inhalation or ingestion may lead to systemic disease, particularly in immunosuppressed patients and chronic alcoholics [61].

Clinical Features

The majority of cases exhibit cutaneous lesions on exposed skin parts. A 1–5 cm nodule results at the inoculation site, with subsequent ulceration and lymphatic invasion. Multiple secondary nodules arise along the lymphatic drainage pathway, with accompanying regional lymphadenopathy. People with previous immunity may develop limited localized lesions [62]. Immunosuppressed persons may develop systemic disease involving bones, joints, lungs, and meninges [63].

Histopathology

Multinucleated giant cells in the mid-dermis, containing organisms are surrounded by a dense lymphoplasmacytic and histiocytic infiltrate (Fig. 11.8). Organisms are also found in faintly PAS positive eosinophilic material with stellate borders, the so-called Splendore–Hoeppli phenomenon [32].

The epidermis shows pseudoepitheliomatous hyperplasia, with overlying hyperkeratosis, parakeratosis, and ulceration [64].

Secondary nodules seen along lymphatic pathways generally exhibit deep dermal or subcutaneous necrotizing granulomas with peripheral fibrosis [32,61].

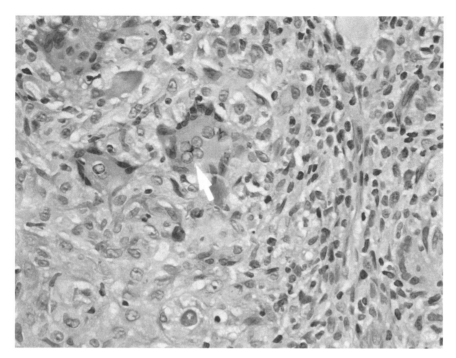

Fig. 11.8 Multinucleated giant cell containing pigmented fungal spores

Diagnosis

Biopsy, currettings, and aspirate of skin lesions reveal oval, 4–6 μm yeasts, rarely forming elongated "cigar bodies" [61] and rare hyphael forms [65]. The organism is dimorphic [66]. Smooth colonies are seen on culturing.

Chromomycoses

Epidemiology

Causative black fungi include *Fonseacea pedrosoi* [67] (commonest in most parts of the world), *Fonseacea compacta* [68], *Phialophora verrucosa, Cladiosporium carrioni,* and rarely *Acrotheca aquaspersa* [69] and *Aureobascidium pullalans* [70].

Disease has a world-wide distribution, affecting commonly adult males, particularly farmers. The organism is found in vegetable matter, wood, and soil.

Clinical Features

Distal extremities [69], especially legs and feet are involved by traumatic inoculation. The resultant papule changes to a pruritic verrucous plaque [71]. Itching leads to secondary bacterial infection with foul-smelling discharge. Dissemination to the CNS has been reported [72].

Histopathology

Tuberculoid granulomas are present in the mid-upper dermis, with overlying chronic inflammation. Marked fibrosis occurs with healing.

Pseudoepitheliomatous hyperplasia, hyperkeratosis and intraepidermal microabscesses are identified in the epidermis. "Sclerotic" or "medlar" bodies, 5–12 µm, round golden brown, thick-walled structures are easily seen on H&E (Fig. 11.9). These represent phenotypically arrested forms between yeast and hyphae.

Diagnosis

Subclassification of inciting organism depends on culture, but is generally not performed as treatment is similar.

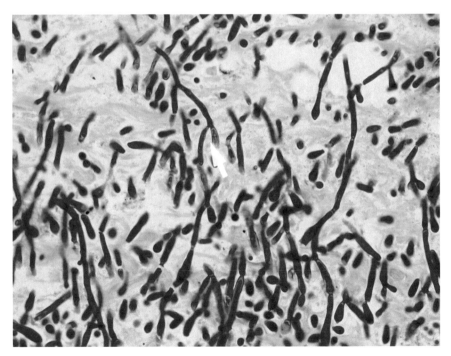

Fig. 11.9 Candida with pseudohyphae, which can closely resemble true-hyphae. The presence of round spores in tissue is helpful in the differential diagnosis from fungi with true hyphae

Cryptococcus associated with HIV infection warrants therapy [73]. Fluconazole is the first line of treatment. In patients unable to tolerate side effects, itraconazole may be substituted. In severe cases, fluctosine can be added to the regimen.

Coccidioidomycosis is self-limited in immunocompetent patients, and requires patient monitoring to ensure resolution of disease [74]. Disseminated disease mandates prolonged therapy, especially in the immunocompromised. Amphotericin B, ketoconazole, fluconazole or itraconazole may be employed. Amphotericin B is necessary in cases with an aggressive course [74].

It has been suggested that blastomycosis may occasionally act as an opportunistic infection in immunocompromised patients, requiring early and aggressive treatment with Amphotericin B [75]. Despite this, many immunocompromised patients have repeated relapses, requiring long-time, sometimes indefinite therapy. Such patients may be maintained on fluconazole or itraconazole.

Even though most patients acquiring sporotrichosis are immunocompetent, spontaneous resolution seldom occurs, necessitating antifungal and local hyperthermia therapy. Itraconazole is the drug of choice for lymphocutaneous sporotrichosis [76]. This may be substituted with fluconazole in patients unable to tolerate side effects. Ketoconazole is not effective against sporotrichosis [77]. Data on effectiveness of terbinafine is too limited and preliminary to determine its effectiveness in sporotrichosis. Amphotericin is not indicated as sporotrichosis generally runs a localized and benign course. Hyperthermia therapy involves daily local application of warm compresses or infra-red heat to maintain a temperature of 42–43°C. Although rarely used, it may be an option in patients who should not be on antifungal medication (e.g. severe liver disease or pregnancy).

Treatment is not indicated in localized pulmonary histoplasmosis, since it runs a self-limited course. Immunosuppression and extremes of age are risk factors for disseminated disease. In these circumstances, mortality of untreated cases is high, but can be reduced to 25% with proper medications [78, 79]. The choices of medication include amphotericin B, itraconazole, ketoconazole, and fluconazole.

Normal immune response, normal bacterial flora and intact mucosal barriers usually inhibit opportunistic fungi. Any disruption in this environment can lead to invasive fungal infection. Risk factors for developing opportunistic fungal infections include: HIV infection, hematologic malignancy, and diabetes mellitus. Other risk factors include treatment with chemotherapy agents, high-dose corticosteroids, and broad spectrum or chronic antibiotics. Hospitalized patients are also at risk for fungal infection with chronic catheterization (vascular and Foley) and intubation. Fungal infections can be especially detrimental to neutropenic patients [80]. Unfortunately empirical or prophylactic antifungal treatment has not been shown to decrease mortality in patients with cancer complicated by neutropenia [80].

There is confusion in current studies in regards to what defines superficial colonization, superficial infection and invasive infection. European and NIH groups have proposed consensuses for fungal infections [81]. Clinical signs of proven fungal infection include histologic evidence of invasive infection on biopsy or autopsy or microbial evidence of infection in two separate, closed, normally sterile body cavities [81]. Probable infections can be defined by positive fungal culture in the setting of host factors (i.e. fever, neutropenia, corticosteriod therapy, or other form of immunosuppression) and clinical factors (including radiographic and symptomatic evidence of infection) [81].

Aspergillosis

Epidemiology

The causative organism is *Aspergillus*. Over 700 species have been isolated, with approximately 19 identified in human infection. The most common species to infect humans are *Aspergillus fumigatus, A. flavus, A. terrus*, and *A. niger* [82]. The conidia of *Aspergillus* are commonly found in the soil and decaying organic matter. Inhalation of the spores is the route of infection for sinus and respiratory infection. To cause primary cutaneous disease, direct contact with the conidia is required [82]. Patients usually are immunocompromised, however, immunocompetent individuals may also be affected.

Aspergillus infection of the skin can be either primary or secondary to hematogenous spread. Acquisition of primary cutaneous infection has been linked to trauma, surgical wounds, and maceration of the skin secondary to tape and catheters [83–86].

Clinical Features

Five different forms of presentation of secondary aspergillosis have been described: (a) isolated necrotizing patch; (b) subcutaneous granuloma or abscess; (c) eruptive maculopapules, sustained, vegetative or with a tendency to necrobiosis; (d) erythematous or exanthemic reactions; and (e) coalescent graulomas with papules and nodules [87].

Histopathology

While identification of *Aspergillus* is difficult on hemotoxylin and eosin stained tissue, PAS and GMS are excellent for revealing the hyphae (Fig. 11.10). *Aspergillus* is easily identified by regular dichotomous branching at 45° angles [82]. The hyphae typically range from 5–10 μm [88]. Hyphal invasion into the tissues is rarely accompanied by a cellular response [82]. However, varying degrees of necro-

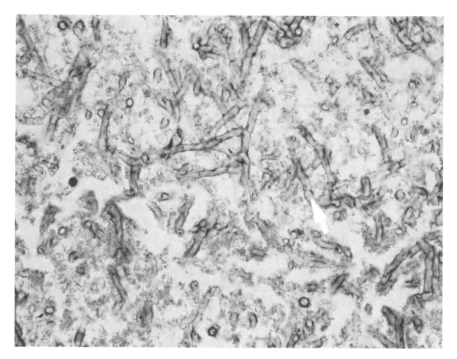

Fig. 11.10 Aspergillus with true branching hyphae

sis and occasional purulent and granulomatous responses (including fungal balls) have been identified [82]. In the granulomatous response, grains can be noted in the suppurative foci. The Splendore–Hoeppli phenomenon is described as these grains surrounded by eosinophilic, amorphous, hyaline-like, homogenous material [89].

Diagnosis

Accurate diagnosis of *Aspergillus* on tissue specimens is not always easy. Other fungi such as *Fusarium* species and *Pseudallescheria boydii* have similar hyphal appearances. Presence of the distinct conidial heads can serve as confirmation of the identity of *Aspergillus* [90]. Follow-up culture is recommended for definitive diagnosis.

Treatment

Itraconzale has uncertain efficacy in *Aspergillus* invasive infections, but is useful in treating patients who are unable to receive amphotericin B [91]. Drawbacks include poor absorption in patients with gastric achlorhydria and mucositis [91]. Serum levels must be measured to ensure that the patient has adequate absorption. A liquid formulation has demonstrated improved bioavailability [91].

Inhaled amphotericin B has been demonstrated to be effective in preventing *Aspergillus* infection, but is not well tolerated by cancer patients [91]. Another study shows that low dose IV amphotericin B significantly reduces mortality for invasive *Aspergillus* in allogeneic transplant recipients and in patients who have a history of fungal infection [91].

Geotrichosis

Epidemiology

The causative agent is *Geotrichum candidum*. It is a rare cause of opportunistic fungal infections. It is found as a saprophyte of the soil, in decaying vegetable matter, and contaminated food. Many people are colonized with *G. candidum*, and positive cultures of the feces or sputum do not necessarily indicate infection [90].

Elderly patients who are immunosupressed (either due to disease or treatment), receive parenteral nutrition, or undergo prolonged treatment with broad-spectrum antibiotics are at increased risk of infection by *Geotrichum candidum* [90]

Clinical Features

Patients with geotrichosis typically present with lesions in the mouth, intestines and other areas, including the skin. Patients often present with non-specific symptoms including fever cough, thick, gray mucoid, or purulent sputum [90].

Histopathology

While identification of *Geotrichum* is difficult on hemotoxylin and eosin stained tissue, PAS and GMS are excellent for revealing the hyphae. Hyphae and arthroconidia have varying sizes (range 10–30 μm) [90]. Hyphal branches are usually at acute angles [90]. Host response is usually minimal.

Diagnosis

Geotrichum candidum grows on cornmeal agar with true hyphae and anthroconidia. Arthroconidia produce hyphal extension from a corner producing structures that resemble hockey sticks [82]. *Geotrichum* does not produce urease, but does assimilate glucose, galactose and xylose, which can be used to distinguish it from the histologically similar *Trichosporon* [82].

On standard medium at 25°C, soft, white colonies usually develop in 2–4 days. These colonies later turn cream-colored and develop grooves that extend from the dense central core. Deep growth is prominent in 37°C cultures.

Treatment

The prognosis of geotrichosis is debatable for this uncommon infection. Reports on mortality vary from minimal if the underlying immunosuppression is resolved, to approximately 75% in immunosuppressed patients [82, 92]. While amphotericin B has provided moderate success in treatment, the current preferred regime includes 5-fluorocytosine and itraconazole [93].

Alternariosis

Epidemiology

The causative agent is the *Alternaria* species. *Alternaria* is a saprophytic fungus causing opportunistic infections [94]. Most cases of cutaneous *Alternaria* infection have been described in immunocompromised patients, most a result of corticosteroid therapy both systemic and local [94]. There has also been an association with Cushing's syndrome [94]. It has also been identified in a patient with idiopathic pulmonary fibrosis [95].

Clinical Features

Cutaneous alternariosis has many presentations, ranging from erythematous scaly plaques to plaques with pustules and ulceration [94–96]. Lesions are typically confined to the extremities and the face [94, 95, 97].

Histopathology

Hematoxylin and eosin staining may demonstrate an intradermal abscess cavity with focal areas of epidermal ulceration [95]. The inflammatory response consists of polymorphonuclear leukocytes, histiocytes, and multinucleated giant cells [95]. PAS and GMS stains can demonstrate broad branching fungal hyphae and large spores both in the abscess cavity and within the giant cells [95].

Diagnosis

Alternaria forms a characteristic chain of multicellular, macroconidia which are separated by horizontal and longitudinal septa [82]. The elongated bead of one conidium extends to the blunted end of the next [82].

The organism can be grown on Sabourand's dextrose agar with cloramphenicol, revealing dark, gray–white colonies with a dark brown underside [95]. Both culture and tissue examination should be utilized in the diagnosis of alternariosis.

Treatment

The proper treatment and the duration of the treatment has remained a point of controversy [96]. However, success has been achieved with itraconazole in addition to the reduction in corticosteroid therapy [95]. The length of time required for successful treatment has been reported to range from 3 months to 1 year [95, 98].

Fusariosis

Epidemiology

The causative agents are *Fusarium* spp. Cutaneous infections, particularly mycotic keratitis and onychomycosis have been attributed to Fusarium [99]. Disseminated infection has been identified in patients with hematologic malignancies, particularly aplastic anemia, lymphoma, and chronic leukemia [82]. Disseminated infections have also been identified in patients status post bone marrow transplant, and patients with extensive burns [82]. Disseminated infections may result from onychomycosis or cutaneous lesions [100].

Clinical Features

Patients with fusariosis may present with lesions ranging from red/gray macules with central ulceration or eschar, papules, pustules, and subcutaneous nodules [100]. Patients with disseminated disease are often neutropenic and may present with pneumonia, fever, skin lesions, and myalgia in addition to fungaemia [101].

Histopathology

Fusarium's septated hyphal branches are scattered throughout the lesion [90]. *Fusarium* cannot be easily distinguished from *Aspergillus* on histology, necessitating culture is necessary for accurate identification [90]. The hyphae can enter the vasculature leading to occlusion and infarction [90]. A PAS fungal stain is helpful in the diagnosis [102].

Diagnosis

Fusarium spp. are the only opportunistic molds that can be recovered easily in the blood of patients recovering from skin infection [103]. The toxins produced by the fungi are believed to cause a tissue breakdown, leading to easy invasion of the vasculature [103]. Due to the rapid progression in immunocompromised patients, rapid blood and wound cultures in addition to histologic examination of tissue is important in the diagnosis [104].

Fusarium produces both micro- and macroconidia. *Fusarium*'s microconidia can be easily confused with *Acremonium*. Examination for the distinctive large, pointed, sickle-form multicellular macroconidia of *Fusarium* can be used to dis-

tinguish the two [82]. On Sabouraud's dextrose agar, Fusarium displays characteristic rose, lavender, or magenta pigmentation on fluffy, granular rapidly growing
colonies [82].

Treatment

Treatment of disseminated disease with antifungal agents has not been effective,
unless the patient's neutropenia is resolved [100]. Some beneficial treatment has
resulted from the combination of granulocyte transfusions, subcutaneous GM-CSF
and amphotericin B [104]. Since Fusarium does not produce fatal infections in the
immunocompetent, it has been suggested that systemic antifungal therapy is not
necessary in this population [105]. Surgical debridement of wounds and removal
of infected lines/catheters can help prevent cutaneous infections from becoming
systemic [105]. Itraconazole has been shown to be effective in patients with onychomycosis [106].

Zygomycosis

Epidemiology

The causative agents are members of the *Zygomycetes* family, including *Mucor*
species, *Rhizopus* species, and *Absidia* species. *Zygomycetes* is an opportunistic
fungus that affect immunocompromised patients and diabetics. It has been rarely
identified in the immunocompetent following to traumatic implantation [107]. Infections typically begin after exposure to airborne spores or ingestion of contaminated
food.

Clinical Features

Patients with cutaneous zygomycosis present with varying appearances ranging
from encrusted erythematous plaques and papules to black necrotic lesions [107,
108]. Among diabetic patients, black eschars with destructive mutilaty of the central
face may occur, termed rhinocerebral mucomycosis. This infection is notorious for
its rapid progression and high disease specific morbidity. Patients with systemic
disease can present with multiple pulmonary lesions and fungus balls in the body
cavities [82]

Histopathology

Characteristic hyphae in the tissues in a background of acute inflammation is virtually diagnostic for *Zygomycetes*. In the skin, widespread granulomatous inflammation and characteristic broad, non-septate hyphae with right angle branching in
the dermis have been described in cases of zygomycosis [107]. However, when
the hyphae are viewed in cross-section a misdiagnosis of coccidiomycosis is possi-

ble [82]. The hyphae do not typically stain well with hematoxylin and eosin, PAS, or GMS stains. *Zygomycetes* have the tendency to invade blood vessels leading to hemorrhagic infarctions and fungus balls in body cavities [82].

Diagnosis

Zygomycetes can be identified as quickly growing, multicolored ill-defined colonies that darken as they mature [82]. Characteristic features include broad, ribbonlike aseptate hyphae with the production of sporangiospores in sporangia [82].

Treatment

Ketoconazole has been shown to be effective in the treatment of cutaneous zygomycosis [109]. Other cases of zygomycosis in the skin have been treated with surgical debridement and amphotericin B [110].

Actinomycosis and Nocardiosis

While *Actinomyces* and *Nocardia* are bacteria, their resemblance to fungi can be confusing in tissue samples and deserve brief discussion.

Epidemiology

The causative agents are *Actinomyces israelii* and *Nocardia asteroides*. *Actinomyces* are very common in the soil, where they exist in the filamentous phase. Actinomycosis typically results from infection stemming from tooth and gingival disease. Cutaneous actinomycosis has been identified in immunocompetent individuals and has been associated with poor oral hygiene [106].

The most common agent of norcardiosis is *Nocardia asteroids*. Inhalation of airborne particles or traumatic implantation into the subcutaneous tissues are the principle routes of infection [82]. Infected individuals are not always immunocompromised and can present with acute, subacute, or chronic disease [82].

Clinical Features

Actinomycosis can cause chronic granulomatous infections commonly in the neck, face, lung, intestine and pelvic area [106]. Cutaneous actinomycosis present as painless, erythematous, suppurative soft lesions and can be nodular that tend to form fistulae [106].

Patients with nocardiosis typically present with fever, productive cough, and infiltrates on chest X-ray [82]. Pneumonia may progress to empyema, fistula tracts, abscesses and granulomas [82]. Approximately 50% of patients develop disseminated disease.

Histopathology

While actinomycosis is not very common in tissues, gram-stained smears reveal the characteristic sulfur colonies. These sulfur colonies are granular microcolonies surrounded by purulent exudate [82]. *A. israelii* colonies are gram-positive rods, with varying sizes, but are significantly smaller than normal fungi [111].

Evidence of *Nocardia* infection in tissues is demonstrated by acute granulocytic inflammation accompanied by necrosis and abscess formation. *Nocardia* is capable of surviving in macrophages, where it inhibits phagosome–lysosome fusion [82]. *Nocardia* is not seen on hematoxylin and eosin stained sections, and PAS staining does not always stain them.

Diagnosis

A. israelii grows blood agar plates in anaerobic culture at 37°C. There is more rapid growth on thioglycolate medium, and *A. israelii* is capable of indole production, esculin and gelatin hydrolysis, and fermentation of carbohydrates [82]. Florescent antibodies are used for identification of different species of actinomyces [82].

GMS, Gram–Weigert, Giemsa, Brown and Brenn Gram stain, and Brown–Hopps Gram stains demonstrate the *Nocardia* well [82]. In tissue, *Nocardia* appears as a thin, beaded, branched filamentous rod. *Nocardia* is acid-fast, which is helpful in distinguishing it from *Actinomyces* [82]. The significance of the presence of *Nocardia* in blood and sputum cultures remains a point of contention; since *Nocardia* is a common component of the normal oral flora and a common contaminant of cultures [112].

Treatment

Actinomycosis is treated with antibiotics, most commonly penicillin, erythromycin and tetracycline and followed by surgery. Nocardiosis is treated with long-term antibiotics, commonly sulfonamides, and surgical drainage if necessary.

References

1. Loo DS. Cutaneous fungal infections in the elderly. Dermatol. Clin. North. Am. 2004; 22: 33–50.
2. Crespo Erchiga V, Ojeda Martos A, Vera Casano A, et al. *Malassezia globosa* as the causative agent of pytiriasis versicolor. Br. J. Dermatol. 2000; 143: 799–803.
3. Gupta AK, Jain HC, Lynde CW, et al. Prevalence and epidemiology of onychomycosis in patients visiting physicians' offices: a multicenter Canadian Survey of 15,000 patients. J. Am. Acad. Dermatol. 2000; 43: 244–8.
4. Habif, TP. Clinical Dermatology: A Color Guide to Diagnosis and Therapy, 4th ed. Mosby, Inc, 2004.
5. Elewski BE. Large-scale epidemiological study of the causal agents of onychomycosis: mycological findings from the Multicenter Onychomycosis Study of Terbinafine. Arch. Dermatol. 1997; 133: 1317–18.
6. Midgley G, Moore MK. Onychomycosis. Rev. Iberoam. Micol. 1998; 15: 113–7.

7. Daniel III CR, Elewski BE. The diagnosis of nail fungus infection revisited. Arch. Dermatol. 2000; 136: 1162–4.

8. Elewski BE, Leyden J, Rinaldi MG, et al. Office practice-based confirmation of onychomycosis: a US nationwide prospective survey. Arch. Intern. Med. 2002; 162: 2133–8.

9. Elewski BE. New developments in cutaneous fungal infections. Curr. Probl. Dermatol. 2000; 12: 81–5.

10. Friedlander SF, Aly R, Krafchik B, et al. Terbinafine in the treatment of *Trichophyton* tinea capitis: a randomized, double-blind, parallel-group, duration- finding study. Pediatrics 2002; 109: 602–7.

11. Lipozencic J, Skerlev M, Orofino-Costa R, et al. A randomized, double-blind, parallel-group, duration- finding study of oral terbinafine and open-label, high-dose griseofulvin in children with tinea capitis due to *Microsporum* species. Br. J. Dermatol. 2002; 146: 816–23.

12. Lesher JL Jr. Oral therapy of common superficial fungal infections of the skin. J. Am. Acad. Dermatol. 1999; 40: S31–4. Review.

13. Faergemann J, Anderson C, Hersle K, et al. Double-blind, parallel-group comparison of terbinafine and griseofulvin in the treatment of toenail onychomycosis. J. Am. Acad. Dermatol. 1995; 32: 750–3.

14. Havu V, Heikkila H, Kuokkanen K, et al. A double-blind, randomized study to compare the efficacy and safety of terbinafine (Lamisil) with fluconazole (Diflucan) in the treatment of onychomycosis. Br. J. Dermatol. 2000; 142: 97–102.

15. De Backer M, De Vroey C, Lesaffre E, et al. Twelve weeks of continuous oral therapy for toenail onychomycosis caused by dermatophytes: a double-blind comparative trial of terbinafine 250 mg/day versus itraconazole 200 mg/day. J. Am. Acad. Dermatol. 1998; 38: S57–63.

16. Hunger RE, Paredes BE, Quattroppani C, et al. Primary cutaneous cryptococcosis in a patient with systemic immunosuppression after liver transplantation. Dermatology 2000; 200: 352–5.

17. Lauerma AI, Jeskanen L, Rantanen T, et al. Cryptococcosis during systemic glucocorticoid treatment. Dermatology 1999; 199: 180–2.

18. Hernandez AD. Cutaneous cryptococcosis. Dermatol. Clin. 1989; 7: 269–74.

19. Williams DM, Krick JA, Remington JS. Pulmonary infection in the compromised host (Part 1). Am. Rev. Respir. Dis. 1976; 114: 359–94.

20. Tomasini C, Caliendo V, Puiatti P, et al. Granulomatous-ulcerative vulvar cryptococcosis in a patient with advanced HIV disease. J. Am. Acad. Dermatol. 1997; 37: 116–7.

21. Murakawa GJ, Kerschmann R. Berger T. Cutaneous cryptococcal infection and AIDS. Report of 12 cases and review of literature. Arch. Dermatol. 1996; 132: 545–8.

22. Sugar AM. Overview: cryptococcosis in patients with AIDS. Myocpathologia 1991; 114: 153–7.

23. Kozel TR, Gotschlich EC. The capsule of *Cryptococcus neoformans* passively inhibits phagocytosis of the yeast by macrophages. J. Immunol. 1982; 129: 1675–80.

24. Hamann ID, Gillespie RJ, Ferguson JK. Primary cryptococcal cellulitis caused by *Cryptococcus neoformans* var *gatti* in an immunocompetent host. Australas J. Dermatol. 1997; 38: 29–32.

25. Patel P, Ramanathan J, Kayser M, Baran J Jr. Primary cutaneous cryptococcosis of the nose in an immunocompetent woman. J. Am. Acad. Dermatol. 2000; 43: 344–5.

26. Hecker MS, Weinberg JM. Cutaneous cryptococcosis mimicking keloid. Dermatology 2001; 202: 78–9.

27. Borton LK, Wintroub BU. Disseminated cryptococcosis presenting as herpetiform lesions in a homosexual man with aquired immunodeficiency syndrome. J. Am. Acad. Dermatol. 1984; 10: 387–90.

28. Picon L, Vaillant L, Duong T, et al. Cutaneous cryptococcosis resembling molluscum contagiosum: a first manifestation of AIDS. Acta Derm. Venereol. 1989; 69: 365–7.

29. Gordon PM, Omerod AD, Harvey G, et al. Cutaneous cryptococcal infection without immunodeficiency. Clin. Exp. Dermatol. 1994; 19: 181–4.

30. Sussman EJ, McMahon F, Wright D, et al. Cutaneous cryptococcosis without evidence of systemic involvement. J. Am. Acad. Dermatol. 1984; 11: 371–4.

31. Narisawa Y, Kojima T, Iriki A, et al. Tissue changes in cryptococcosis: histologic alteration from gelatinous to suppurative tissue response with asteroid body. Mocopathologia 1989; 106: 113–9.
32. Hirsh BC, Johnson WC. Pathology of granulomatous disease. Mixed inflammatory granulomas. Int. J. Dermatol. 1984; 23: 585–97.
33. Ro JY, Lee SS, Ayala AG. Advantage of Fontana Masson in capsule-deficient cryptococcal infection. Arch. Pathol. Lab. Med. 1987; 111: 53–7.
34. Farmer SG, Komorowski RA. Histologic response to capsule-deficient *Cryptococcus neoformans*. Arch. Pathol. 1973; 96: 383–7.
35. Naka W, Masuda M, Konohana A, et al. Primary cutaneous cryptococcosis and *Cryptococcus neoformans* serotype D. Clin. Exp. Dermatol. 1995; 20: 221–5.
36. Pappagianis D. Coccidioidomycosis. Semin. Dermatol. 1993; 12: 301–9.
37. Stevens DA. Coccidioidomycosis. N. Engl. J. Med. 1995; 332: 1077–82.
38. Quimby SR, Connolly SM, Winkelmann RK, et al. Clincopathologic spectrum of specific cutaneous lesions of disseminated coccidioidomycosis. J. Am. Acad. Dermatol. 1992; 26: 79–85.
39. Hobbs E. Coccidioidomycosis. Dermatol. Clin. 1989; 7: 227–39.
40. Bronnimann DA, Galgiani JN. Coccidioidomycosis. Eur. J. Clin. Microbiol. Infect. Dis. 1989; 8: 466–73.
41. Fish DG, Ampel NM, Galgiani JN, et al. Coccidioidomycosis during human immunodeficiency virus infection. A review of 77 patients. Medicine (Baltimore) 1990; 69: 384–91.
42. Prichard JC, Sorotzkin RA, James RE III. Cutaneous manifestations of disseminated coccidioidomycosis in the acquired immunodeficiency syndrome. Cutis 1987; 39: 203–5.
43. Schwartz RA, Lamberts RJ. Isolated nodular cutaneous coccidioidomycosis. The initial manifestion of disseminated disease. J. Am. Acad. Dermatol. 1981; 4: 38–46.
44. Bayer AS, Yoshikawa TT, Galpin JE, Guze LB. Unusual syndromes of coccidioidomycosis: diagnostic and therapeutic considerations: a report of 10 cases and review of the English literature. Medicine (Baltimore) 1976; 55: 131–52.
45. Levan NE, Huntington RW Jr. Primary cutaneous coccidioidomycosis in agricultural workers. Arch. Dermatol. 1965; 92: 215–20.
46. Ampel NM, Wieden MA, Galgiani JN. Coccidioidomycosis: clinical update. Rev. Infect. Dis. 1989; 11: 897–911.
47. DiTomasso JP, Ampel NM, Sobonya RE, et al. Bronchoscopic diagnosis of pulmonary coccidioidomycosis. Comparison of cytology, culture and transbronchial biopsy. Diagn. Microbiol. Infect. Dis. 1994; 18: 83–7.
48. Pappagianis D, Zimmer BL. Serology of coccidioidomycosis. Clin. Microbiol. Rev. 1990; 3: 247– 68.
49. Carman WF, Frean JA, Cerwe-Brown HH, et al. Blastomycosis in Africa. A review of cases diagnosed between 1951 and 1987. Mycopathologia 1989; 107: 25–32.
50. Tenenbaum MJ, Greenspan J, Kerkering TM. Blastomycosis. Crit. Rev. Microbiol. 1982; 9: 139–63.
51. Malak JA, Farah FS. Blastomycosis in Middle East. Report of suspected case of North American blastomycosis. Br. J. Dermatol. 1971; 84: 161–6.
52. Bradsher RW. Blastomycosis. Clin. Inf. Dis. 1992; 14: S82–90.
53. Pladson TR, Stiles MA, Kuritsky JN. Pulmonary histoplasmosis. A possible risk in people who cut decayed wood. Chest 1984; 86: 435–8.
54. Dijkstra JWE. Histoplasmosis. Dermatol. Clin. 1989; 7: 251–7.
55. Goodwin RA, Owens FT, Snell JD, et al. Chronic pulmonary histoplasmosis. Medicine (Baltimore) 1976; 55: 413–52.
56. Witty LA, Steiner F, Curfman M, et al. Disseminated histoplasmosis in patients receiving low-dose methotrexate therapy for psoriasis. Arch. Dermatol. 1992; 128: 91–3.
57. Studdard J, Sneed WF, Taylor MR Jr, et al. Cutaneous histoplasmosis. Am. Rev. Respir. Dis. 1976; 113: 689–93.

58. Cohen PR, Bank DE, Silvers DN, et al. Cutaneous lesions of disseminated histoplasmosis in human immunodeficiency virus-infected patients. J. Am. Acad. Derm. 1990; 23: 422–8.
59. Williams AO, Lawson EA, Lucas AO. African histoplasmosis due to *Histoplasma duboisii*. Arch. Pathol. 1971; 92: 306–18.
60. Davies SF. Histoplasmosis: update 1989; Semin. Respir. Infect. 1990; 5: 93–104.
61. Belknap BS. Sporotrichosis. Dermatol. Clin. 1989; 7: 193–202.
62. Shiraishi H, Gomi H, Kawada A, et al. Solitary sporotrichosis lasting for 10 years. Dermatology 1999; 198: 100–1.
63. Purvis RS, Diven DG, Drechsel RD, et al. Sporotrichosis presenting as arthritis and subcutaneous nodules. J. Am. Acad. Dermatol. 1993; 28: 879–84.
64. Urabe H, Honbo S. Sporotrichosis. Int. J. Dermatol. 1986; 25: 255–7.
65. Mayberry JD, Mullins JF, Stone OJ. Sporotrichosis with demonstration of hyphae in human tissue. Arch. Dermatol. 1966; 39: 65–7.
66. Binford DH, Dooley JR. Sporotrichosis. Pathology of Tropical and Extraordinary diseases, Vol. 2; Bunford CH, Connor DH, eds. Washington: Armed Forces Institute of Pathology, 1976, pp 574–7.
67. Rajendran C, Ramesh V, Misra RS, et al. Chromoblastomycosis in India. Int. J. Dermatol. 1997; 36: 29–33.
68. Sharma NL, Sharma RC, Grover PS, et al. Chromoblastomycosis in India. Int. J. Dermatol. 1999; 38: 846–51.
69. Fukushiro R. Chromomycosis in Japan. Int. J. Dermatol. 1983; 22: 221–9.
70. Redondo-Bellon P, Idoate M, Rubio M, et al. Chromoblastomycosis produced by *Aureobasidium pullulans* in an immunosuppressed patient. Arch. Dermatol. 1997; 133: 663–4.
71. Tomecki KJ, Steck WD, Hall GS, et al. Subcutaneous mycoses. J. Am. Acad. Dermatol. 1989; 21: 785–90. Review.
72. Bansal AS, Prabhakar P. Chromomycosis: a twenty-year analysis of histologically confirmed cases in Jamaica. Trop. Geogr. Med. 1989; 41: 222–6.
73. Saag MS, Graybill RJ, Larsen RA, et al. Practice guidelines for the management of cryptococcal disease. Infectious Diseases Society of America. Clin. Infect. Dis. 2000; 4: 710–8.
74. Galgiani JN, Ampel NM, Catanzaro A, et al. Practice guideline for the treatment of coccidioidomycosis. Infectious Diseases Society of America. Clin. Infect. Dis. 2000; 4: 658–61.
75. Pappas PG, Threlkeld MG, Bedsole GD, et al. Blastomycosis in immunocompromised patients. Medicine (Baltimore) 1993; 72: 311–25.
76. Conti Diaz IA, Civila E, Gezuele E, et al. Treatment of human cutaneous sporotrichosis with itraconazole. Mycoses 1992; 35: 153–6.
77. Dismukes WE, Stamm AM, Graybill JR, et al. Treatment of systemic mycoses with ketoconazole: an emphasis on toxicity and clinical response in 52 patients. National Institute of Allergy and Infectious diseases collaborative antifungal study. Ann. Intern. Med. 1983; 98: 13.
78. Dismukes WE, Bradsher RW Jr, Cloud GC, et al. Itraconazole therapy for blastomycosis and histoplasmosis. NIAID Mycoses Study Group. Am. J. Med. 1992; 93: 489–97.
79. Wheat J, MaWhinney S, Hafner R, et al. Treatment of histoplasmosis with fluconazole in patients with acquired immunodeficiency syndrome. National Institute of Allergy and Infectious Diseases Acquired Immunodeficiency Syndrome Clinical Trials Group and Mycoses Study Group. Am. J. Med. 1997; 130: 223–32.
80. Gotzsche, PC, Johansen HK. Meta-analysis of prophylactic or empirical antifungal treatment vs. placebo or no treatment in patients with cancer complicated by neutropenia. Brit. Med. J. 1997. 314: 1238–44.
81. Ascioglu S, Rex JH, de Pauw B, et al. Defining opportunistic invasive fungal infections in immunocompromised patients with cancer and hematopoetic stem cell transplants: an international consensus. Clin. Infect. Dis. 2002; 34: 7–14.
82. Koneman EW, Allen SD, Janda WM, Schrenkengerger PC, Winn WC Jr. Color Atlas and Textbook of Diagnostic Microbiology, 5th ed. New York: Lippincott, Williams and Wilkins, 1997.

83. Allo MD, Miller J, Townsend T, et al. Primary cutaneous aspergillosis associated with Hickman intravenous catheters. New Eng. J. Med. 1987; 317: 1105– 8.
84. Romero LS, Hunt SJ, Hickman catheter associated primary cutaneous aspergillosis in a patient with the acquired immunodeficiency syndrome. Int. J. Dermatol. 1995; 34: 551–3.
85. Stiller MJ, Teperman L, Rosenthal SA, et al. Primary cutaneous infection by *Aspergillus ustus* in a 62-year-old liver transplant recipient. J. Am. Acad. Dermatol. 1994; 31: 344–7.
86. Pla MP, Berenguer J, Arzuaga JA, et al. Surgical wound infection by Aspergillus fumigatus in liver transplant recipients. Diagn. Microbiol. Infect. Dis. 1992; 15: 703–6.
87. Findlay GH, Roux H, Simson I. Skin manifestations in disseminated aspergillosis. Brit. J. Dermatol. 1971; 85 (Suppl.): 94–7.
88. Koneman EW and Roberts GD "Mycotic Disease" in Henry JB, ed. Clinical Diagnosis and Management by Laboratory Methods, 18th ed. Philadelphia: Saunders, 2001; pp. 1099–157.
89. Sugar, AM. Agents of Mucormycosis and Related Species. Mandell, Douglas, and Bennett's Principles and Practice of Infectious Diseases, 5th ed. New York: Churchill Livingstone, Inc., 2000, p. 2692.
90. Chandler FW and Watts JC. Pathologic Diagnosis of Fungal Infections. Chicago: ASCP Press, 1987.
91. Vusirikala M. Supportive care in hematologic malignancies. In Greer JP, Foerster J, Lukens JN, et al., eds. Wintrobe's Clinical Hematology, 11th ed. Philadelphia: Lippincott, Williams and Wilkins, 2004, pp. 2102–13.
92. Fouassier M, Joly D, Cambon M, et al. Geotrichum capitatum infection in a neutropenic patient. Apropos of a case and review of the literature. Revue Med. Intern. 1998; 19: 431–3.
93. Listemann H, Schonrock-Nabulsi P, Kuse R, et al. Geotrichosis of oral mucosa. Mycoses 1996; 39: 289– 91.
94. Machet L, Jan V, Machet MC, et al. Cutaneous alternariosis: role of corticosteroid-induced cutaneous fragility. Dermatology 1996; 193: 342–4.
95. Ioannidou DJ, Stefanidou MP, Maraki SG, et al. Cutaneous alternariosis in a patient with idiopathic pulmonary fibrosis. Int. J. Dermatol. 2000; 39: 293–5.
96. Acland KM, Hay RJ, Groves R. Cutaneous infection with *Alternaria alternata* complicating immunosuppression: successful treatment with itraconazole. Br. J. Dermatol. 1998; 138:354–6.
97. Iwatsu T. Cutaneous alternariosis. Arch. Dermatol. 1988; 124(12): 1822–5.
98. Lespessailles E, Kerdraon R, Michenet P, et al. Alternaria infection of the skin and joints. A report of two cases involving the hand. Rev. Rhum, Engl, Ed. 1999; 66(10): 509–11.
99. Rippon JW. Medical Mycology: The pathogenic fungi and the pathogenic Actinomycetes, 3rd ed. Philadelphia: WB Saunders, 1988, p. 482.
100. Bodey GP, Boktour M, Mays S, et al. Skin lesions associated with Fusarium infection. J. Am. Acad. Dermatol. 2002; 47: 659–66.
101. Frediank H. Hyalohyphomycoses due to *Fusarium* spp.—two case reports and review of the literature. Mycoses 1995; 38(1): 69–74.
102. Collins MS, Rinaldi MG.Cutaneous infection in man caused by *Fusarium moniliforme*. Sabouraudia 1977; 15: 151–60.
103. Anaissie E, Legrand C, Hachem R, et al. Recovery of *Fusarium* sp from the bloodstream using a rabbit model of systemic fusariosis. Abstracts from the Annual Meeting of the American Society of Microbiology 1990; 90: 413 (abstr F-28).
104. Peltroche-Llacsahuanga H, Manegold E, Kroll G, et al. Case report. Pathohistological findings in a clinical case of disseminated infection with *Fusarium oxysporum*. Mycoses 2000; 43(9–10): 367–72.
105. Musa MO, Al Eisa A, Halim M, et al. The spectrum of *Fusarium* infection in immunocompromised patients with hematological malignancies and in non- immunocompromised patients: a single institution experience over 10 years. Br. J. Haematol. 2000; 108(3): 544–8.

106. Romano C, Massai L, De Alo GB, et al. A Case of Primary Cutaneous Actinomycosis. Acta Derm. Venereol. 2002; 82: 144–5.
107. Song WK, Park HJ, Cinn YW, et al. Primary cutaneous mucormycosis in a trauma patient. J. Dermatol. 1999; 26(12):825–8.
108. Adriaenssens K, Jorens PG, Meuleman L, et al. A black necrotic skin lesion in an immuno-compromised patient. Diagnosis: cutaneous mucormycosis. Arch. Dermatol. 2000; 136: 1165–70.
109. Kobayashi M, Hiruma M, Matsushita A, et al. Cutaneous zygomycosis: a case report and review of Japanese reports. Mycoses 2001; 44: 311–15.
110. Wu CL, Hsu WH, Huang CM, et al. Indolent cutaneous mucormycosis with pulmonary dissemination in an asthmatic patient: survival after local debridement and amphotericin B therapy. J. Formos Med. Assoc. 2000; 99: 354–7.
111. Tortora GJ, Funke B, Case CL. Microbiology: An Introduction, 5th ed. Addison-Wesley, 1995.
112. Esteban J. Zaparadiel J, Soriano F. Two cases of soft-tissue infection caused by *Arcanobacterium haemolyticum*. Clin. Infect. Dis. 1994; 18: 35–6.

Chapter 12

Xerosis and Pruritus in the Elderly—Recognition and Management

Robert A. Norman

Xerosis and Pruritus Overview

Dry skin is known as xerosis. The condition is characterized by pruritic, dry, cracked and fissured skin with scaling. Xerosis occurs most often on the legs of elderly patients, but may be present on the hands and trunk. Xerotic skin appears like a pattern of cracked porcelain. These cracks or fissures result from epidermal water loss. The skin splits and cracks deeply enough to disrupt dermal capillaries, and bleeding fissures may occur. Itching or pruritus occurs leading to secondary lesions. Scratching and rubbing activities produce excoriations, an inflammatory response, lichen simplex chronicus (leather-like skin) and even edematous patches [1]. Subsequently, environmental allergens and pathogens can easily penetrate the skin increasing the risk of allergic and irritant contact dermatitis as well as infection. Allergic and irritant contact dermatitis may be a cause for a persistent and possibly more extensive dermatitis despite therapy [1]. Eczematous changes can occur with a delayed hypersensitivity response even in advanced age [2]. Secondary infection is an inherent risk with any break in the skin barrier.

Dry skin, or xerotic eczema, can be labeled as xerosis, eczema craquele, dyshidrotic eczema or asteatotic eczema. Incidence increases with age and is common in the elderly. Symptoms may include pruritus without rash and may be intense, although generally a sporadic occurrence.

Common areas involved are the anterolateral lower legs (most commonly affected), back and flanks, abdomen and waist and arms. Areas spared generally include the axilla, groin, face and scalp.

Provocative factors include cold, dry weather, such as winter or air conditioning exposure. Palliative factors are warm, humid weather. Signs include mild changes such as faint reticulate pinkness, with fine scale or cracks seen with tangential light.

Moderate to severe changes include dramatic deep redness and cracking and skin may appear as cracked porcelain (eczema craquele) or as nummular eczema-type lesions.

Management includes topical agents such as alpha-hydroxy acid moisturizers (e.g., Eucerin Plus) applied after warm water soaks or steroid ointment (triamcinolone for 4–5 days). For dyshidrotic eczema of the hands the management includes applying moisturizing lotions 10–20 times daily and petroleum jelly at bedtime under glove.

Research Findings

I completed a study of the nursing home patients in our extensive treatment group, and found the two most common problems overwhelmingly to be xerosis and pruritus (Table 12.1—includes age and gender distribution). Given these results, I focus here on the recognition and treatment of these entities. Of ultimate importance is the comprehensive treatment of these problems to prevent stasis dermatitis and ulcer formation.

Xerosis

Prevalence and Predisposing Factors

Xerosis preys upon the elderly. This is primarily due to the fact that aged individuals have decreased sebaceous and sweat gland activity. This reduced activity predisposes the aged skin to moisture depletion. There are a number of situations that deplete the skin's moisture. For example, xerosis tends to relapse in the winter when

Table 12.1 Most common diagnoses (Includes gender and age distribution)

Diagnosis	ICD 9 CM code	N^1	% Male	Mean age (SD)[2]
Pruritus and other related diseases	698.0–698.9	1002	31.34	78.9 (14.1)
Diseases of the sebaceous glands (xerosis = 772)	706.0–706.8	813	29.53	80.6 (13.5)
Other dermatoses[2]	702.0–702.8	546	25.74	84.1 (9.8)
Basal or squamous cell carcinoma of the skin	173.0–173.9	353	29.28	84.5 (10.3)
Scabies	133.0	220	35.35	78.0 (14.7)
Contact dermatitis and other eczema	692.0–692.9	218	37.56	77.1 (14.3)
Erythematosquamous dermatitis	690	216	48.36	75.6 (16.5)
Disorders of the sweat gland	705.0–705.9	166	35.98	78.3 (14.0)
Non-thrombocytopenic purpura	287.2	145	24.65	84.8 (8.0)
Stasis dermatitis with varicosites	454.1	135	21.05	81.3 (11.3)
Candidiasis	112.0–112.9	80	21.79	80.5 (13.3)
Cellulitis, unspecified site	682.9	77	27.27	79.3 (14.1)
Dermatophytosis	110.0–110.9	71	27.12	78.4 (14.4)
Other hypertrophic and atrophic conditions of the skin[3]	701	47	24.12	83.9 (18.1)

[1] Total sample size = 1556.
[2] SD = standard deviation.
[3] specified and unspecified hypertropic and atrophic conditions, keratoderma.

a lower humidity environment predominates [3]. Another situation involves the daily use of cleansers and/or bathing without replacing natural skin emollients [4].

Additionally, pre-existing disease states, therapies and medications make the aged individual more susceptible to xerosis. Some of these pre-existing situations include radiation, end-stage renal disease [5], nutritional deficiency (especially zinc and essential fatty acids) [6], thyroid disease and neurological disorders with decreased sweating, anti-androgen medications, diuretic therapy, human immunodeficiency virus and malignancies [7].

Pathology

In healthy skin, skin cells called corneocytes detach from neighboring cells to be lost to the environment and are replaced by younger cells from the deeper layers. This orderly process leads to corneocytes or skin cell loss from the skin surface and is called desquamation. Desquamation is controlled primarily by two intercellular components called corneodesmosomes and lipids. The intercellular actions of these two components provide for the maintenance of tissue thickness. Corneodesmosomes bind the corneocytes to maintain intercellular cohesion and tissue integrity. For effective desquamation corneodesmosomes must eventually be broken down. This process is called corneodesmolysis.

In healthy skin, corneodesmolysis is totally effective in eliminating the corneodesmosomes [3]. This is not the case with xerotic skin. Corneodesmosomes persist and disturb the orderly desquamation process. In chronic and acute dry skin conditions, this disturbed process is manifested by the formation of visible, powdery flakes on the skin surface [8].

Another important consideration is that free water is necessary to control the corneodesmolysis process. Adequate lipid content is required to retain the free water. Inadequately hydrated skin cannot provide this free water. Therefore, deficits in both skin hydration and lipid content play a key role in xerosis [3]. Consequently, the skin's inability to retain moisture and provide an effective barrier directly impacts the development of xerosis in aged skin [9, 10].

Treatment

Once the stage is set for xerosis development, the scenarios of flaking, fissuring, inflammation, dermatitis and infection develop. The xerotic vicious cycle needs to be broken to disable the process and prevent complications [11, 12]. This is precisely the goal of xerosis treatment—break the xerotic cycle.

To achieve this goal, keratolytics, moisturizers and steroids are the primary components of xerosis treatment. The keratolytic effect of ammonium lactate 12% lotion is effective in reducing the severity of xerosis. Several studies have demonstrated this benefit [13, 14]. Individuals with sensitive skin may not tolerate some products formulated with alpha-hydroxy acids (AHAs) due to unacceptable levels of stinging and irritation. In this case, a sensitive skin-variant formulation should be substituted [15]. Liberal use of moisturizers reduce scaling and enhance the corneodesmosome degradation process [16–18]. Additional treatment via application of topical steroids (Classes III–VI) is recommended in moderate to severe cases [4]. Antipruritics should be added if disturbing pruritus is present [12].

Other additional management suggestions include the following:

- Reduced frequency of bathing with lukewarm (not hot) water
- Minimal use of a non-irritant soap such as Cetaphil soap, Oil of Olay, Dove
- Avoidance of harsh skin cleansers
- Applying moisturizer of choice directly on skin that is still damp
- Avoiding friction from washcloths, rough clothing and abrasives
- Using air humidification in dry environments [4, 19]

Aged skin is very susceptible to the development of xerosis. The vicious cycle of the xerotic process preys on the elderly, making them an easy target for xerosis-related complications. The treatment goal focuses on breaking the xerotic cycle to prevent secondary complications.

Pruritus

A perceived itching sensation is known as pruritus. Characteristic features of pruritus include scratching and inflammation. The condition is often associated with other underlying diseases. Itching is thought to be induced by the effect of histamine on the touch propreoceptors and is mediated exclusively by the peripheral nervous system. Itching evokes the desire to scratch. Scratching produces an immunology-based inflammatory response. Pruritus can be psychogenic in origin. However, there are a number of dermatological and metabolic conditions that involve pruritus. Xerosis is the most common underlying dermatological condition. Other dermatological conditions include infestations, infection (fungal, bacterial or viral), lichen planus, nodular prurigo, dermatitis, eczema and miliaria. Underlying metabolic conditions which can produce pruritus include renal failure, HIV, diabetes mellitus, thyroid disease, parathyroid disease, hypervitaminosis A, iron-deficiency anemia, neuropathy, hepatic disease, malignancy and drugs.

Initial treatment focuses on relief of pruritus. The specific etiology is then determined. To maximize effectiveness, pruritus treatment strategy is then tailored to the specific underlying condition.

Description

Pruritus is a perceived itching sensation. The propreoceptors of touch are thought to be responsible for the itching sensation. Cutaneous histamine effects induce itch and are mediated exclusively by the peripheral nervous system [20]. Itching evokes the desire to scratch [21, 22]. Scratching is an itch-associated response and produces inflammation, which is an immunologic response [23, 24].

Pruritic skin diseases are the most common dermatological problem in the elderly [25]. Xerosis is the most common underlying problem associated with pruritus [25, 26]. Other common dermatological conditions associated with pruritus are identified in Table 12.1 [27]. In addition to common skin conditions, other pruritogens include drug therapy, psychological causes and many systemic diseases.

Pathology

There is little understanding of the pathophysiology of pruritus. Pruritus is known to be a feature of inflammation. Inflammation is the result of activation of the body's immune response, normally to an antigen. Involved skin cells have IgE molecules on their surface. The main physiological role of IgE is to trigger acute inflammation [23]. Release of compounds such as histamine and heparin (vasoactive amines) occurs [28]. Histamine causes small blood vessels to dilate and heparin acts as an anticoagulant. Skin blood vessel walls have lymphocyte receptors on their surface, aiding the migration of lymphocytes from the blood into the tissues [29]. The inflammatory stage is set. With repetitive rubbing, scratching and touching (induced by a foreign body or self), inflammatory and pigmentary cutaneous manifestations occur [27]. Some of these manifestations include excoriations, prurigo nodularis and lichen simplex chronicus [27, 30, 31].

Clinical Work-Up and Initial Treatment

Immediate relief of pruritus is the focus of initial treatment efforts. The goal of these efforts is to dull the inflammatory response [32]. Treatment regimens for pruritus and products recommended are highly variable [26]. Furthermore, pruritus relief evaluation is subjective since valid itch measurement techniques are needed for the evaluation of antipruritic therapies [21]. Mild pruritus may respond to non-pharmacologic measures such as avoiding hot water and irritants, maintaining proper humidity, using cool water compresses, trimming the nails and behavior therapy. Topical symptomatic treatments include moisturizers, emollients, tar compounds, topical corticosteroids, topical anesthetics such as benzocaine or dibucaine and pramoxine HCl (alone or combined with menthol, petrolatum or benzyl alcohol) [33].

Once temporary pruritic relief is obtained, efforts should focus on finding the underlying cause [27]. This process begins with a thorough history, physical exam and laboratory result evaluation. The goal of pruritus therapy is to optimize treatment efficacy by tailoring the treatment to underlying etiology. For example, topical doxepin cream has been shown to be very effective in pruritus associated with eczematous dermatitis [32]. It can be used alone for acute pruritus or with corticosteroids in chronic conditions [33]. Other treatments include localized ultraviolet B phototherapy and intralesional injections of corticosteroid [33]. For pruritus associated with atopic dermatitis, Zafirlukast is very effective [34]. With cholestatic and uremic-related pruritus, serotonin type 3 (5-HT3) receptor antagonists are useful [35]. Fluvoxamine has some effectiveness in reducing psychogenic excoriation from scratching [36]. Other medication/measures employed to treat generalized pruritus include odansetron (5 HT3 antagonist) and transcutaneous nerve stimulation [27].

In patients with HIV, systemic therapies such as indomethacin, pentoxifylline and hydroxyzine with or without doxepin at night have been more beneficial than topical steroids [33]. Danazol has proven to be a good alternative for patients with severe refractory pruritus associated with myeloproliferative and other systemic disorders [37]. One study of patients on hemodialysis who received either fish oil, olive oil or safflower oil documented an improved patient perception of symptoms of pruritus [38]. Due to the presence of reduced stratum corneum hydration, simple emollient therapy may relieve the pruritus in patients on maintenance dialysis [39]. Other drug treatments used include activated charcoal, antihistamines, capsaicin cream, amitryptilline tablets at night and cholestyramine [31, 40]. Cooling lotions such as camphor and menthol have been effectively used [31, 40]. Avoidance of fragrance soap, irritating chemicals and hot water helps reduce pruritus, especially in elderly patients who have the xerotic changes of aging.

Allergic skin disorders in the elderly, which may arise from contact with or ingestion of offending allergens, must be distinguished from other causes of itching in the elderly such as xerosis, itching due to systemic disease and bullous disease. Elderly people have decreased cell-mediated immunity and may be harder to sensitize under experimental conditions. However, they have had many years to acquire allergic responses and develop contact dermatitis frequently. Patch testing is an important tool to diagnose contact allergy in the elderly. Particularly attention should be paid to patients at high risk of contact dermatitis, such as those with chronic lower extremity dermatitis or ulcers due to venous stasis. A knowledge of the common sensitizers is important, especially when prescribing topical medications to high-risk patients. Dressings used to treat stasis ulcers, contact allergy to dental prostheses and medications used to treat ocular disease are common in the elderly as a result of increased usage and exposure. Allergic non-eczematous dermatoses caused by ingested allergens are much more commonly due to medications than food in the elderly. In particular, urticarial skin reactions are often associated with the administration of antibacterials, non-steroidal anti-inflammatory drugs (NSAIDs), antidepressants or opioids. Systemic reaction to anticonvulsants, gold, allopurinol or diuretics commonly result in morbilliform rashes. The administration of tetracyclines, diuretics, NSAIDs and antihyperglycemic agents can result in phototoxic reactions. Multiple medication intake in the elderly can make diagnosis of drug allergy difficult because diagnosis is most commonly accomplished by observing clinical response once the medication is withdrawn. Clinical improvement from lichenoid cutaneous reactions may take several months following withdrawal of the offending drug [41].

Summary

The pathophysiology of xerosis is related to abnormal keratin production; elderly have decreased skin fatty acids that result in decreased skin barrier and hydration.

The perceived itch of pruritus induces scratching and subsequently immunologically mediated inflammation. The condition is often associated with several underlying dermatological and systemic diseases. However, pruritus can be psychogenic in origin. Xerosis is the most common underlying dermatological condition. Several infectious, metabolic, hepatic, hematological and other systemic conditions are associated with pruritus. Immediate relief of pruritus is the initial treatment goal. After initial pruritic relief, a thorough history, physical examination and laboratory testing work-up is necessary to find the underlying treatable cause including genetic predisposition. Once the underlying etiology is uncovered, an effective pruritic treatment strategy is tailored to etiology.

References

1. Anderson C, Miller F. Xerosis [Online], September 28, 2000. Available: http://www.emedicine.com/derm/topic538.htm.
2. Aoyama H, Tanaka M, Hara M, Tabata N, Tagami H. Nummular eczema: an addition of senile xerosis and unique cutaneous reactivities to environmental aeroallergens [From Karger Online abstracts, ISSN: 1018-8665]. Dermatology 1999; 199(2): 135–9. Available: http://www.online.karger.com/library/karger/renderer.
3. Harding R, Mayo C, Rawlings A. Stratum corneum lipids: the effect of ageing and the seasons [Online from MedScape Medline, ISSN: 0340-3696]. Arch. Dermatol. Res. 1996; 288(12): 765–70. Available: http://www.medscape.com/server-java/MedLineApp?/member-search/.
4. Huntley, A. Eczematous diseases [Online from Matrix Dermatology Resources in Other Skin Diseases, Dermatology 420: Ecematous Diseases], 1998. Available: http://matrix.ucdavis.edu/tumors/eczema/eczema.htm.
5. Nunley, JR. Xerosis [Online], 2001. Available: http://www.emedicine.com/derm/" \l "section~introduction".
6. Weismann K, Wadskov S, Mikkelsen HI, Knudsen L, Christensen KC, Storgaard L. Acquired zinc deficiency dermatosis in man. Arch. Dermatol. [Online Abstract from Entrz-PubMed] 1978; 114(10): 1509–11. Available: http://www.ncbi.nlm.nih.gov:80/entrez/query.
7. Rowe A, Mallon E, Rosenberger P, Barrett M, Walsh J, Bunker C. Depletion of cutaneous peptidergic innervation in HIV-associated xerosis. J. Invest. Dermatol. [From PubMed Abstracts, Item PMID: 10084303], 1999; 112(3): 284–9. Available: http://www.ncbi.nlm.nih.gov/entrez/query.
8. Simon M, Bernard D, Minondo AM, Camus C, Fiat F, Corcuff P, Schmidt R, Serre G. Persistence of both peripheral and non-peripheral corneodesmosomes in the upper stratum corneum of winter xerosis skin versus only peripheral in normal skin [Online Serial from Medline Abstracts ISSN:0022-202X]. J. Invest. Dermatol. 2001; 116(1): 23–30. Available: www.medscape.com/server-java/MedLineApp?/member-search.
9. Engelke M, Jensen J, Ekanayake-Mudiyanselage S, Proksch E. Effects of xerosis and ageing on epidermal proliferation and differentiation [Online Abstract from Medscape, ISSN 007-0963]. Br. J. Dermatol. 1997; 137(2): 219–25. Available: http://www.medscape.com/server-java/MedLineApp?/member-search.
10. Paepe K, Derde M, Roseeuw D, Rogiers V. Incorporation of ceramide 3B in dermatocosmetic emulsions: effect on the transepidermal water loss of sodium lauryl sulphate-damaged skin [Online from Synergy Abstracts]. J. Eur. Acad. Dermatol. Venereol. 2000; 14(4): 272–9. Available: http://www.blackwell-synergy.com/Journals/member/searchresults.asp.
11. Seidenari S, Giusti G. Objective assessment of the skin of children affected by atopic dermatitis [Online From Entrez-PubMed, PMID: 8651017]. Acta Dermato-venereol. 1995; 75: 429–33. Available: http://www.ncbi.nlm.nih.gov/entrez/query.

12. Thaipisuttikul Y. Pruritic skin diseases in the elderly [Online Abstract From Entrez-PubMed, PMID: 9575676]. J. Dermatol. 1998; 25(3): 153–7. Available: http://www.ncbi.nlm.nih.gov/entrez/query.

13. Jennings M, Alfieri D, Ward K, Lesczczynski C. Comparison of salicylic acid and urea versus ammonium lactate for the treatment of foot xerosis. A randomized, double blind, clinical study [Online from MedScape Medline, ISSN: 8750-7315]. J. Am. Podiatr. Med. Assoc. 1998; 88(7): 332–6. Available: http://www.medscape.com/server-java/MedLineApp?/member-search/.

14. Kempers S, Katz H, Wildnauer R, Green B. An evaluation of the effect of an alpha hydroxy acid-blend skin cream in the cosmetic improvement of symptoms of moderate to severe xerosis, epidermolytic hyperkeratosis, and ichthyosis [Online Abstract from MedScape Medline, ISSN: 0011-4162]. Cutis 1998; 61(5): 347—50. Available: http://www.medscape.com/server-java/MedLineApp?/member-search.

15. Wolf B, Paster A, Levy S. An alpha hydroxy acid derivative suitable for sensitive skin [Online Abstract from Medscape Medline, ISSN: 1076-0512]. Dermatol. Surg. 1996; 22(5): 469–73. Available: http://www.medscape.com/server-java/MedLineApp?/member-search.

16. Gammal C, Pagnoni A, Kligman A, Gammal S. A model to assess the efficacy of moisturizers—the quantification of soap-induced xerosis by image analysis of adhesive-coated discs (D-Squames) [Online Abstract from Medscape Medline, ISSN: 0307-6938]. Clin. Exp. Dermatol. 1996; 21(5): 338—43. Available: http://www.medscape.com/server-java/MedLineApp?/member-search.

17. Harding C, Watkinson I, Rawlings I, Scott I. Dry skin, moisturization and corneodesmolysis [Online]. Int. J. Cosmet. Sci. 2000; 22(1): 21–52. Available: http://www.blackwell-synergy.com/Journals/member/.

18. Rawlings A, Harding C, Watkinson A, Banks J, Ackerman C, Sabin R. The effect of glycerol and humidity on desmosome degradation in stratum corneum [Online Abstract from Medscape Medline, ISSN: 0340-3696]. Arch. Dermatol. Res. 1995; 287(5): 457–64. Available: http://www.medscape.com/server-java/MedLineApp?/member-search.

19. Lazar A, Lazar P. Dry skin, water, and lubrication [Online Abstract from PubMed]. Dermatol. Clin. 1999; 9(1): 45–51. Available: http://www.ncbi.nlm.nih.gov:80/entrez/query.

20. Johansson O, Virtanen M, Hilliges M. Histaminergic nerves demonstrated in the skin. A new direct mode of neurogenic inflammation [Online Serial from Medline Abstracts, ISSN: 0906-6705]. Exp. Dermatol. 1995; 4(2): 93–6. Available: http://www.medscsape.com/server-java/MedLineApp?/member-search.

21. Wahlgren C. Measurement of itch [Online Serial from Medline Abstracts, ISSN: 0278-145X]. Semin. Dermatol. 1995; 14(4): 277–84. Available: http://www.medscsape.com/server-java/MedLineApp?/member-search.

22. Woodward D, Nieves A, Spada C, Williams L, Tuckett R. Characterization of a behavioral model for peripherally evoked itch suggests platelet-activating factor as a potent pruritogen [Online Serial from Medline Abstracts, ISSN: 0022-3565]. J. Pharmacol. Exp. Ther. 1995; 272(2): 758–65. Available: http://www.medscsape.com/server-java/MedLineApp?/member-search.

23. Seidenari S, Giusti G. Objective assessment of the skin of children affected by atopic dermatitis [Online from Entrez-PubMed, PMID: 8651017]. Acta Dermato-venereol. 1995; 75: 429–33. Available: http://www.ncbi.nlm.nih.gov/entrez/query.

24. Yamaguchi T, Maekawa T, Nishikawa Y, Nojima H, Kaneko M, Kawakita T, Miyamoto T, Kuraishi Y. Characterization of itch-associated responses of NC mice with mite-induced chronic dermatitis [Online Serial from Medline Abstracts, ISSN: 0923-1811]. J. Dermatol. Sci. 2001; 25(1): 20–8. Available: http://www.medscsape.com/server-java/MedLineApp?/member-search.

25. Thaipisuttikul Y. Pruritic skin diseases in the elderly [Online Abstract from Entrez-PubMed, PMID: 9575676]. J. Dermatol. 1998; 25(3): 153–7. Available: http://www.ncbi.nlm.nih.gov/entrez/query.

26. Fleischer A Jr. Pruritus in the elderly: management by senior dermatologists [Online Serial from Medline Abstracts, ISSN: 0190-9622]. J. Am. Acad. Dermatol. 1993; 28(4): 603–9. Available: http://www.medscsape.com/server-java/MedLineApp?/member-search.

27. Leung C. Pruritus. In Handbook of Dermatology & Venereology, 2nd ed., Chap. 2 [Online, I.S.B.N. 962 3340303]. Available: http://www.hkmj.org.hk/skin/.

28. Rukwied R, Lischetzki G, McGlone F, Heyer G, Schmelz M. Mast cell mediators other than histamine induce pruritus in atopic dermatitis patients: a dermal microdialysis study [Online Serial from Medline Abstracts, ISSN: 0007-0963]. Br. J. Dermatol. 2000; 142(6): 1114–20. Available: http://www.medscsape.com/server-java/MedLineApp?/member-search.

29. Graham J. Itching (Pruritus) [Online]. Napier University Department of Biological Sciences Honours Project, 1997. Available: http://www.biol.napier.ac.uk/BWS/COURSES/ projects/eczema/itching.htm.

30. Kosko D. Dermatologic manifestations of human immunodeficiency virus disease [Online Serial from Medline Abstracts, ISSN: 1088-5471]. Lippincotts Prim. Care Pract. 1997; 1(1): 50–61. Available: http://www.medscsape.com/server-java/MedLineApp?/member-search.

31. Robertson K, Mueller B. Uremic pruritus [Online Serial from Medline Abstracts, ISSN: 0271-0749]. J. Health Syst. Pharm. 1996; 53(18): 2159–70. Available: http://www.medscsape.com/server-java/MedLineApp?/member-search.

32. Drake L, Millikan L. The antipruritic effect of 5% Doxepin cream in patients with eczematous dermatitis: Doxepin Study Group [Online Serial from Medline Abstracts, ISSN: 0003-987X]. Arch. Dermatol. 1995; 131(12): 1403–8. Available: http://www.medscsape.com/server-java/MedLineApp?/member-search.

33. Herting R. Dermatology: Pruitis. In University of Iowa Family Practice Handbook, 3rd ed., Chap. 13, pp. 1–13 [Online]. Available: http://www.vh.org/Providers/ClinRef/ FPHandbook/Chapter13/01-13.html.

34. Zabawski E, Kahn M, Gregg L. Correspondence: treatment of atopic dermatitis with Zafirlukast [Online]. Dermatol. Online J. 1999; 5(2): 10. Available: http://dermatology.cdlib.org/ DOJvol5num2/editorials/zafirlukast.html.

35. Weisshaar E, Ziethen B, Gollnick H. Can a serotonin type 3 (5-HT3) receptor antagonist reduce experimentally-induced itch? [Online Serial from Medline Abstracts, ISSN: 1023-3830]. Inflamm. Res. 1997; 46(10): 412. Available: http://www.medscsape.com/server-java/MedLineApp?/member-search.

36. Arnold L, Mutasim D, Dwight M, Lamerson C, Morris E, McElroy S. An open clinical trial of fluvoxamine treatment of psychogenic excoriation [Online Serial from Medline Abstracts, ISSN: 0271-0749]. J. Clin. Psychopharmacol. Semin. Dermatol. 1999; 19(1): 15–18. Available: http://www.medscsape.com/server-java/MedLineApp?/member-search.

37. Kolodny L, Horstman L, Sevin B, Brown H, Ahn Y. Danazol relieves refractory pruritus associated with myeloproliferative disorders and other diseases [Online Serial from Medline Abstracts, ISSN: 0361-8609]. Am. J. Hematol. 1996; 51(2): 112–6. Available: http://www.medscsape.com/server-java/MedLineApp?/member-search.

38. Peck L. Essential fatty acid deficiency in renal failure: can supplements really help? [Online Serial from Medline Abstracts, ISSN: 0002-8223]. J. Am. Diet Assoc. 1997; (10 Suppl 2): S150–3. Available: http://www.medscsape.com/server-java/MedLineApp?/member-search.

39. Morton C, Lafferty M, Hau C, Henderson I, Jones M, Lowe J. Pruritus and skin hydration during dialysis [Online Serial from Medline Abstracts, ISSN: 0931-0509]. Nephrol. Dial. Transplant. 1996; 11(10): 2031–6. Available: http://www.medscsape.com/server-java/MedLineApp?/member-search.

40. Oakley A. The itching patient [Online Dermatology GP Lecture 3]. N. Z. Dermatol. Soc. 2001. Available: http://dermnetnz.org/home.htm.

41. Nedorost ST, Stevens SR. Diagnosis and treatment of allergic skin disorders in the elderly. Drugs Aging 2001; 18(11): 827–35.

Chapter 13
Sarcoidosis in Aging Skin

Amor Khachemoune and Carlos Rodríguez

Introduction

Sarcoidosis is an idiopathic multisystem granulomatous inflammatory disease which commonly presents with manifestations in the lungs, skin, eyes and lymph nodes, although various organs may be affected. Cutaneous involvement is seen in approximately one-third of patients with systemic illness [1], and isolated skin disease occurs in roughly one-fourth of all patients [2]. The hallmarks of sarcoidosis include an accumulation of mononuclear phagocytes and infiltration of affected tissues by noncaseating granulomas (NCGs). Several eponyms have been used to characterize skin involvement in the disease, such as "Boeck's sarcoidosis," "Darier–Roussy sarcoidosis," "lupus pernio of Besnier," "Heerfordt's disease," and "Löfgren's syndrome," as well as more visually descriptive terms including papular, macular, annular, psoriasiform, verrucous, hypomelanotic, ichthyosiform, lymphedematous, and so forth. Labeled one of the "great imitators," cutaneous sarcoidosis may exhibit a myriad of different morphologic lesions and pose a challenge to accurate diagnosis. This chapter will discuss the background of cutaneous sarcoidosis with an emphasis on elderly patients, as well as the principal morphologic forms of skin lesions in relation to differential diagnostic considerations. A brief summary on treatment options will also be presented.

Epidemiology

Sarcoidosis occurs worldwide with a roughly equal incidence of 1–40/100,000 in both sexes [3], with individuals under 40 years of age being most commonly affected [4]. A second peak in incidence occurs in women aged 45–65 years [5,6], and in Europeans the age at disease onset tends to average in the fifth decade [3]. A much greater incidence of sarcoidosis is seen in blacks (particularly females) in the United States and South Africa, as well as in Scandinavian and Irish populations [7]. In Europe, white individuals are more commonly affected, as are western Europeans [3]. African-American patients generally present at a younger age than individuals of other ethnic groups, and may experience a more widely involved and advanced disease course, while in whites the opposite tends to occur [8]. The incidence of sarcoidosis in those older than 60 years of age at diagnosis has been estimated at approximately 8% [9, 10]; however, it has been suggested that the paucity of cases reported among older patients may actually be an underestimate of the true incidence, when compared to more common diseases afflicting the elderly such as pulmonary tuberculosis or lung carcinoma [10]. Cutaneous sarcoidosis tends to occur with greater frequency in elderly females than in males [10–12].

Clinicopathologic Characteristics

The precise etiology of sarcoidosis is unknown. However, immune dysregulation has been implicated, likely due to persistence of a low-virulence antigen incompletely cleared by the immune system, resulting in a chronic T-cell response with granuloma formation. Postulated antigens consist of infectious agents including Mycobacteria, viruses and fungi; environmental triggers such as metals, pollens and dust; as well as auto-antigens [3, 8].

An accumulation of CD4+ T cells and increased levels of interleukin 2 (IL-2) occur at sites of disease activity, along with elevated levels of T_H1 cytokines including interferon, and increased production of tumor necrosis factor (TNF) and TNF receptors [13]. Elevated B-cell activity and immunoglobulin production have also been noted, and increased antigen presenting cells and circulating immune complexes may also play a role [13, 14]. Genetic susceptibility has also been postulated to play an etiologic role, as familial clusters of the disease correlating with certain class I and II HLA alleles on chromosome 6 have been documented, including HLA-B8, HLA-A1 and HLA-D3 [3, 8, 14].

Although patients most commonly present with bilateral hilar lymphadenopathy, pulmonary infiltration, and skin or eye lesions, organ involvement in sarcoidosis can range from localized to widespread, mild to severe, and cause a self-limited to chronic disease course, depending on the impact of NCG formation on involved organ systems. In addition to pulmonary and cutaneous disease, sarcoidosis can manifest with ocular, lymph node, bone marrow, endocrine, hepatic, cardiac, musculoskeletal, neurologic and renal involvement. Roughly 5% of cases are asymptomatic and discovered incidentally by chest radiograph, while systemic and pulmonary symptoms are noted in approximately 45 and 50% of cases, respectively [13]. One-third of sarcoidosis patients develop lymphadenopathy, roughly 25–50% develop ocular disease, and approximately 5–10% experience neurologic or cardiac involvement [3, 14].

The extent of cutaneous lesions in sarcoidosis does not seem to correlate well with the extent of systemic involvement, but the mode of disease onset may be more closely associated with its course and prognosis [15, 16]. Patients who experience an acute onset of illness with development of erythema nodosum generally undergo a more self-limited course and spontaneous resolution of their disease, while those who experience a more insidious onset have a greater likelihood of developing progressive pulmonary fibrosis [17]. Spontaneous remission of disease occurs in approximately two-thirds of all patients, while approximately 1–6% experience a fatal course with death secondary to severe cardiac or pulmonary involvement [3]. Morbidity as a direct consequence of sarcoidosis results from pulmonary symptoms including shortness of breath, ocular disease resulting in scarring and possible blindness, as well as cutaneous disfigurement.

Amongst the geriatric population of sarcoidosis patients, shortness of breath is generally the most common presenting complaint [12], though approximately 34% of elderly patients experience asymptomatic disease [18]. No single test can accurately diagnose sarcoidosis, which is often confirmed using a combination of clinical, radiologic and histologic evidence. Laboratory values indicative of the disease include hypercalcemia, hypercalciuria and elevated angiotensin converting enzyme (ACE) level, resulting from secretion of 1,25-vitamin D and ACE by NCGs, as well as elevated levels of alkaline phosphatase seen with hepatic involvement.

Chest radiographs are of central importance in patient work-up, which typically reveal bilateral hilar lymphadenopathy with or without perihilar calcifications. Bronchoalveolar lavage with an inverted CD4/CD8 ratio greater than 3.5 has a specificity of 94% for sarcoidosis [3]. Patient work-up should also include an electrocardiogram to rule out unsuspected or symptomatic arrhythmias, in addition to pulmonary function tests in symptomatic patients [3, 13]. Eosinophilia, false positive rheumatoid factor (RF) and antinuclear antibody (ANA) levels, skin anergy to common antigens, as well as elevated erythrocyte sedimentation rate (ESR) may also be found. Other less commonly employed studies include high-resolution computed tomography (HRCT) scans and the highly specific Kveim test. Whole-body gallium-67 scanning may demonstrate the "lambda" and "panda" patterns of increased uptake in the hilar lymph nodes and lacrimal/parotid glands, respectively [3]. Lesional biopsy of skin, lung, or lymph nodes demonstrating presence of NCGs is required for diagnosis in most cases [13].

Histopathology

Skin manifestations in sarcoidosis are categorized into specific lesions, which demonstrate NCGs on biopsy, and nonspecific lesions, which reveal a reactive change. Punch or incisional wedge biopsy should be performed to obtain a histologic sample that includes the dermis with or without subcutaneous tissue, and when clinically appropriate, biopsy specimens should be stained and cultured to exclude infectious causes of granuloma formation including mycobacteria and fungi.

With the exception of erythema nodosum, which is nonspecific for sarcoidosis and demonstrates septal panniculitis, the histologic findings in typical sarcoid lesions are characterized by the presence of circumscribed granulomas of epithelioid cells with little or no caseating necrosis. Granulomas are generally located in the superficial dermis but may extend throughout the entire dermal layer and into the subcutis. These granulomas are often referred to as "naked tubercles" because they demonstrate only a minimal lymphocytic infiltrate at their margins

Fig. 13.1 Histology: 10×.
Scanning magnification of
noncaseating sarcoid
granuloma (naked
granuloma)

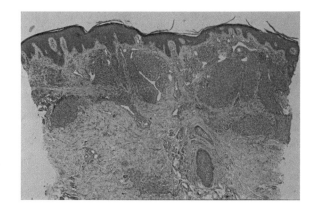

Fig. 13.2 Histology: 200×.
Magnified view of sarcoid
granuloma in Fig. 13.1

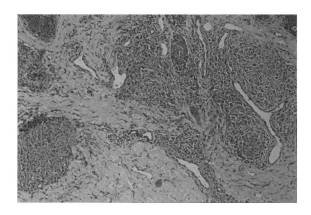

(Fig. 13.1 and 13.2). Fibrosis, if present, begins at the periphery and progresses toward the center of the lesions. Islands of epithelioid cells may include a few Langhans giant cells, which, in turn, may enclose star-shaped eosinophilic asteroid bodies, as well as Schaumann bodies, which are round laminated structures with peripheral calcification. In considering the differential diagnosis of sarcoidosis based on histopathologic findings alone, several other granulomatous dermatitides should be considered, including granuloma annulare, necrobiosis lipoidica diabeticorum, annular elastolytic giant cell granuloma, Crohn's disease and rheumatoid nodules. Other possible entities include granulomatous mycosis fungoides, Hodgkin's disease, granulomatous rosacea, cheilitis granulomatosa, and sarcoidal reaction to an underlying lymphoma or other malignancy [19–21].

Clinical Presentations and Differential Diagnoses

Cutaneous lesions in sarcoidosis tend to be asymptomatic and are most likely to manifest at disease onset [2, 7]. They may be divided into specific and nonspecific types. Nonspecific lesions are reactive processes. Specific lesions demonstrate

NCGs histologically, however their clinical appearances may vary dramatically and thus be misleading from a diagnostic standpoint. Sarcoidosis should be included in the differential diagnosis of any granulomatous skin lesion without an apparent diagnosis [14]. Generally, cutaneous involvement does not bear any relation to prognosis or extent of illness, with the exceptions of erythema nodosum, which correlates with a better prognosis and spontaneous disease resolution, and lupus pernio, which has been associated with more debilitating osseous and pulmonary involvement [8, 14]. Stadnyk et al. [10] did not note any particular cutaneous features more distinctive in the elderly when compared to younger patients, and indicated that tissue biopsy be routinely performed for diagnosis in older individuals with suspicious cutaneous lesions. The discussion below divides the various manifestations of sarcoidosis based on morphologic characteristics of the diverse array of skin lesions encountered. (Table 13.1)

Specific Lesions

Small papules or maculopapules are the most common specific cutaneous findings in sarcoidosis [8, 22]. A variety of different colors may be seen, including skin-colored papules, hyper- or hypopigmented lesions, and red, brown and violaceous tones (Fig. 13.3). These generally asymptomatic lesions occur commonly on the

Table 13.1 Differential diagnosis of cutaneous sarcoidosis by morphologic forms of specific lesions.

Morphology	Differential diagnosis
Papules	Xanthelesma, acne rosacea, granulomatous rosacea, syringoma, trichoepithelioma, secondary lues, polymorphous light eruption, adenoma sebaceum, perioral dermatitis, lupus miliaris disseminatus faciei
Nodules	Furunculosis, B-cell lymphoma, cutaneous T cell lymphoma (CTCL), leukemia cutis, epidermal inclusion cysts, morphea, lipomas, metastatic carcinomas, foreign body granulomas
Plaques	Lupus vulgaris, discoid lupus erythematosus (DLE), psoriasis, nummular eczema, lichen planus, granuloma annulare, necrobiosis lipoidica, morphea, CTCL, Kaposi's sarcoma, leprosy, leishmaniasis, gyrate erythema
Alopecia	DLE, lichen planopiliaris, pseudopelade, alopecia neoplastica, secondary syphilis
Ulcerative lesions	Vascular insufficiency, ulcerated neoplasms, pyoderma gangrenosum
Miscellaneous descriptions of specific sarcoid lesions	Ichthyosiform, psoriasiform, pityriasis-like, infiltration of scars, hypopigmented, verrucous, lichenoid, erythrodermic, mutilating, morpheaform, perforating, umbilicated; nodular finger tip lesions, plaques of palms and soles; penile, scrotal and vulvar papules and plaques; folliculitis, eruptive, lichenoid, chelitis-like, annular elastocytic, erythema annulare centrifugum-like

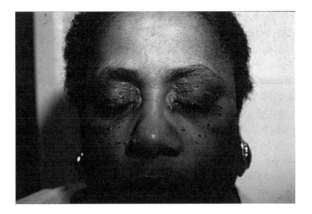

face in a solitary or confluent arrangement, but may be seen on the neck, upper back and extremities as well [8]. Diascopic examination of papules demonstrates a characteristic "apple-jelly" color, which corresponds microscopically to granuloma formation, but this is not seen exclusively in sarcoidosis. Papular and macular lesions are very common in African-American women (Fig. 13.4) and may be associated with a lower incidence of systemic involvement and a better overall prognosis [3, 23].

Disorders within the papular or maculopapular morphologic group which may be mimicked by sarcoidosis include xanthelesma, acne rosacea, granulomatous rosacea, syringoma, trichoepithelioma, secondary lues, polymorphous light eruption, adenoma sebaceum, perioral dermatitis and lupus miliaris disseminatus faciei [3, 23, 24]. Granulomatous acne rosacea may appear essentially identical to papular sarcoidosis, both clinically and histologically, in which careful history, physical

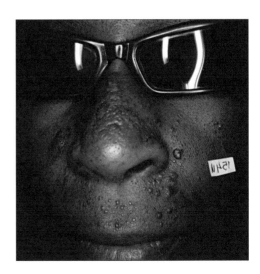

Fig. 13.4 Multiple papules
involving the nose, nasal sulci
and upper lip in an
African-American patient

examination, and characteristic laboratory findings are needed to make an accurate diagnosis. Papular lesions generally leave no scarring upon resolution [3].

Sarcoidosis may also present with subcutaneous nodular lesions, a manifestation known as Darier–Roussy sarcoidosis. Lesions are firm, painless, mobile nodules measuring up to 2 cm in diameter, typically appearing on the trunk and extremities in single and multiple arrangements, involving the subcutis alone with no dermal infiltration [8, 14]. The skin surface shows no inflammatory change. Nodules tend to appear later in the course of illness [22], and may be associated with more advanced disease and visceral involvement [25]. Disease entities which may be confused with nodular sarcoidosis include furunculosis, cutaneous T- and B-cell lymphomas, leukemia cutis, epidermal inclusion cysts, morphea, lipomas, metastatic carcinomas and foreign body granulomas [23, 24]. Laboratory tests detecting hypercalcemia, hypercalciuria, and elevated angiotensin-converting enzyme (ACE) levels, in addition to biopsy, may help point the clinician toward the correct diagnosis. Nodular lesions are usually chronic and may produce scarring [3].

Plaques of various colors may occur on the face, trunk, extremities and buttocks in both single and multiple configurations; the latter tending to demonstrate a more symmetric and possibly annular arrangement. These sarcoid lesions indicate deeper granulomatous involvement of the skin and may be found in any area of the body. Angiolupoid sarcoidosis is a subtype within the plaque group which demonstrates large telangiectatic blood vessels within lesions. Plaque-like and annular forms may be associated with more chronic disease, higher risk of systemic involvement and a poorer prognosis when compared to papular lesions [3, 23].

Morphologically similar entities mimicked by sarcoidosis include lupus vulgaris, discoid lupus erythematosus, psoriasis, nummular eczema, lichen planus, granuloma annulare, necrobiosis lipoidica, morphea, cutaneous T-cell lymphoma, Kaposi's sarcoma, leprosy, cutaneous leishmaniasis and gyrate erythema [23, 24]. Lesions may heal with scarring, and plaque involvement of the head and neck may produce a cicatricial alopecia, in which case differential entities to be considered include chronic cutaneous lupus erythematosus, lichen planopiliaris and pseudopelade, as well as alopecia neoplastica and secondary lues [3, 23, 24, 26].

Lupus pernio is the most characteristic presentation of sarcoidosis, manifesting as indolent red to violaceous indurated shiny nodules or plaques resembling an acute cold injury (pernio) (Fig. 13.5). These most frequently involve the central face, particularly the alar rim of the nose, and are most common in African-American women with longstanding disease [3, 8]. Lesions in this area may infiltrate the nasal mucosa and upper respiratory tract and cause ulceration along with possible airway obstruction [27] (Fig. 13.6). A significant association with upper airway involvement and bone cysts has been noted, as has a more chronic disease course with a less favorable prognosis [23]. The cosmetic effects of lupus pernio may be quite distressing to patients and prompt them to seek medical attention.

Several more rare, although specific, manifestations of sarcoidosis may be encountered, including an ichthyotic scaling process on the lower extremities [28], or ulcerative lesions mimicking vascular insufficiency [23]. Scaling psoriasiform or pityriasis-like plaques on the trunk have been described [28], as have infiltration

Fig. 13.5 Lupus pernio

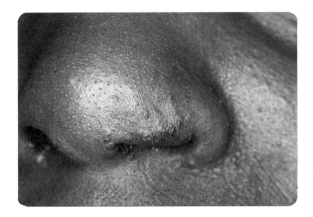

of scars, tattoos or injection sites creating red to purple indurated lesions [3, 8] (Fig. 13.7). Other less common atypical presentations of sarcoidosis include hypopigmented, verrucous, lichenoid, erythrodermic, mutilating, morpheaform, perforating and umbilicated forms [8]. Several of these more rare manifestations may mimic lymphomas, solid organ malignancies, HIV, syphilis, mycobacterial infections, iatrogenic connective tissue disorders, malnutrition, thyroid and parathy-

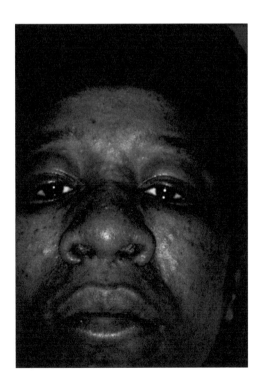

Fig. 13.6 Involvement of the nasal mucosa in a patient with lupus pernio

Fig. 13.7 Sarcoid lesions arising within a scar on the leg

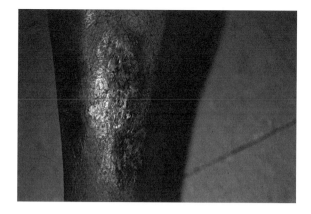

roid diseases. Case reports of nodular finger tip lesions; plaques of palms and soles; penile, scrotal and vulvar papules and plaques (Fig. 13.8); and lupus erythematosus-like, umbilicated papules have also been described, as have folliculitis-like, eruptive, lichenoid, chelitis-like, annular elastocytic, and erythema annulare centrifugum-like processes [4, 14, 29–33].

Nonspecific lesions

Nonspecific lesions are reactive processes, with erythema nodosum (EN) being the most common manifestation. EN occurs in approximately 3–25% of patients with systemic sarcoidosis, usually during the acute phase in the setting of Löfgren's syndrome (acute onset of EN in conjunction with bilateral hilar lymphadenopathy, fever, arthralgias and/or arthritis and uveitis) [34]. This reactive pattern is seen more frequently among Scandinavian patients, as well as in Irish and Puerto Rican females [3]. Although EN is a rather common finding for dermatologists, sarcoidosis as a cause of EN is uncommon.

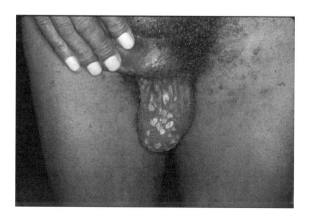

Fig. 13.8 Scrotal involvement with sarcoid papules

Clinically, EN presents with a rather abrupt onset of 1–5 cm tender, warm, erythematous nodules, most commonly the anterior tibial surfaces, as well as on the ankles and knees bilaterally. Nodules may become confluent and form erythematous plaques. EN is known to go through a play of colors. Initially, the nodules demonstrate a bright red color and are slightly elevated. Subsequently, a livid red or purplish color with flattening of lesions follows within several days. Finally, a bruise-like appearance ("erythema contusiformis") with yellow to greenish tone ensues. Ulceration is not seen in EN, and the nodules and plaques generally heal without atrophy or scarring, thus differentiating the process from erythema induratum. Bouts of EN are often associated with a fever of 38–39°C, fatigue, malaise, arthralgia and even arthritis of the ankle joints, headache, abdominal pain, vomiting, cough or diarrhea [35]. The eruption generally lasts from 3 to 6 weeks, and recurrences are the exception. Löfgren's syndrome is frequently seen as an early manifestation of sarcoidosis in northern Europe, particularly in Scandinavia [36]. This presentation, however, is not entirely specific for sarcoidosis, as infectious etiologies such as tuberculosis, coccidioidomycosis, histoplasmosis and others, as well as various drug exposures and malignancies (particularly lymphomas) should be considered [35, 37, 38].

Other nonspecific manifestations of sarcoidosis include erythema multiforme, erythroderma, pruritus, calcinosis cutis, nail clubbing, prurigo, and leonine facies [1, 4, 29].

Treatment

Cutaneous involvement in sarcoidosis is typically asymptomatic and not life-threatening. The major indication for treatment of skin lesions is disfigurement, and therapy is guided by disease severity and progression. Corticosteroids, either in topical, intralesional or systemic forms, are the mainstay of therapy.

Limited cutaneous disease may respond to very high potency topical corticosteroids, topical steroids under occlusive dressing, or monthly intralesional triamcinolone (3–10 mg/ml/month). Additional therapeutic options include psoralen ultraviolet A (PUVA) and medium-dose ultraviolet (UV-A1) phototherapy [39]. PUVA has been reported successful in treatment of erythrodermic and hypopigmented sarcoid lesions, while pulsed-dye and CO_2 laser therapy may be more effective in patients with lupus pernio [40, 41]. Surgical excision with grafting, as well as the use of new skin substitutes, have been used in treatment of ulcerative sarcoidosis [42, 43].

Large or diffuse lesions, as well as those resistant to topical therapy, may require systemic treatment. Glucocorticoids are the agents of choice, the typical adult dose being 20–40 mg/d for 4–6 weeks, followed by a slow taper over several months. Cutaneous sarcoidosis may respond to relatively low doses of prednisone, including every-other-day regimens [29].

To avoid long-term steroid-induced morbidity in chronic disease, nonsteroidal immunosuppressive agents may also be administered. Antimalarials are commonly employed in less severe cases, but may take 3–6 months to demonstrate any effect. Hydroxychloroquine may be administered using a daily or alternate-day dose of 200–400 mg. Chloroquine is typically prescribed at 250 mg/d for long-term suppression, but Zic et al. [44] recommend an initial 14-day course of 500 mg/d. Methotrexate has been an effective agent in both chronic cutaneous and lung disease, the typical regimen consisting of 15–25 mg/wk in three divided doses at 12-h intervals. Baughman and Lower [45] found that 16 of 17 patients noted improvement in cutaneous lesions treated with methotrexate. Twelve patients were treated with minocycline at 200 mg/d for a median duration of 12 months, and a clinical response was observed in 10 patients, with complete resolution in 8 and partial responses in 2 patients [46]. Allopurinol has been effective at doses of 100–300 mg/d administered over a several month treatment course [47,48].

Other agents employed in the treatment of sarcoidosis, with potentially more severe side effects, include azathioprine, chlorambucil, cyclophosphamide, cyclosporine and isotretinoin. Infliximab, an anti-human TNF-α monoclonal antibody, has recently shown promising results in complicated cases [49], as have thalidomide and mycophenolate mofetil [45,50,51].

References

1. Samstov AV. Cutaneous sarcoidosis. Int. J. Dermatol. 1992; 31: 385–91.
2. Hanno R, Needelman A, Eiferman RA, Callen JP. Cutaneous sarcoidal granulomas and the development of systemic sarcoidosis. Arch. Dermatol. 1981; 117: 203–7.
3. Gould KP, Callen JP (October 22, 2003), Sarcoidosis, [Online], eMedicine, Available from http://www.emedicine.com/derm/topic381.htm [accessed March 6, 2004]
4. Sharma OP. Sarcoidosis of the skin. In Freedberg IM, Fitzpatrick TB, eds. Fitzpatrick's Dermatology in General Medicine, 5th ed. New York: McGraw-Hill, 1999, pp. 2099–106.
5. Chestnutt AN. Enigmas in sarcoidosis. West J. Med. 1995; 162: 519–26.
6. Hillerdal G, Nou E, Osterman K, Schmekel B. Sarcoidosis: epidemiology and prognosis. A 15-year European study. Am. Rev. Respir. Dis. 1984; 130: 29–32.
7. Newman LS, Rose CS, Maier LA. Sarcoidosis. N. Engl. J. Med. 1997; 336: 1224–34.
8. English JC, Patel PJ, Greer KE. Sarcoidosis. J. Am. Acad. Dermatol. 2001; 44: 725–43.
9. Henke CE, Henke G, Elveback LR, et al. The epidemiology of sarcoidosis in Rochester, Minnesota: a population-based study of incidence and survival. Am. J. Epidemiol. 1986; 123: 840–5.
10. Stadnyk AN, Rubinstein I, Grossman RF, et al. Clinical features of sarcoidosis in elderly patients. Sarcoidosis 1988; 5: 121–3.
11. Longcope WT, Freiman DG. A study of sarcoidosis; based on a combined investigation of 160 cases including 30 autopsies from the Johns Hopkins Hospital and Massachusetts General Hospital. Medicine 1952; 31: 1–132.
12. Margolis ML, Israel HL. Sarcoidosis in older patients-clinical characteristics and course. Geriatrics 1983; 38: 121–8.
13. Shorr AF. (March 17, 2004), Sarcoidosis, [Online], eMedicine, Available from http://www.emedicine.com/med/topic2063.htm [accessed March 6, 2004]
14. Giuffrida TJ, Kerdel FA. Sarcoidosis. Dermatol. Clin. 2002; 20: 435–47.

15. Veien NK, Stahl D, Brodthagen H. Cutaneous sarcoidosis in caucasians. J. Am. Acad. Dermatol. 1987; 16: 534–40.
16. Elgart ML. Cutaneous lesions of sarcoidosis. Prim Care 1978; 5: 249–62.
17. Johns CJ, Scott PP, Schonfeld SA. Sarcoidosis. Annu. Rev. Med. 1989; 40: 353–371.
18. Siltzbach LE, James DG, Neville E, et al. Course and prognosis of sarcoidosis around the world. Am. J. Med. 1974; 57: 847–52.
19. Sina B, Goldner R, Burnett JW. Granulomatous panniculitis and Hodgkin's disease. Cutis 1984; 33: 403–4.
20. Howard A, White CR Jr. Non-infectious granulomas. In Bolognia J, Rapini R, J Jorrizzo, eds. Dermatology, 1st ed. CV Mosby, 2003, pp. 1455–69.
21. Weedon D. Skin Pathology, 2nd ed. New York: Churchill-Livingstone, 2002.
22. Mana J, Marcoval J, Graells J, et al. Cutaneous involvement in sarcoidosis. Relationship to systemic disease. Arch. Dermatol. 1997; 133: 882–8.
23. Young RJ, Gilson RT, Yanase D, Elston DM. Cutaneous sarcoidosis. Int. J. Dermatol. 2001; 40: 249–53.
24. Katta R. Cutaneous sarcoidosis: a dermatologic masquerader. Am. Fam. Phys. 2002; 65: 1581–4.
25. Kalb RE, Epstein W, Grossman ME. Sarcoidosis with subcutaneous nodules. Am. J. Med. 1988; 85: 731–36.
26. Takahashi H, Mori M, Muraoka S, et al. Sarcoidosis presenting as a scarring alopecia: report of a rare cutaneous manifestation of systemic sarcoidosis. Dermatology 1996; 193: 144–6.
27. Jorizzo JL, Koufman JA, Thompson JN, et al. Sarcoidosis of the upper respiratory tract in patients with nasal rim lesions: a pilot study. J. Am. Acad. Dermatol. 1990; 22: 439–43.
28. Zax RH, Callen JP. Granulomatous reactions. In Sams WM Jr, Lynch PJ, eds. Principles and Practices of Dermatology, 2nd ed. New York: Churchill Livingstone, 1996, pp. 629–39.
29. Russo G, Millikan LE. Cutaneous sarcoidosis: diagnosis and treatment. Compr. Ther. 1994; 20: 418–22.
30. Banse-Kupin L, Pelachyk JM. Ichthyosiform sarcoidosis. Report of two cases and a review of the literature. J. Am. Acad. Dermatol. 1987; 17: 616–20.
31. Cather JC, Cohen PR. Ichthyosiform sarcoidosis. J. Am. Acad. Dermatol. 1999; 40: 862–5.
32. Nathan MP, Pinsker R, Chase PH, Elguezabel A. Sarcoidosis presenting as lymphedema. Arch. Dermatol. 1974; 109: 543–4.
33. Tomoda F, Oda Y, Takata M, et al. A rare case of sarcoidosis with bilateral leg lymphedema as an initial symptom. Am. J. Med. Sci. 1999; 318: 413–14.
34. Burov EA, Kantor GR, Isaac M. Morpheaform sarcoidosis: report of three cases. J. Am. Acad. Dermatol. 1998; 39: 345–8.
35. Requena L, Requena C. Erythema nodosum. Dermatol. Online J. 2002; Jun;8(1): 4.
36. Löfgren S. Primary pulmonary sarcoidosis. I. Early signs and symptoms. Acta Med. Scand. 1953; 145: 424–31.
37. Marie I, Lecomte F, Levesque H, et al. Lofgren's syndrome as the first manifestation of acute infection due to chlamydia pneumoniae: a prospective study. Clin. Infect. Dis. 1999; 28: 691–2.
38. Löfgren S. Erythema nodosum studies on etiology and pathogenesis in 185 adult cases. Acta Med. Scand. 1946; 174: S1–197.
39. Mahnke N, Medve-Koenigs K, Megahed M, Neumann NJ. Medium-dose UV-A1 phototherapy. Successful treatment of cutaneous sarcoidosis. Hautarzt 2003; 54: 364–6.
40. Cliff S, Felix RH, Singh L, Harland CC. The successful treatment of lupus pernio with the flashlamp pulsed dye laser. J. Cutan. Laser Ther. 1999; 1: 49–52.
41. Young HS, Chalmers RJ, Griffiths CE, August PJ. CO_2 laser vaporization for disfiguring lupus pernio. J. Cosmet. Laser Ther. 2002; 4: 87–90.
42. Collison DW, Novice F, Banse L, Rodman OG, Kelly AP. Split-thickness skin grafting in extensive ulcerative sarcoidosis. J. Dermatol. Surg. Oncol. 1989; 15: 679–83.

43. Streit M, Bohlen LM, Braathen LR. Ulcerative sarcoidosis successfully treated with apligraf. Dermatology 2001; 202: 367–70.
44. Zic JA, Horowitz DH, Arzubiaga C, King LE Jr. Treatment of cutaneous sarcoidosis with chloroquine. Review of the literature. Arch Dermatol 1991; 127: 1034–40.
45. Baughman RP, Lower EE, du Bois RM. Sarcoidosis. Lancet 2003; 361: 1111–18.
46. Bachelez H, Senet P, Cadranel J, Kaoukhov A, Dubertret L. The use of tetracyclines for the treatment of sarcoidosis. Arch. Dermatol. 2001; 137: 69–73.
47. Baughman RP. Therapeutic options for sarcoidosis: new and old. Curr. Opin. Pulm. Med. 2002; 8: 464–9.
48. Brechtel B, Haas N, Henz BM, Kolde G. Allopurinol: a therapeutic alternative for disseminated cutaneous sarcoidosis. Br. J. Dermatol. 1996; 135: 307–9.
49. Serio RN. Infliximab treatment of sarcoidosis. Ann. Pharmacother. 2003; 37: 577–81.
50. Kouba DJ, Mimouni D, Rencic A, Nousari HC. Mycophenolate mofetil may serve as a steroid-sparing agent for sarcoidosis. Br. J. Dermatol. 2003;148: 147–8.
51. Baughman RP, Judson MA, Teirstein AS, Moller DR, Lower EE. Thalidomide for chronic sarcoidosis. Chest 2002; 122: 227–32.

Chapter 14

Inflammatory Scaling Dermatoses (Psoriasis)

Charles Camisa

Introduction

Psoriasis is the prototype for the inflammatory scaling dermatoses, also known as the *papulosquamous skin diseases*. The differential diagnosis includes seborrheic dermatitis, lichen planus, secondary syphilis, pityriasis rosea, drug eruption, tinea corporis, and cutaneous T-cell lymphoma. The experienced clinician can usually recognize the classic morphology of psoriasis, but appropriate diagnostic tests including skin biopsy may be necessary to confirm the diagnosis of less common variants of psoriasis and to rule out the other considerations.

Definition

Psoriasis is a common inflammatory scaling dermatosis with a bilateral symmetric distribution and may be associated with a seronegative spondyloarthropathy. It affects 1–3% of the world's population with no gender preference. Up to one-third of patients develop psoriatic arthritis (PSA). The mean age of onset of psoriasis is about 30 years with a possible range from newborn to 100 years. We have also observed in the clinic that the extent and severity of psoriasis increases with age. In the United States, primary care physicians initially see about 60% of the estimated 150,000 new cases of psoriasis each year, but dermatologists encounter 80% of the total 3 million office and hospital visits per year [1].

Pathophysiology

The pathogenesis of psoriasis is unknown, but more is known about the pathophysiology of psoriasis than perhaps of any other skin disease. The clinical expression or *lesion* of psoriasis is the result of inflammation in the dermis and vascular changes leading to hyperproliferation and abnormal differentiation of the epidermis. These changes are triggered by the proper combination of genes, environmental factors (e.g., trauma and climate), associated conditions (e.g., infections and emotional stress), and concomitant medications. Lithium, anti-malarials, beta-adrenergic blockers, calcium channel blockers, angiotensin-converting enzyme inhibitors, interferons, and ethanol have all been reported to induce or aggravate pre-existing psoriasis.

Signs and Symptoms

Plaque-type psoriasis

There are several clinical variants of psoriasis. The most common type by far is called "plaque-type" or psoriasis vulgaris found in 75–80% of patients. The typical morphology is a 1-cm or larger well-demarcated red round or oval plaque surmounted by white to silvery scales (Fig. 14.1). The lesions can occur anywhere, but the most commonly involved areas are the elbows, knees, scalp, sacrum, intergluteal cleft, and genitalia. The face is frequently spared. About 70% of patients complain

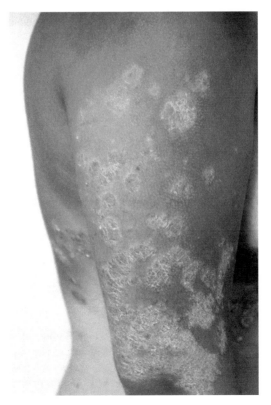

Fig. 14.1 Psoriasis vulgaris

of pruritus and skin pain or burning. Active psoriasis demonstrates the Koebner phenomenon or isomorphic response whereby normal skin injured by trauma or surgery develops psoriasis.

Guttate psoriasis

In guttate or eruptive psoriasis, 0.1–1.0 cm, red, droplet-shaped lesions appear predominantly on the trunk and proximal extremities. Guttate psoriasis may be the initial presentation of psoriasis or represent an acute flare of pre-existing plaque-type psoriasis. In either instance, there is frequently an antecedent history of an upper respiratory infection, pharyngitis, or tonsillitis, particularly due to Streptococcus. The guttate variant accounts for about 18% of all cases of psoriasis.

Pustular psoriasis

Pustular psoriasis accounts for about 2% of cases and may be localized to palms and soles, glabrous skin (annular), or become generalized (von Zumbusch type). The age of onset of pustular psoriasis is about 50 years.

Clinically, it is characterized by groups of tiny sterile pustules that develop on a background of bright red skin. They may coalesce into lakes of pus followed by desquamation. The pressure-bearing areas of palms and soles are most often affected, and lesions may be observed in all stages of evolution from clear vesicles, to yellow pustules, to dry reddish-brown macules. Palmoplantar pustular psoriasis is highly associated with cigarette smoking (nearly 100%) and extraordinarily recalcitrant to therapy. Patients with generalized pustular psoriasis (GPP) are acutely ill and may require admission to hospital. A recent review indicated that GPP in patients with preceding plaque-type disease was more likely to be triggered by systemic corticosteroid treatment, whereas those with no prior history of psoriasis were more likely preceded by infection.

Erythrodermic psoriasis

Psoriatic erythroderma is the least common form of psoriasis accounting for about 1% of cases. The mean age of onset is 50 years with a male predominance. It usually develops during the course of chronic plaque-type psoriasis in adults, but it may also be the first manifestation of psoriasis. In that case, the differential diagnosis includes drug eruption, seborrheic dermatitis, pityriasis rubra pilaris, and Sezary syndrome. Skin biopsies are essential but may not show specific changes at this stage. Precipitating factors include the inappropriate or excessive use of potent topical and systemic corticosteroids as well as systemic illnesses, emotional stress, and alcoholism.

Nail psoriasis

The nails are involved in up to 50% of patients with psoriasis. In patients with PSA, the prevalence is more than 80%, and may be a helpful clue to diagnosis. The most common manifestation is pitting of the nail plate.

Fingernails are affected more often than toenails. Other signs of nail psoriasis are yellow–brown spots in the nail bed (*oil droplet sign*), thickening of the nail plate, and separation of the distal nail from the nail bed (onycholysis) (Fig. 14.2). It is important to remember that all of these nail changes may closely mimic onychomycosis, especially in toenails, and that both conditions may coexist.

Psoriatic arthritis (PSA)

PSA is a destructive arthropathy and enthesopathy that affects up to one-third of patients with psoriasis. Arthritis occurs after the onset of skin disease in the majority of cases. PSA and rheumatoid arthritis (RA) have some clinical features in common. Most patients with PSA have asymmetric oligoarticular arthritis, followed in frequency by symmetric arthritis and spondyloarthritis. Radiographic changes in the sacroiliac joints and cervical spine help to differentiate PSA from RA. The severity of skin involvement does not correlate with severity of PSA, however, distal interphalangeal joint involvement is likely to be associated with dystrophy of the

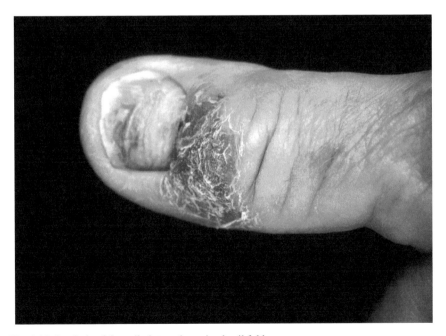

Fig. 14.2 Psoriasis of the nail plate and proximal nail fold

adjacent nail. Although many of the systemic agents used to manage psoriasis are also effective for PSA, the specific treatment of PSA is beyond the scope of this chapter.

Treatment

There are many effective treatments for psoriasis. These are traditionally organized into a "level" or "step ladder" approach according to the severity of the skin disease as judged by inflammation, thickness, scaling, and estimated body surface area (BSA) involvement, symptoms, and quality of life parameters.

With the exception of palmoplantar pustular psoriasis many patients with mild to moderate disease (< 10% BSA) can be managed with a combination of topical therapy, natural sunlight, or tanning booth. Because this approach is less effective for patients with moderate to severe disease, these patients should consult a dermatologist.

Bland emollients or lubricants should be tried on mild cases first, followed by keratolytic creams or gels. Non-responders are treated with a medium to high-potency corticosteroid combined with either calcipotriene or tazarotene. The efficacy of the latter two agents is enhanced by the addition of the corticosteroid, and their inherent irritation potential is mitigated (Table 14.1).

Natural sunlight and tanning beds are mildly therapeutic and may be combined with the topical therapies listed in Level 1. Coal tar products combined with the UVA in a tanning bed or sunlight may cause stinging or a smarting sensation of the skin. Phototherapy with UVB or PUVA is very effective and can markedly improve the majority of cases (Table 14.2). However, maintenance is usually necessary to prevent flaring. The disadvantages are that the treatment requires special equipment

Table 14.1 Level 1: Topical Therapy

Emollients: Eucerin$^{®}$ cream, Aquaphor$^{®}$ ointment, Vaseline$^{®}$
Keratolytics: salicylic acid, lactic acid, urea
Coal tar: gel, oil, and ointment
Corticosteroids: fluocinolone 0.025%, fluocinonide 0.05%, bethamethasone 0.1%, triamcinolone 0.1%.
Calcipotriene
Tazarotene 0.05, 0.1%

Table 14.2 Level 2: Phototherapy

Natural sunlight
Tanning booth (UVA 320–400 nm)
Ultraviolet-B (broad-band 290–320 nm)
Ultraviolet-B (narrow-band 311 nm)
Excimer laser (308 nm)
Psoralen and ultraviolet A (PUVA)

Table 14.3 Level 3: FDA-approved oral systemic therapy

Acitretin: Teratogenic, increases lipids, rarely hepatotoxic; works best in combination with UVB or PUVA

Methotrexate: Myelosuppressive, causes liver fibrosis, and rarely pneumonitis. Antimetabolite most prescribed by dermatologists; dose weekly with daily folic acid supplement.
Monitor blood counts and liver functions; perform serial liver biopsies.

Cyclosporine: Nephrotoxic, causes hypertension; many drug interactions. Dose intermittently for 12 weeks to reduce toxicity. Monitor creatinine and blood pressure

Table 14.4 Level 4: Non-FDA-approved oral systemic therapy

Hydroxyurea
Calcitriol
Mycophenolate mofetil
6-Thioguanine

Table 14.5 Level 5: Non-FDA-approved oral systemic therapy that also helps PSA

Sulfasalazine
Azathioprine
Tacrolimus
Leuflonamide

Table 14.6 Level 6: Biologic Immunomodulators

Alefacept
Efalizumab
Etanercept *t*
Infliximab *t*
Adalimumab *t*

t, Tumor necrosis factor inhibitor

and safety training, and there are potential risks of causing burning and skin cancer. Levels 3–6 treatments would likely be used in collaboration with a specialist (Tables 14.3,14.4,14.5,14.6).

The Level 6 biologic immunomodulators represent the new paradigm of treatment of moderate to severe psoriasis in the twenty first century. These drugs are monoclonal antibodies, ligand receptors, or fusion proteins that are designed to antagonize cell–cell communication, memory-effector T-cell function, and the action of proinflammatory cytokines. They are all administered by the parenteral route. The tumor necrosis factor inhibitors are also expected to be highly active in PSA as disease modifying anti-rheumatic drugs.

Seborrheic Dermatitis

Definition

Seborrheic dermatitis is a common inflammatory scaling dermatosis that occurs in a distribution corresponding to a high concentration of sebaceous glands, namely the scalp, face, and trunk. The two peak incidences are in infants and adult life. Seborrheic dermatitis has been observed in association with AIDS, Parkinson's disease, stroke victims, and other chronic neurological conditions. *Dandruff* is a non-inflammatory scaling condition of the scalp that is considered to be a mild manifestation of seborrheic dermatitis.

Pathophysiology

The cause of seborrheic dermatitis is multifactorial [2]: sebum, climatic conditions, emotional or physical stressors, and the presence of *Pityrosporum ovale*, a lipophilic yeast which normally inhabits skin.

Signs and Symptoms

In babies, whose sebaceous glands are stimulated by maternal androgens, seborrheic dermatitis manifests as yellow greasy adherent scale on the scalp called "cradle cap" or in the diaper area.

In adults, the typical lesions are yellow–red papules, and patches with greasy scale in the following characteristic locations: scalp, eyebrows, eyelid margins, nasolabial folds (Fig. 14.3), the moustache, beard and sideburn areas (if there is hair there), behind the ears, and the mid-chest area. The differential diagnosis includes psoriasis, and it is helpful to compare the clinical morphologies. Psoriasis tends to be well demarcated with dry white–silvery scales, whereas seborrheic dermatitis is more diffuse with yellow greasy scales and sometimes exudation. At times it is impossible to separate the two entities on clinical growths, and it is appropriate to use the term "sebo-psoriasis".

Seborrheic dermatitis may also affect the groin, axillae, and submammary area and cause an intertriginous dermatitis to be differentiated from inverse psoriasis and candidiasis.

Treatment

Dandruff or mild seborrheic dermatitis is usually well controlled with regular use (2–3 times weekly) of therapeutic shampoos containing selenium sulfide (1, 2.5%), zinc pyrithione, coal tar, ketoconazole (1, 2%), or ciclopirox. Inflammatory scalp conditions with pruritus may require the addition of a medium potency topical cor-

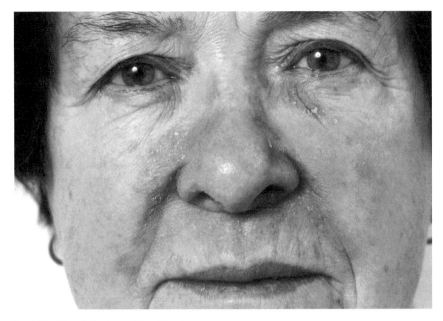

Fig. 14.3 Seborrheic dermatitis of the face

ticosteroid in an oil or hydroalcoholic vehicle, e.g. fluocinolone 0.01%, betamethasone valerate 0.1%, fluocinonide 0.05%, applied at bedtime.

Facial dermatitis and intertriginous dermatitis usually responds well to either the topical anti-yeast medicines ketoconazole cream 2% or ciclopirox gel 0.77% or the non-fluorinated topical corticosteroids such as hydrocortisone (1%, 2.5%) and desonide 0.05%. Once daily, applications of the anti-yeast and the anti-inflammatory creams may be necessary for slow responders. In the past few years, there has been a proliferation of creams, gels, and cleansers containing sodium sulfacetamide 10% and sulfur 5% as adjunctive therapy for seborrheic dermatitis.

For the most severe or recalcitrant cases of seborrheic dermatitis, a 1-week course of itraconazole 400 mg daily or fluconazole 200 mg daily, may "jump-start" therapy by temporarily eradicating the population of *P. ovale* in the skin.

Patients should understand that seborrheic dermatitis is a chronic relapsing condition and is not curable. They should treat the skin disease intermittently for a few weeks until it clears and re-treat as necessary. Regular scalp maintenance may help to prevent facial outbreaks.

Lichen Planus

Definition

Lichen planus (LP) is a common inflammatory scaling disorder that affects about 1% of the world's population [3]. LP is a disease of middle age with an average

age of onset of about 50. Childhood LP is unusual but may occur in a familial setting. The distribution of LP skin lesions is characteristic: flexor surfaces of the wrists, ankles, lumbrosacral spine, genitalia, and neck. Although not unique in this regard, LP is remarkable because it has a tendency to involve the entire integument producing specific clinical and histologic lesions of skin, mucous membranes, hair follicles, and the nail apparatus.

Pathophysiology

The etiology of lichen planus is unknown, but it is believed to result from a cell-mediated immune response directed against the basal cell layer of epithelium [4]. Histologically, a dense band-like infiltrate of lymphocytes is distributed along the basement membrane zone.

Lichen planus-like rashes may occur as hypersensitivity reactions to many different drugs prescribed for hypertension, diabetes, and arthritis. The association of LP with hepatitis C virus infection is controversial.

Signs and Symptoms

The typical skin lesion of LP is a violaceous, flat-topped, angulated, papule that is usually quite pruritic (Fig. 14.4). Notwithstanding, excoriations of LP are usually not seen. It may show fine white striae on the surface of a papule or plaque.

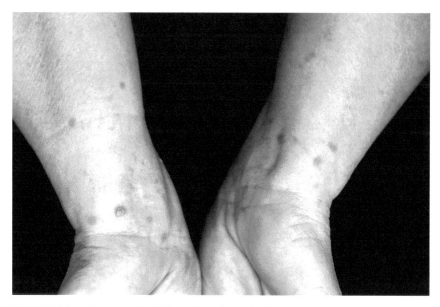

Fig. 14.4 Lichen planus papules of the volar surfaces of wrists

The Koebner phenomenon occurs in LP as it does in psoriasis. The differential diagnosis includes psoriasis, pityriasis rosea, drug reaction, and secondary syphilis.

Thick hypertrophic lesions of LP on the shins may resemble chronic eczematous dermatitis, prurigo nodularis, lupus erythematosus, and keratoacanthomas.

Therefore, a skin biopsy is usually necessary to confirm the diagnosis. LP of the skin is usually self-limited and resolves on average within 2 years of onset, leaving dark brown post-inflammatory hyperpigmentation in its wake.

Oral LP, on the other hand, is much less likely to remit. Lesions may appear as a network of asymptomatic white lines or painful red erosions (Fig. 14.5). Oral LP has been associated with candidiasis, hypersensitivity reactions to silver amalgam fillings, and rarely, oral squamous cell carcinoma.

Treatment

Topical and systemic corticosteroids are the mainstay of therapy, particularly for pruritic disease. Examples of the former are fluocinonide 0.05% and clobetasol 0.05% ointments applied twice daily for 4 weeks with at least 1 week off to avoid cutaneous atrophy. Oral anti-histamines and emollients containing anti-pruritics such as menthol, camphor, and pramoxine may be used adjunctively. For resistant or generalized LP, a burst of prednisone 60 mg daily tapered over a 4-week period or an intramuscular injection of a long-acting corticosteroid such as Kenalog® or triamcinolone acetonide suspension 80 mg induces remission. Relapses of LP

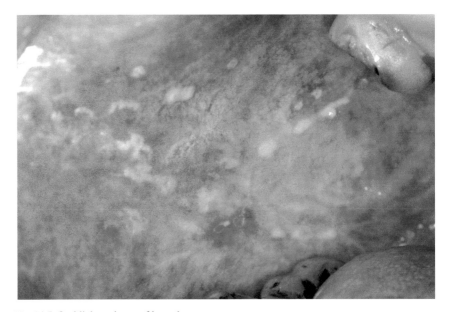

Fig. 14.5 Oral lichen planus of buccal mucosa

are common. Numerous other oral medications have been used empirically by dermatologists for LP with variable results: azathioprine, cyclosporine, cyclophosphamide, dapsone, griseofulvin, hydroxychloroquine, levamisole, photochemotherapy, retinoids, and thalidomide. Topical tacrolimus 0.1% ointment applied twice daily has shown modest improvement of oral but not cutaneous LP. The follow-up of oral LP requires cancer surveillance and removal of additional risk factors such as tobacco and alcohol habits.

Eczema (Dermatitis)

Definition

Superficial inflammation of the skin, referred to as eczema or dermatitis, is the most common reaction pattern seen by dermatologists. The morphology and the histopathology are virtually identical for all of the forms of eczema [2] described below, but the causes may differ.

The clinical changes range from acute, to subacute to chronic. In the acute stage the skin is red, edematous, vesicular and possibly weeping. Subacute lesions are usually not exudative but show some crusting and scaling on the surface (Fig. 14.6). Chronic rubbing and scratching leads to lichenification (accentuation of normal skin folds), thickening of the skin, and alterations in pigmentation. Chronic eczema may be plaque-like (lichen simplex chronicus) or nodular (prurigo nodularis).

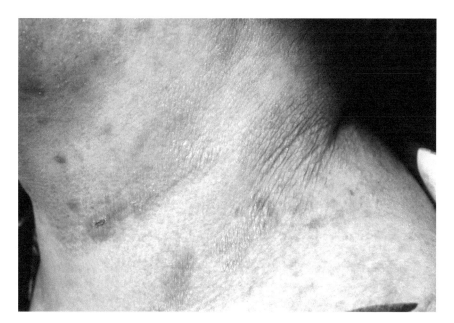

Fig. 14.6 Subacute eczema on side of the neck

Histopathology of all forms of eczema shows edema between epidermal cells called *spongiosis* and collections of lymphocytes and eosinophils surrounding superficial dermal capillaries to varying degrees. Pruritus is the *sine qua non* of eczema; all forms of eczema are more or less itchy. Unlike psoriasis and lichen planus, scratching makes the itch of eczema feel better temporarily and fits of uncontrolled excoriations may lead to bleeding and secondary bacterial infections. In the following sections, the most common clinical forms of eczema will be covered separately: atopic, contact, nummular, stasis, dyshidrosis, photodermatitis. Treatment, which is similar for all, will be covered in the final section.

Atopic Dermatitis

Atopic dermatitis (AD) runs in families: about 70% of patients have a family history of atopy which includes dermatitis, rhinitis, and asthma. Patients have an exaggerated response to heat, cold and low humidity, and altered vascular response to pressure and injections of histamine and cholinergic and sympathomimetic agents. Intermittent exacerbations of AD occur during their lifetime in 30–80% of patients when under physical or emotional stress [2]. About one-third of relapses are secondary to bacterial infection. Eyelid, retroauricular and, hand dermatitis are the most common residuals in adult-life. Several immunologic abnormalities are associated with AD: elevated serum IgE in 80% of patients, eosinophilia during exacerbations, and reduced cell-mediated immune response which leads in turn to a higher prevalence of warts, herpes simplex, and molluscum contagiosum. Dermatitic skin is colonized by *S.aureus,* and patients may become sensitized to the bacterial antigens. The following associated features are more prominent in children but may be seen in adults: ichthyosis vulgaris manifesting as extremely dry skin of arms and legs and hyperlinear palms, Dennie–Morgan lines (extra infraorbital skin folds), and keratosis pilaris.

Contact Dermatitis

Contact dermatitis is the result of environmental exposure of skin to a chemical or chemicals that are either irritants or allergens. *Irritant contact dermatitis* accounts for about 80% of cases. The irritant may be simply repeated hand-washing with soap and warm water. Occupations with higher risk of irritant hand dermatitis are food service, health care, child care, and hair styling. Other irritants besides detergents include organic solvents, oils, acids or alkaline chemicals, oxidants, fiberglass, and wood dust. The hands, dorsal and palmar surfaces, are most often affected.

Atopic individuals are predisposed to irritant contact dermatitis and may be forced to avoid or change certain activities or occupations. *Allergic contact dermatitis* is a delayed type hypersensitivity reaction to a chemical, usually a small molecule. Poison ivy or oak dermatitis is the most familiar paradigm of the mechanism of ACD. After the first exposure to the skin of *Toxicodendron* resin or oleoresin, it takes 2–3 weeks for the immune system to become *sensitized*. When the next exposure to the allergen occurs, it takes 12–48 hours to *elicit* a reaction in the skin depending on the amount of allergen exposure and the sensitivity of the individual. Besides poison ivy there are many common allergens in everyday use at home and in occupations that can cause sensitization and ACD, for example, fragrances, preservatives, hair dye, rubber, leather additives, nickel, formaldehyde and over-the-counter topical medicaments such as neomycin, bacitracin, hydrocortisone, and benzocaine. Owing to their increase in use, allergy to natural rubber latex in gloves has become an occupational hazard for doctors, dentists, and their assistants. About 10% of health care workers are sensitized and 1–2% are symptomatic [5]. Patients who require frequent bladder catheterization, are also at high risk for sensitization to latex.

Natural rubber latex protein may cause immediate IgE-mediated hypersensitivity reactions that may range in severity from contact urticaria to anaphylaxis.

In ACD, the dorsal surfaces of the hands and forearms and the face are most commonly affected. Plant dermatitis is distinctly linear in distribution (Fig. 14.7). The dermatitis may be localized to the anatomic site where the chemicals is repeatedly applied, for example, ears/nickel in earrings; tops of feet/leather or rubber shoes; incisional wound/neomycin in antibiotic ointment; eyelids/preservative in cosmetic. About half of eyelid dermatitis is due to ACD, and one quarter is AD.

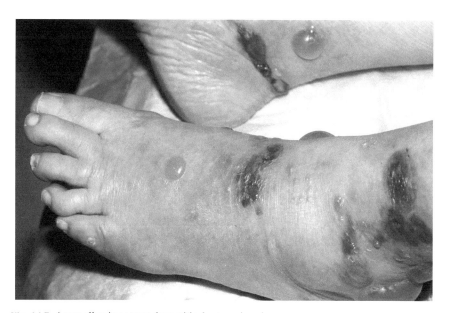

Fig. 14.7 Acute allergic contact dermatitis due to poison ivy

Nummular Dermatitis

Nummular dermatitis is a form of eczema of unknown cause, which begins on the legs or trunk of adults. The primary lesions are 1–5 cm in diameter, coin-shaped with a tendency to central clearing [6]. They are red and scaly, and sometimes vesicular and crusted. They are always exquisitely pruritic and may become impetiginized from scratching. Occasionally, there is a history of atopy or an antecedent emotional stressor. The eruption may become generalized. When there are few lesions, the differential diagnosis of tinea corporis, psoriasis, and Bowen's disease (squamous cell carcinoma *in situ*) must be considered. Nummular dermatitis has a well-deserved reputation as being "treatment-resistant". It tends to be chronic and reoccur in the same locations.

Stasis Dermatitis

Stasis dermatitis is a form of eczema that develops on the lower legs and ankles of adults who have a history of varicose veins, trauma or surgery to the leg, or one or more episodes of thrombophlebitis. The condition may begin as excessive dryness of the skin, followed by a pattern of superficial fissures, called eczema craquele. Subacute dermatitis develops with dependent edema of the ankles. When the condition is chronic, post-inflammatory hyperpigmentation develops, and there is risk of ulcer formation after mild trauma to the malleoli (Fig. 14.8). The dermatitis is itchy,

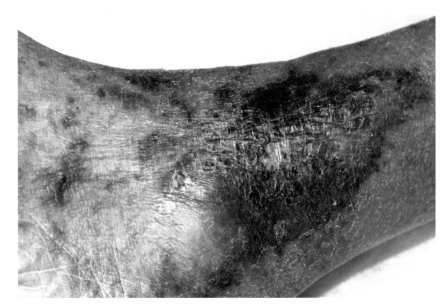

Fig. 14.8 Chronic venous stasis dermatitis of the ankle with post-inflammatory hyperpigmentation

but if the patient complains of pain, bacterial cellulitis and deep vein thrombosis must be ruled out. Eczema is also commonly seen around scars where vein grafts were harvested on the legs.

Dyshidrosis

Dyshidrotic eczema is also known as pompholyx. It may be associated with hyper-hidrosis of the palms and soles, but the sweat glands function normally. About 50% of patients have a history of atopy. The eruption is distinctive: 0.1–0.5 cm superficial clear vesicles resembling tapioca appear on the sides of the fingers, palms and soles. The lesions are usually, but not always, pruritic. Superficial desquamation follows the resolution of the blisters. The differential diagnosis includes allergic contact dermatitis, localized pustular psoriasis, and inflammatory dermatophyte infection.

Diagnosis

The diagnosis of eczema is usually made on clinical grounds based on morphology and distribution. In rare instances a skin biopsy of a nummular lesion or a vesico-pustule on the palm or sole may be needed to rule out Bowen's disease or psoriasis. Potassium hydroxide preparations in search of fungal hyphae should be examined on scaly lesions and blister fluid, particularly if they do not respond to topical corticosteroids or get worse. Culture and sensitivity for bacteria may be performed on exudates and pus. In cases where ACD is suspected, except for plant dermatitis, allergy patch testing should be performed. A standard allergen screening patch test battery is commercially available (TRUE Test®). The tray consists of 23 allergen patches and one negative control which contain 42 unique allergens and 4 complex mixtures. Collectively, the TRUE test allergens identify 28% of clinically relevant allergens in patients with documented ACD [7]. A negative TRUE test, however, does not rule out ACD. Thus, many patients require testing to an expanded panel of allergens to include unusual chemicals specifically identified from their occupations, hobbies, and medicaments. The diagnosis of latex allergies is based on positive radioallergosorbent test (RAST) and/or skin prick test.

Treatment

There are several basic tenets of therapy that may be applied to all forms of eczema based on the stage of evolution. There are caveats for the specific types of eczema.

General

Acute weeping eczema is treated with astringent and antiseptic compresses such as Burow's (aluminum acetate 1:40) for 20 min 2–3 times daily until exudation stops, followed by application of medium to high potency corticosteroid cream twice daily.

After 2 weeks, a weaker steroid or a bland emollient such as Cetaphil®, Eucerin®, or Aquaphor® may be applied.

For chronically relapsing eczema, a program of 2 week cycles of topical steroid followed by 1 week off theoretically prevents skin atrophy and tachyphylaxis.

Pruritus

Anti-histamines of the H1-blocking sedating type may be helpful in the early stages, e.g. diphenhydramine, hydroxyzine, and doxepin.

Secondary infection

If localized superficial infection (impetigo) is suspected, it is usually caused by Gram-positive organisms. Topical mupirocin three times daily is recommended.

Avoid neomycin in Neosporin® because it can sensitize inflamed skin. If superficially infected eczema becomes generalized, or there is clinical evidence of soft tissue cellulitis, then a full course of oral antibiotics with good anti-staphylococcal coverage is prescribed, e.g. dicloxacillin, cephalexin, clindamycin, or ciprofloxacin.

Caveats

Atopic Dermatitis

While topical steroids and occasional bursts of systemic steroids (e.g. Medrol® dose pack, Kenalog® 40 mg IM injection) have historically been the mainstay, some cases are well-maintained on the newer topical immunomodulators such as pimecrolimus 1% (Elidel®) cream or tacrolimus 0.1% (Protopic®) ointment. Both are safe for the face and intertriginous areas. Severe, generalized or recalcitrant cases should be referred to a dermatologist where modalities such as ultraviolet light (UVB or PUVA) or immunosuppressive therapy, for example, azathioprine or cyclosporine, may be utilized. Measures taken to reduce contact with house dust mites, such as impermeable mattress dust covers, may improve the dermatitis.

Contact Dermatitis

Acute allergic contact dermatitis often requires a course of systemic corticosteroids. For poison ivy dermatitis, administer a 4-week course of prednisone tapering from 60 mg daily or I.M. Kenalog® 60 mg. Remove or reduce direct contact with the irritating or allergenic substances. If possible, have the patient reduce hand washing, or use waterless cleanser or milder bar or liquid soaps such as Cetaphil®, Purpose®, and Oil of Olay®. Moisturize frequently with Vanicream®

or Theraseal®. Wear white cotton liner gloves under latex or plastic gloves for food handling, dishwashing, and other wet work.

Nummular Dermatitis

Treat for secondary infection on an empiric basis. Use high potency corticosteroid ointment, for example, clobetasol 0.05% or halobetasol 0.05%, twice daily for 4 weeks before switching to lower strength corticosteroids and emollients. If the response is poor, treat with systemic steroids as for acute allergic contact dermatitis (above).

Stasis Dermatitis

Treat with medium potency ointment such as triamcinolone acetonide 0.1% twice daily for 4 weeks. Replace with 1 or 2.5% hydrocortisone ointment. Support or compression stockings (10–30 mm Hg based on severity) improve ankle swelling and dermatitis when worn during the day.

Dyshidrosis

Combine potent topical steroid once daily with pimecrolimus or tacrolimus once daily. It may require bursts of systemic steroid to break the cycle of blistering. Patients who have a positive patch to nickel may respond to a reduced nickel diet or a course of disulfiram (Antabuse, 200 mg daily for 8 weeks). For recalcitrant cases, consult a dermatologist for possible bath PUVA treatment of the hands and feet.

Photodermatitis

Simply stated, photodermatitis refers to a skin eruption occurring as a reaction to a chemical or drug, either ingested or applied to skin followed by exposure to light, usually long-wave ultraviolet (UVA) or visible light [8]. The reaction may be either *phototoxic* or *photoallergic.*

By definition, toxic or irritant reactions are related to concentration of the chemical and can occur in everyone, whereas allergic reactions are not concentration-dependent and are much less common.

Moreover, the individual must first be sensitized in order for an allergic reaction to develop upon subsequent exposures. Clinically, phototoxic dermatitis first appears erythematous and edematous or vesicular, and develops hyperpigmentation upon resolution. Photoallergic dermatitis is eczematous.

Examples of systemic drugs that cause photosensitivity are amiodarone, furosemide, phenothiazines, sulfonamides, and thiazides.

Photoirritant contact dermatitis is most commonly caused by synthetic or naturally occurring furocoumarins in the form of psoralens used therapeutically by dermatologists or from the juice of lime, lemon, bergamot, fig, parsnip, and celery.

Photoallergic contact dermatitis can be caused by PABA and benzophenone in sunscreens, musk ambrette in colognes, and anti-bacterial agents in soaps. The only way to confirm the diagnosis of photoallergic contact dermatitis is by photo-patch testing. Referral to a dermatologist experienced with this technique is necessary.

Another conundrum to consider is whether a patient has airborne contact dermatitis or photoallergic contact dermatitis. The distribution on the face, arms, and hands is similar for both, however, more submental, upper eyelid, and post-auricular sparing may be noted in photoallergic dermatitis. Airborne contact dermatitis may be irritant (e.g, fiberglass, sawdust) or allergic (e.g. smoke from burning poison ivy or ragweed).

References

1. Camisa C, ed. Handbook of Psoriasis, 2nd ed. Oxford: Blackwell Publishing, 2004.
2. Arndt KA, Bowers KE. Manual of Dermatologic Therapeutics, 6th ed. Philadelphia: Lippincott Williams and Wilkins, 2002.
3. Boyd AS, Neldner KH. Lichen Planus. J. Am. Acad. Dermatol. 1991; 25: 593–619.
4. Camisa C, Rindler JM. Diseases of the oral mucous membranes. Curr. Probl. Dermatol. 1996; 8: 45–96.
5. Taylor JS, Erkek E. Latex allergy: diagnosis and management. Dermatol. Ther. 2004; 17: 289–301.
6. Habif TP, Campbell JL, Quitadamo MJ, Zug KA. Skin Disease Diagnosis and Treatment. St. Louis: Mosby, 2001.
7. Belsito DV. Patch testing with a standard allergen ("screening") tray: rewards and risks. Dermatol. Ther. 2004; 17: 231–39.
8. Deleo VA. Photocontact Dermatitis. Dermatol. Ther. 2004; 17: 279–88.

Chapter 15

The Cutaneous Manifestations
of Nutritional Deficiencies

Robert R. Haight and Robert A. Norman

This article reviews the cutaneous manifestations of nutritional deficiencies. There have been reports of malnutrition states presenting with dermatologic problems [1]. Nutritional deficiencies may result from a number of conditions that effect intake, absorption, or metabolism of the nutrient. While the findings will be discussed as they apply to the individual nutrients, it is important to remember that multiple vitamin deficiencies are more common than isolated vitamin deficiencies [2].

Importance of Recognizing Nutritional Deficiencies in the Elderly

Nutritional deficiencies are very common in the elderly. This is probably because elderly are both less likely to have an adequate intake of nutrients and they are more likely to have many of the conditions that interfere with their absorption and metabolism. An estimated 55% of the hospitalized elderly and 85% of the institutionalized elderly are undernourished. It is also estimated that 50% of the elderly do not receive the RDA of vitamins and minerals [3]. In a 1979 study, the elderly were found to have diets deficient in vitamin B6, niacin, vitamin B12, folate, thiamine, and vitamin C [4].

Vitamin C Deficiency

Vitamin C is also known as ascorbic acid. Humans cannot make vitamin C so they must get it from their diets. In the United States, it is restricted to specific populations: the urban poor, alcoholics, the elderly, and patients with chronic diseases [3]. The requirement for vitamin C is increased in smokers and patients taking aspirin, sulfinpyrozone, indomethacin, phenylbutazone, tetracycline, oral contraceptives, corticosteroids, and chlorcyclizine [5]. Scurvy is the classic disease of vitamin C deficiency. The symptoms of scurvy typically appear after 30–90 days of inadequate intake [6, 7]. Vitamin C is necessary for proper collagen formation, iron metabolism, and tyrosine synthesis [2]. It is necessary for hair growth and stability [2]. Vitamin C activates propyl and lysyl hydroxylase for the hydroxylation

R.A. Norman (ed.), *Diagnosis of Aging Skin Diseases,*
© Springer-Verlag London Limited 2008

of procollagen. Without vitamin C, there is little hydroxylation of proline residues, intracellular procollagen increases, and few triple helical structures are secreted [7]. The result of deficiency is vessel walls that are pliable and rupture easily.

The cutaneous manifestations of vitamin C deficiency include: perifollicular hemorrhages, petechiae, gingival bleeding, splinter hemorrhages, and impaired wound healing. There is follicular keratosis with coiled hairs on the upper arms, back, buttocks, and lower extremities earlier [8]. The petechiae, perifollicular hemorrhage, ecchymoses, and gingival hypertrophy occur later [8]. The hyperkeratosis and perifollicular hemorrhages are typically on the posterior thighs, anterior forearms, and abdomen [5]. This may resemble keratosis pilaris [5]. Petechiae then spreads to the other hair-bearing parts of the body [2]. Ecchymoses develop in areas of trauma or irritation [2]. There is malaise, fatigue, weight loss, depression, epistaxis, diarrhea, and weakness [3,7]. Hemathrosis, periosteal hemorrhages, peripheral edema, mental depression, and a normochromic normocytic anemia may occur [3,6,9]. The subperiosteal hemorrhages may produce painful shin nodules [5]. Anemia does not occur in experimental vitamin C deficiency [2]. A megaloblastic anemia seen in scurvy may be due to an altered folate metabolism [7]. Sjögren's syndrome, xerostomia, keratoconjunctivitis sicca, and enlargement of the submandibular or parotid glands are sometimes seen [6]. Biopsy of the dermis shows perivascular edema, blood vessels with endothelial cells protruding into the lumina, and red blood cell extravasation [7]. The laboratory diagnosis is based on the level of ascorbic acid in the plasma or leukocytes [10]. Scurvy improves in less than 1 week with 300–1000 mg of vitamin C per day [10].

Thiamine Deficiency

Thiamine is also known as vitamin B_1. It is a coenzyme in many cellular metabolic processes including the pentose phosphate shunt and is required for the metabolism of branched-chain amino acids and carbohydrates, collagen repair, and fatty acid synthesis [5,10]. Alcoholism is the major risk for thiamin deficiency [2]. The majority of the cases of thiamine deficiency in the western world occur in alcoholics or patients with chronic diseases [2]. Pure thiamine deficiency is very rare [4]. It is often associated with a deficiency of niacin and riboflavin [9]. Thiaminase, an enzyme found in raw fish, or malabsorption may also be responsible [2].

Early thiamine deficiency produces anorexia, irritability, apathy, and generalized weakness. Chronic thiamine deficiency produces beriberi, which may present with cardiovascular or peripheral neuropathy symptoms. In alcoholics, chronic thiamine deficiency produces Wernicke–Korsakoff syndrome. Strachan's syndrome has an orogenital dermatitis, a sensorial neuritis, and amblyopia [2]. Skin findings are not a major manifestation of thiamine deficiency [6] and the cutaneous findings of thiamine deficiency are the least distinctive of the B vitamins [4, 5]. An increase in seborrheic dermatitis-like lesions may be associated with beriberi [6]. There is an association with non-specific buccal mucosal vesicles that resemble those of early herpes simplex or aphthous stomatitis [5]. The diagnosis can be made by a functional enzymatic assay of transketolase activity before and after thiamine pyrophosphate administration [10].

Riboflavin Deficiency

Riboflavin is also known as vitamin B_2. Riboflavin is part of the coenzymes, FMN and FAD, which are involved in a number of oxidation–reduction reactions. It is important for the metabolism of carbohydrates, fats, and proteins [10]. Riboflavin is involved in the synthesis of vitamin B_6 [5]. Riboflavin deficiency is almost always due to a dietary deficiency and often occurs along with a deficiency of other water-soluble vitamins [10]. It also occurs in alcoholism and hepatic cirrhosis [6]. Borate poisoning results in an acute deficiency of vitamin B_2 [6].

The primary manifestations of riboflavin (B2) deficiency are mucocutaneous lesions [2]. These include oral lesions—angular stomatitis (pelèche), cheilosis, atrophic glossitis with a magenta tongue, and pharyngitis—and skin—seborrhea and genital dermatitis [9, 10]. The facial lesions resemble seborrheic dermatitis around the eyes, ears, and nose [2]. Facial creases and wrinkles around the eyes and nose are often involved in the dermatitis in the elderly [5]. The scrotum and vulva may be hyperpigmented [2]. The skin findings are similar to those seen in niacin deficiency, B_6 deficiency, essential fatty acid deficiency, or zinc deficiency [6, 7]. There may also be conjunctivitis [9] or corneal vascularization [5]. The laboratory diagnosis is made by the measurement of red cell or urinary riboflavin levels or erythrocyte glutathione activity with and without the addition of FAD [10].

Niacin Deficiency

Niacin is also known as vitamin B_3. Two thirds of the niacin is produced from tryptophan in a reaction requiring B_1, B_2, and B_6. Since vitamins B_1, B_2, and B_6 are involved in NAD production, a deficiency of these vitamins may also cause pellagra [6]. The other third comes from the diet [2]. Pellagra may be due to the deficiency of B vitamins (classically niacin) or tryptophan. Niacin is part of the coenzymes NAD and NADP. These compounds are necessary for numerous reactions at the cellular level [6]. Niacin deficiency is one of the most common vitamin deficiencies in the elderly [5]. In North America, niacin deficiency is most often seen in patients with alcoholism or chronic disease. Chronic diarrhea, a diet grossly lacking in protein, anorexia nervosa, or a diet heavily based on corn may also produce a deficiency of niacin. Niacin in corn is bound so washing it in lime-water releases it [7]. Drugs that affect tryptophan or NAD metabolism such as isoniazid, dopa, pyrazinamide, 6-mercaptopurine, 5-fluorouracil, hydantoin, ethionamide, prothionamid, phenobarbital, azathioprine, and chloramphenicol may cause a niacin deficiency picture [6]. Hartnup disease, a congenital defect in tryptophan absorption [2], and carcinoid syndrome which effects tryptophan metabolism [5, 9] may produce a pellagra picture.

Pellagra has a classic triad of dermatitis, dementia, and diarrhea. Pellagra may present with only cutaneous signs [5]. The cutaneous manifestations of pellagra may be divided into four basic categories: a dermatitis in sun-exposed areas, a perianal and genital dermatitis, lichinification and hyperpigmentation on osseous prominences, and a seborrheic eczema-like dermatitis [6]. The skin has been described as smooth and edematous [9]. Early manifestations of pellagra include: anorexia, weakness, irritability, weight loss, abdominal pain, and vomiting [10]. This is followed by stomatitis and bright-red glossitis and then a pigmented scaling rash on the sun-exposed areas [10]. This dermatitis actually occurs in areas exposed to sunlight, heat, friction, or pressure [8]. Photosensitivity is a major feature of the dermatitis [4]. Early there is a symmetric itching and painful erythema on the face, neck (Casal's necklace), back, and dorsum of the hands (gauntlet of pellagra). There is erythema on the nose and cheekbones [9]. There is a silvery scale on the ears [9]. The erythema typically disappears in the winter and returns in the spring [2]. There may be vesicles and bullae, which crust and scale. The skin eventually becomes lichinified and covered with dark scales and crust. The affected areas are sharply demarcated from normal skin. The skin findings do not correlate with the severity of the internal manifestations of pellagra [6]. Skin biopsy shows epidermal atrophy of the malpighian layer with orthokeratosis and hyperkeratosis [2]. The laboratory diagnosis of niacin deficiency is usually based on decreased levels of 2-methyl nicotinamide and 2-pyridone in the urine [10].

Pyridoxine Deficiency

Pyridoxine is also known as vitamin B_6. It is involved in neurotransmitter and heme synthesis as well as the metabolism of glycogen, amino acids, lipids, steroids, and spingoid bases. It is also involved in the conversion of tryptophan to niacin and linoleic acid to arachidonic acid [5, 10]. Pyridoxine deficiency is seen in alcoholism, uremia, and hepatic cirrhosis [6]. Alcoholics have an inadequate intake and abnormal liver storage of vitamin B_6 [2]. Drugs that effect pridoxal-5-phosphate such as isoniazid, hydralazine, cyclosporine, penicillamine, and oral contraceptives may cause a deficiency of vitamin B_6. Consumption of excessive protein-rich canned foods can cause a pyridoxine deficiency [9]. Pyridoxine deficiency is more common in the elderly [5].

The cutaneous findings show similarities to those of essential fatty acid deficiency or B vitamin deficiency especially pellagra [5]. Cutaneous findings of B_6 deficiency are seborrheic dermatitis, glossitis, stomatitis, and cheilosis [10]. The seborrheic dermatitis is typically seen on the face, neck, shoulders, perianal region, and perineum [6]. Severe deficiency causes generalized weakness, irritability, peripheral neuropathy, depression, and confusion [10]. Polyneuropathy and gastrointestinal manifestations are common [2]. The cutaneous findings clear promptly with replacement therapy [5]. The laboratory diagnosis of a vitamin B_6 deficiency is usually based on a low plasma 5ʹ-pyridoxal phosphate level [10].

Vitamin B₁₂ Deficiency

Vitamin B_{12} is also known as cobalamin. Vitamin B_{12} deficiency is more common in the elderly [5]. Vitamin B_{12} is the only vitamin that can be obtained solely from animal sources [5]. Its absorption involves intrinsic factor, R protein, and transcobalamins I, II, and III [2]. The deficiency of B_{12} is usually due to digestive malabsorption [9]. This is often from a defect in hydrochloric acid or intrinsic factor, intestinal disease, a defect in the exocrine pancreas, *Diphyllobothrium latum* infection, celiac disease, or Imerslund–Gäsbeck disease [2,7]. Because the body stores are relatively large, it typically takes 3–6 years to develop a deficiency [7]. Vitamin B_{12} is involved in DNA, protein, lipid, and carbohydrate metabolisms [5].

The megaloblastic anemia and neurologic findings are probably the best-known findings of B_{12} deficiency [2]. Vitamin B_{12} deficiency has been reported to result in hyperpigmentation of the oral mucosa and skin of the forearms, elbows, palmar creases and periunguinal area, knees, and feet [11]. Vitamin B_{12} deficiency results in a decrease of the reduced glutathione level. Reduced glutathione inhibits tyrosinase, which is involved in melanogenesis. The increase in tyrosinase activity causes the hyperpigmentation [2]. There are two other theories regarding the hyperpigmentation in B_{12} deficiency. A deficiency of folate could elevate the level of biopterin, which is involved in melanin synthesis [7]. Megaloblastic changes in the keratinocytes might result in redistribution in melanin [7]. If the deficiency is severe enough to produce pernicious anemia, there are usually cutaneous findings [4,5]. Hunters' glossitis is a bright-red painful tongue found in most cases of megaloblastic anemia [2]. There is a lemon yellow pallor to the skin everywhere except for the hands and feet [4]. There may be brown reticular hyperpigmentation on the finger pulps, brown molting on the nape of the neck, axillae, and lateral abdominal area, or macular pigmentation on the face, hands, and feet [9]. There may be stomatitis, glossitis, and glossodynia [4]. In addition to pernicious anemia the non-cutaneous findings include metal deterioration. Biopsy of the pigmented areas shows atrophic epidermis and melanin pigmentation of the basal cell layer without an increase in the number of melanocytes. The keratinocytes have an increase in nuclear size [2]. The skin lesions and fatigue resolve with supplementation [7,11]. The neurologic deficits may not resolve [7].

Folic Acid

Folic acid is a B vitamin. Folate is involved in the metabolism of amino acids, DNA, purines, and pyrimidines [2]. The requirement for folate increases in pregnancy, prematurity, long-term dialysis, hemolytic anemia, leukemia, myeloid proliferation, myelosclerosis, and exfoliative dermatitis [2,9]. Drugs such as phynytoin, barbiturates, methotrexate, and pyrimethamine can cause a folic acid deficiency [2]. The absorption of folate is reduced in vitamin B_{12}deficiency [2].

A skin hyperpigmentation is seen that is similar to the one observed in vitamin B_{12}deficiency [2, 9]. Deficiency of folate produces cheilitis, glossitis, and mucosal erosions. There is a well-known megaloblastic anemia in folic acid deficiency. The serum level of folate is considered more reliable than the erythrocyte level, which is dependant on the availability of vitamin B_{12}.

Biotin

Biotin is a slightly water-soluble and alcohol-soluble vitamin [2]. Biotin acts as a CO_2carrier and it is involved in fatty acid synthesis and gluconeogensis [10]. Clinical biotin deficiency is rare because it is widely distributed in nature [4]. Avidin, a protein found in raw egg whites, prevents the absorption of biotin by binding to it [4]. Biotin deficiency may occur with total parenteral nutrition [2]. There are also neonatal and infantile genetic biotin deficiencies [7].

The cutaneous findings of biotin deficiency are scaling, seborrheic, and erythematous rash around the eyes, nose, mouth, and extremities [10]. Biotin deficiency is also associated with perioralfacial dermatitis, xeroderma, glossitis, cheilitis, and alopecia [5]. The skin lesions may be similar to ichthyosis or generalized seborrheic dermatitis [2, 9]. The symptoms include nausea, depression, lethargy, muscle pain, elevated cholesterol, hallucinations, paresthesias, and anorexia [6, 10]. On biopsy there are atrophic sebaceous glands, hair follicles, dilated sweat glands, and perivascular inflammation [2].

Vitamin E Deficiency

Dietary deficiency of vitamin E does not exist. It is seen in malabsorption diseases. Vitamin E deficiency is associated with poor wound healing [3]. It has also been associated with seborrheic dermatitis-like eruption and a shortened erythrocyte survival [9].

Vitamin D Deficiency

Vitamin D is required for calcium absorption. A deficiency results in osteomalacia or rickets. Although the skin is involved in the synthesis of vitamin D there are no skin findings associated with its deficiency.

Vitamin A Deficiency

Vitamin A is available from animal sources (retinyl esters) or it may be synthesized from provitamin carotenoids in plants (retinal) [5, 7]. Vitamin A is involved in the growth and differentiation of epidermal and mesenchymal cells [6]. It is also involved in carbohydrate metabolism and glycoprotein synthesis [9]. Vitamin A circulates bound to retinal-binding proteins and is stored in the liver [9]. Cirrhosis, diabetes, and thyrotoxicosis alter vitamin A absorption and storage [2]. Hypothyroidism and diabetes interfere with the conversion of carotenoids to active vitamin A [5].

A deficiency may affect the skin, eyes, mucous membranes of the gastrointestinal, respiratory, and urogenital tracts, and the immune system [6]. Nyctalopia, impairment of dark adaptation, and hemeralopia, inability to see in bright light, are the earliest sign of vitamin A deficiency [5, 7]. Vitamin A deficiency is associated with a follicular hyperkeratosis, phrynoderma, and generalized xerosis [6]. This needs to be differentiated from pityriasis rubra pilaris and lichen spinulosus [6]. The follicular hyperkeratosis may actually be due to a coexistent B vitamin deficiency. There is poor wound healing [8]. There is atrophy of the sebaceous glands and sweat glands and horny plugging of follicles on the limbs, back of the neck, and shoulders that causes the skin to be rough [2]. Keratotic papules first appear on the anterolateral thighs and posterolateral upper arms and spread to the extensor surfaces of the upper extremities, shoulders, abdomen, back, and buttocks. They appear on the face and posterior neck later [5]. Vitamin A deficiency also causes hemeralopia (night blindness), xerophthalmia, and blindness [6,9]. In severe cases there may be xerosis conjunctivae, Bitot's spots, xerosis corneae, and keratomalacia of the cornea [5]. The deficiency syndrome is usually apparent when the serum vitamin A levels are less than 30 mcg/dl which corresponds to the exhaustion of the hepatic stores. [5]. The diagnosis is confirmed by a low plasma retinal concentration [6]. The ocular changes respond rapidly and the skin changes require 2–3 months [2].

Vitamin K Deficiency

Vitamin K is required for the synthesis of coagulation factors II, VII, IX, and X and proteins S and C in the liver [2]. Approximately half of the vitamin K comes from the diet and the other half is synthesized by intestinal flora [7]. It occurs in anorexia nervosa, on antibiotic use, bilairy diseases, liver disease, and on cholestyramine use [2]. Coumarin is an anti-vitamin K agent that inhibits K-2, 3-epoxide reductase and prevents the recycling of the inactive form [7]. Vitamin K deficiency causes disorders of coagulation. The signs and symptoms are those of hemorrhage. Nodular purpura may be seen in adults [9]. The prothrobin time and partial thromboplastin time are prolonged.

Zinc Deficiency

Zinc plays a role in immunologic function and the regulation of DNA and RNA polymerases. It is part of more than 200 metalloenzymes [5]. Zinc deficiency may be seen in alcoholism, anorexia nervosa, a vegetarian diet, gastrointestinal disorders, malignancies, chronic renal disease, or long-term total parenteral nutrition [4, 9].

Acrodermatitis enteropathica is an autosomal recessive disorder in zinc absorption seen in children. This is characterized by alopecia, dermatitis, and diarrhea [4]. The distribution of the eruption on the face, hands, feet, and anogenital area is unique [9]. The cutaneous lesions are patches and plaques that become vestibulobullous, pustular, erosive, crusted lesions. The initial cutaneous lesions are perioral and anogenital. Early findings of zinc deficiency include: anemia, photophobia, mental depression, and eczematous eruptions on the hands, feet, and anogenital regions. There are flat grayish bullous lesions surrounded by red-brown erythema on the finger flexor creases and palms as well as angular stomatitis and paronychia [8]. Later, there are lesions on the scalp, hands, feet, and trunk. There is poor wound healing. Hyperkeratosis, parakeratosis, pereche, paronychia may occur. The chronic lesions tend to be seen where there is repeated pressure or trauma [8]. The lesions are well demarcated, thickened, and brownish. Lichinification and scaling may develop [8]. There may be slow hair growth or alopecia. The nails may have Beau's lines [8]. Marginal zinc deficiencies cause an increased susceptibility to infection, impaired wound healing, and aggravation of existing skin disorders [5]. Zinc deficiency also produces diarrhea, alopecia, muscle wasting, depression, and irritability [10]. Skin biopsy shows acanthosis, pallor and dyskeratosis of keratinocytes, microvesicles, subcorneal pustules, and vacuolar alteration of the dermoepidermal junction. There are lymphohistiocytic perivascular infiltrates in the dermis [9]. Plasma zinc concentration is the most reliable indication of the body stores but it is not always accurate [5]. Two to three weeks of oral supplementation should correct all but the most severe cases [5].

Starvation

Starvation findings are seen in chronic wasting, anorexia nervosa, and underfeeding. The dermatologic findings resemble those of aging [5]. The skin is thin, dry, inelastic, pallid, grayish, and cold [5]. There may be hyperpigmentation on the face, around the mouth, eyes, and malar area [5]. The nails are brittle and fissured and the hair is thin, dry, dull, and fragile [5]. There may also be lanugo hairs [5].

Kwashiorkor

Kwashiorkor is due to a diet low in protein and high in calories from carbohydrates. The dermatologic findings include: hyperpigmentation, hypopigmentation, petechial hemorrhage, hyperkeratosis, scaling of the skin, and cutaneous ulcers [9]. The face, hands, and feet are often spared [9]. There can be superficial desquamation, loss of large areas of skin, linear fissures, depigmentation, and thinning of the hair [9]. Flag sign is alternating bands of dark and pale hair due to alternating periods of adequate and inadequate nutrition [9]. The nails may be thin and soft [9]. Non-cutaneous findings include edema, hypoalbuminemia, hepatospenomegaly, muscle wasting, behavioral changes, and diarrhea [9].

Essential Fatty Acid Deficiency

Linoleic acid is the fundamental essential fatty acid. It is converted to arachidonic acid which then can be used to form prostiglandins and leukotrienes [9]. In the skin, linoleic acid is required for proper lamellar granule formation [7]. The dermatologic findings include diffuse erythema, xerosis, scaling, diffuse alopecia involving the scalp and eyebrows with lightening of the remaining hair [5, 9]. There is also poor wound healing, brittle nails, and capillary fragility [5]. The non-cutaneous findings might include: fatty liver, anemia, thrombocytopenia, poor wound healing [7]. Biopsy shows acanthosis, hyperkeratosis, hypergranulosis, increased intradermal cell spaces, and vacuolated epidermal cells [9]. The diagnosis of an essential fatty acid deficiency is confirmed by a triene–tetraene (5,8,11-eicosatrienoic acid to arachidonic acid) ratio of greater than 0.4 [7].

Conclusions

The cutaneous findings of nutritional deficiencies are often not significantly different from those from other causes. A number of nutritional deficiencies may present with cutaneous manifestations. Table 15.1 reviews the cutaneous and non-cutaneous findings of many of the nutritional disorders discussed in this article. Since it may

Table 15.1 The cutaneous findings and non-cutaneous findings

Deficiency	Cutaneous findings	Non-cutaneous findings
Vitamin C	Perifollicular hemorrhages, petechiae, ecchymoses, gingival bleeding, gingival hypertrophy, splinter hemorrhages, impaired wound healing, follicular keratosis	Malaise, fatigue, weight loss, depression, epistaxis, diarrhea, weakness, hemathrosis, periosteal hemorrhages, peripheral edema, mental depression, normaochromic normocytic anemia, megaloblastic anemia, Sjögren's syndrome, xerostomia, keratoconjunctivitis sicca, enlargement of submandibular or parotid glands, hypotension
Thiamine	Seborrheic dermatitis-like lesions, non-specific buccal mucosal vesicles	Anorexia, irritability, apathy, generalized weakness, beriberi (cardiovascular or peripheral neuropathy symptoms), Wernicke–Korsakoff syndrome

(continued)

Table 15.1 (continued)

Deficiency	Cutaneous findings	Non-cutaneous findings
Riboflavin	Angular stomatitis (pelèche), cheilosis, atrophic glossitis with a magenta tongue, pharyngitis, seborrhea and genital dermatitis.	Conjunctivitis, corneal vascularization
Niacin	Dermatitis in sun-exposed areas, perianal and genital dermatitis, lichinification hyperpigmentation on osseous prominences, seborrheic eczema-like dermatitis, stomatitis, bright-red glossitis, Casal's necklace, gauntlet of pellagra	Anorexia, weakness, irritability, weight loss, abdominal pain, vomiting, diarrhea
Pyridoxine	Seborrheic dermatitis, glossitis, stomatitis, cheilosis	Generalized weakness, somulance, irritability, peripheral neuropathy, depression, confusion, polyneuropathy, anorexia and other gastrointestinal manifestations
B_{12}	Hyperpigmentation of the oral mucosa and skin of the forearms, elbows, palmar creases and periunguinal area, knees and feet, Hunters' glossitis, lemon yellow pallor to the skin, glossodynia, stomatitis	Megaloblastic anemia, neurologic findings, metal deterioration
Folic acid	Skin hyperpigmentation similar to B_{12}, cheilitis, glossitis, mucosal erosions	Megaloblastic anemia
Biotin	Scaling, seborrheic, and erythematous rash around the eyes, nose, mouth, and extremities, xeroderma, perioralfacial dermatitis, glossitis, cheilitis, alopecia	Nausea, depression, lethargy, muscle pain, elevated cholesterol, hallucinations, paresthesias, anorexia
Vitamin E	Poor wound healing, seborrheic dermatitis-like eruption	Shortened erythrocyte survival
Vitamin D	None	Osteomalacia or rickets
Vitamin A	Follicular hyperkeratosis, phrynoderma, generalized xerosis, poor wound healing	Nyctalopia, hemeralopia, xerophthalmia, blindness, xerosis conjunctivae, Bitot's spots, xerosis corneae, keratomalacia of the cornea
Vitamin K	Signs and symptoms of hemorrhage	Disorders of coagulation
Zinc	Alopecia, patches, plaques, eczematous eruptions on the hands, feet, and anogenital regions, angular stomatitis, paronychia, poor wound healing, Beau's lines, aggravation of existing skin disorders	Diarrhea, anemia, photophobia, mental depression, muscle wasting, irritability, anorexia
Essential fatty	Diffuse erythema, xerosis, scaling, diffuse alopecia, poor wound healing, brittle nails, capillary fragility	Fatty liver, anemia, thrombocytopenia, poor wound healing

Recall that combined nutritional deficiencies are more common than isolated ones.

be difficult to detect an early nutritional deficiency based on a history alone the clinician must be alert to other suggestions. It is easy to imagine a skin lesion with a nutritional etiology being treated without consideration of the underlying cause. This would be a tragedy because these disorders respond at least to some degree to replacement therapy. Prompt detection may be the key to avoiding more serious problems. It is also important to keep in mind that the dermatologic finding associated with nutritional deficiencies often overlap and these deficiencies often coexist. For this reason, the clinician will often need to consider multiple deficiencies.

References

1. Mac Donald A, Forsyth A. Nutritional deficiencies and the skin. Clin. Exp. Dermatol. 2005; 30(4): 388–90.
2. Barthelemy H, Chouvet B, Cambazard F. Skin and mucosal manifestations in vitamin deficiency. J. Am. Acad. Dermatol. 1986; 15(16): 1263–74.
3. Schneider JB, Norman RA. Cutaneous manifestations of endocrine-metabolic disease and nutritional deficiency in the elderly. Dermatol. Clin. 2004; 22: 23–31.
4. Neldner KH. Nutrition, aging and the skin. Geriatrics 1984; 32(2): 69–88
5. Ryan AS, Goldsmith LA. Nutrition and the skin. Clin. Dermatol. 1996; 14: 389–406.
6. Fuchs J. Alcoholism, malnutrition, vitamin deficiencies, and the skin. Clin. Dermatol. 1999; 17: 457–61.
7. Miller SJ. Continuing medical education: nutritional deficiency and the skin. J. Am. Acad. Dermatol. 1989; 21(1): 1–30.
8. Oumeish OY. Nutritional skin problems in children. Clin. Dermatol. 2003; 21: 260–3.
9. Delahoussaye AR, Jorizzo JL. Cutaneous manifestations of nutritional disorders. Dermatol. Clin. 1989; 7(3): 559–70.
10. Braunwald E, Fauci AS, Kasper DL, Hauser SL, Longo DL, Jameson JL. Harrison's Principles of Internal Medicine, 15th ed. New York: McGraw-Hill, 2001.
11. Mori K, Ando I, Kukita A. Generalized hyperpigmentation of the skin due to vitamin B12 deficiency. J. Dermatol. 2001; 28(5): 282–5.

Chapter 16

Infestations, Bites and Stings in Aging Skin

Dirk M. Elston[1]

Introduction

Infestations, bites and stings are common in older patients. Increased morbidity and mortality in these patients is often related to pre-existing cardiac disease. Scabies infestation often presents with atypical manifestations in this population. A high index of suspicion is required. In extended care facilities, epidemics of scabies are common. A single patient with crusted scabies may cause infestation of an entire ward. This chapter reviews recent information about infestations, bites and stings in this population.

Infestation

Scabies infestation is a significant source of morbidity among older patients, especially nursing home residents. It is also a problem in hospitals, where entire wards can become infested when one patient with crusted scabies is admitted. Manifestations of scabies infestation are protean, including papules, pustules, burrows, nodules, urticarial papules and plaques. Most younger patients with scabies experience severe pruritus, but pruritus is variable among older patients. Pruritus may be moderate or non-existent in the face of a massive parasite burden. Patients with deficient cellular immunity may not feel the urge to scratch. Those with neurologic dysfunction may not be able to scratch. Even in those who excoriate widely, excoriations often predominate over burrows, and the clinical appearance may resemble prurigo nodularis. Patients with Norwegian scabies are often older, debilitated or immunocompromised. A high index of suspicion is required, or the diagnosis will be missed. Demonstration of mites, eggs or scybala (mite feces) is diagnostic. Dermoscopy has been used as an alternative to traditional scabies slide preparations for confirmation of the diagnosis. A triangular or chevron-shaped structure is visible, which corresponds to the anterior section of the mite, consisting of the mouth parts and the two pairs of front legs [1].

---

[1] The author once served as a consultant to Merck, the manufacturer of invermectin.

R.A. Norman (ed.), *Diagnosis of Aging Skin Diseases,*
© Springer-Verlag London Limited 2008

Scabies infestation may produce bullous lesions filled with eosinophils, mimicking bullous pemphigoid [2]. Direct immunofluorescence testing may be positive in patients with bullous scabies, reinforcing the misdiagnosis of bullous pemphigoid [3]. As pemphigoid commonly affects older patients, a high index of suspicion for scabies infestation must be maintained.

The host's immune response plays a role in determining the clinical manifestations of scabies infestation. Normal human peripheral blood mononuclear cells and dendritic cells react to whole body extracts of *Sarcoptes scabiei* [4]. Patients with crusted scabies are commonly immunosuppressed, often with a decrease in cell-mediated immunity. There is evidence of an altered immune response to scabies antigens in these patients. Specifically, patients with crusted scabies demonstrate pronounced IgE response to scabies mites, whereas patients with ordinary scabies do not. An IgG response is also noted, but neither of these antibody responses appears to provide any protection against infestation. In one study, serum from patients with crusted scabies showed strong IgE binding to scabies proteins. IgG binding was also identified. In contrast, only three of seven patients with ordinary scabies showed any IgE binding. Their antibody binding was also weaker [5].

A variety of treatment options are available for scabetic infestation, including 5% permethrin cream, 1% lindane (gamma benzene hexachloride) lotion and 5–10% precipitated sulfur in petrolatum. Permethrin is first-line therapy. It is applied over the entire body surface overnight, but the head and neck do not require treatment unless there is clinical evidence of involvement in these sites. Lindane must be used with caution in those with a defective cutaneous barrier and is contraindicated in patients with neurologic disease, especially those with a history of seizures. In a widely reported study of 1146 individuals who received lindane, a statistically significant increase in incidence of cancer was demonstrated: 43 cases were observed, in contrast to 30.2 expected. There was also some evidence of a dose–response relationship. However, at least some of the cancers were due to associated morbidities. Four of the cancer patients had Kaposi's sarcoma due to AIDS. Four others had other strong risk factors for their cancer. Despite the statistical association, this study provided no convincing evidence of carcinogenicity of lindane [6]. Lindane remains an acceptable second-line agent for the treatment of scabies.

Crotamiton has an antipruritic effect and may be useful as an adjunctive therapy. Unfortunately, the rate of treatment failure is higher than with other agents, and the product should usually not be used alone. Malathion, allethrin and benzyl benzoate are used outside of the United States.

Ivermectin, the only effective oral treatment, is not approved for scabies in the United States. It has some potential for neurotoxicity and should be used with caution in those with a defective blood–brain barrier. The convenience of oral dosing is an advantage to ivermectin [7], but must be weighed against the risks of therapy. Treatment failures occur, even after multiple doses, and ivermectin resistance has been documented among some sarcoptes mites. Cinical and in vitro evidence of ivermectin resistance was demonstrated in two patients with multiple recurrences of crusted scabies who had received 30 and 58 doses of ivermectin, respectively [8].

Older patients may be infested with more than a single parasite, especially in conditions of poverty or homelessness. Ectoparasites may be the most apparent infestation, but intestinal parasites may produce or exacerbate nutritional deficiency and have a significant impact on long-term health. Ectoparasites such as fleas and lice may be present along with scabies. Ivermectin is an antiparasitic drug with a fairly broad spectrum. In patients concomitantly infected with intestinal helminths and a variety of ectoparasites, two doses of ivermectin (200 microg/kg) at an interval of 10 days cured most parasitic infections. The cure rates for ectoparasitoses were 100% for cutaneous larva migrans, 99% for pediculosis, 88% for scabies and 64% for tungiasis. Cure rates for intestinal parasites were 100% for strongyloidiasis and enterobiasis, 99% for ascariasis, 84% for trichuriasis, 68% for hookworm disease and 50% for hymenolepiasis. Ivermectin may be useful in patients with polyparasitism or when public health measures aim to reduce the prevalence of ectoparasites and intestinal helminthiases [9].

During outbreak of scabies in nursing home, staff and visitors who have close physical contact with residents should be treated. Therapy targeted only at those with symptoms is seldom effective. Close contacts should be treated regardless of the presence of symptoms. Laundry workers in the facility may also require treatment, especially if there are patients with crusted scabies in the facility.

Although canine scabies can affect humans, this is rare. Even among Australian populations who live in close association with their dogs, hypervariable microsatellite markers have shown that the mites on humans were genetically distinct from those on the dogs. *S. scabiei* var. hominis can also be differentiated from *S. scabiei* var. canis by mitochondrial DNA. Using these methods, some gene flow has been demonstrated between scabies mite populations on humans and dogs, but it is extremely rare [10]. This suggests that, even in patients with exposure to canine scabies, control of human scabies endemics must focus on human-to-human transmission.

Renal transplant recipients suffer from a wide variety of skin ailments related to chronic immune suppression. Cutaneous malignancy is the most common problem, but infections and infestation are also common. In a study of 104 renal transplant recipients presenting with infections and infestations, two presented with scabies [11]. Their manifestations may be altered by their immunosuppression. Specifically, itching may be minimal, and crusted scabies may occur.

Reactive perforating collagenosis is commonly associated with diabetes mellitus and renal failure. Excoriations associated with scabies have been reported to give rise to lesions of reactive perforating collagenosis in the setting of diabetes. The characteristic umbilicated lesions arise at sites of excoriation. Treatment for scabies allows for control of the perforating disorder [12].

Demodex mites have been implicated in the pathogenesis of rosacea. Demodectic lesions may appear as confluent facial erythematous papules, pustules and abscesses. Biopsy will demonstrate a variable perifollicular infiltrate with lymphocytes, histiocytes and many *Demodex folliculorum* mites. Topical sulfur is often effective, applied either as 5–10% precipitated sulfur in petrolatum or as a combination of sulfur and sulfacetamide. Ivermectin, lindane, permethrin and benzyl benzoate have also been used. Topical metronidazole is generally ineffective, but oral metronidazole has been reported to be effective in demodectic abscesses that were unresponsive to topical agents [13].

Bites and Stings

The hand–foot syndrome was originally described in association with sickle cell crisis, then as a manifestation of chemotherapy toxicity, anemia and thalassemia. Fire ant stings may produce the hand–foot syndrome in older patients. Both hands and both feet are red, swollen and may be tender. Classic sterile pustular fire ant skin lesions in rosettes may be present [14]. It is important to recognize cases of hand–foot syndrome related to stings, as this can prevent a needless and extensive evaluation.

Ant stings may be fatal in those with severe allergy. In one series of fatal ant sting reactions, all of those who died were males between ages 40 and 80. All had a history of allergy to the ant venom. None of the deceased carried injectable adrenaline and most died within 20 min of a single sting. Cardiopulmonary comorbidities were present in all cases [15]. Ant venom immunotherapy is available for many species, and an allergist should evaluate all patients with severe allergic reactions.

Bees, wasps and hornets are members of the order Hymenoptera. Hymenopterid stings can lead to acute myocardial infarction, especially in those with pre-existing coronary disease. The development of shock and the therapeutic use of epinephrine may also cause acute myocardial infarction. Silent presentation of acute myocardial infarction has been reported after a sting in the absence of any pharmacological intervention [16]. An ECG may be advisable even when symptoms of an allergic reaction are not present. The risk of recurrence of severe sting reactions is high, with 1/12 patients experiencing recurrent anaphyaxis, and 1/50 requiring hospital treatment or adrenaline in any 1-year period [17]. All patients with severe hymenopterid allergy should be evaluated by an allergist. Immunotherapy can prevent severe reactions and has a positive impact on the quality of life [18]. Rush immunization schedules have been developed for those with a significant risk of exposure [19]. Extensive skin and soft tissue necrosis may also occur following hymenoptera stings. Surgical debridement and skin grafting may be required [20].

Scorpion and spider toxins can cause cardiac decompensation in older patients. Scorpion venom causes adrenergic discharge and cardiotoxicity [21]. The risk varies by species, with severe toxicity noted in many Asian species. In the United States, *Centruroides exilicauda* is the most dangerous scorpion, especially for children and older patients with existing cardiovascular disease. Acute myocardial injury has been reported in relation to bites by the Sydney funnel-web spider (*Atrax robustus*) [22].

Lyme disease is an important vector-borne disease in both the United States and Europe. Mosquito-borne encephalitis is a problem in many parts of the United

States, and tick-borne encephalitis is a significant problem in central Europe [23]. In older patients, these conditions may be mistaken for other infectious diseases or for non-infectious causes of neuronal dysfunction or dementia. Patients in highly endemic areas are at high risk of re-exposure to ticks and reinfection [24]. Gardening, golfing and other leisure activities are risks for exposure. The use of permethrin on clothing, repellents and prompt tick removal are important to reduce the risk of recurrent disease.

West Nile virus was first recognized in the United States in 1999. Since then, the geographic distribution has widened progressively, with westward extension of the range of the virus. Elderly persons are at risk for more severe illness [25]. Mosquito control programs, avoidance of exposure to bites and the use of repellents can decrease the incidence of disease in this population.

After years of hard work, older individuals often retire and find the time to travel. Their travels may take them to areas of the world where malaria is endemic. Malaria infections, especially falciparum infections, can be fatal if not diagnosed and treated promptly. The risk is higher in patients with pre-existing cardiac or renal disease. Any person who develops fever or flu-like symptoms after travel to a malarious area should be considered to have malaria until proven otherwise. Laboratory investigation should include blood smears. In a recent survey by the Centers for Disease Control, the majority of US civilians who acquired infection abroad were found not to have taken the appropriate chemoprophylaxis regimen for the country where they acquired malaria [26]. Anyone traveling to a malarious area should consult a knowledgeable physician and take the recommended chemoprophylaxis regimen, without missing a dose. Personal protective measures to prevent mosquito bites, including repellents, appropriate clothing and mosquito netting, are also important measures to prevent infection.

Necrotizing fascitis usually occurs after a perforating trauma, but may also be caused by mosquito bites [27]. The patient experiences pain, swelling and a dusky bluish-red discoloration. Bullae may form. The area becomes gangrenous, usually by the fifth day, and the death rate is high. Common pathogens include beta-hemolytic streptococci, coliform bacteria, enterococci, pseudomonas and fungi. Effective treatment requires early detection, surgical debridement, microbicides and supportive care.

Lare typical CD30-positive cells may be found in bite reactions, and the histology may mimic lymphomatoid papulosis or anaplastic large cell lymphoma [28]. Careful clinicopathologic correlation is required. Conversely, individuals with existing lymphoma or chronic lymphocytic leukemia may exhibit exaggerated responses to arthropod bites and stings. Abnormal reactions should prompt an investigation for underlying disease.

Older individuals often have comorbidities that put them at risk for severe reactions to bites and stings. Aging skin often manifests infestation in a different fashion from younger skin. Physicians caring for older patients should become knowledgeable about the special manifestations and risks of bites, stings and infestations in this population.

References

1. Prins C, Stucki L, French L, Saurat JH, Braun RP. Dermoscopy for the in vivo detection of *Sarcoptes scabiei*. Dermatology 2004; 208(3): 241–3.
2. Brar BK, Pall A, Gupta RR. Bullous scabies mimicking bullous pemphigoid. J. Dermatol. 2003; 30(9): 694–6.
3. Shahab RK, Loo DS. Bullous scabies. J. Am. Acad. Dermatol. 2003; 49(2): 346–50.
4. Arlian LG, Morgan MS, Neal JS. Extracts of scabies mites (Sarcoptidae: *Sarcoptes scabiei*) modulate cytokine expression by human peripheral blood mononuclear cells and dendritic cells. J. Med. Entomol. 2004; 41(1): 69–73.
5. Arlian LG, Morgan MS, Estes SA, Walton SF, Kemp DJ, Currie BJ. Circulating IgE in patients with ordinary and crusted scabies. J. Med. Entomol. 2004; 41(1): 74–7.
6. Friedman GD. Lindane and cancer in humans: a false alarm? Pharmacoepidemiol. Drug Saf. 1997; 6(2): 129–34.
7. Santoro AF, Rezac MA, Lee JB. Current trend in ivermectin usage for scabies. J. Drugs Dermatol. 2003; 2(4): 397–401.
8. Currie BJ, Harumal P, McKinnon M, Walton SF. First documentation of in vivo and in vitro ivermectin resistance in *Sarcoptes scabiei*. Clin. Infect. Dis. 2004; 39(1): e8–12.
9. Heukelbach J, Wilcke T, Winter B, Sales de Oliveira FA, Saboia Moura RC, Harms G, Liesenfeld O, Feldmeier H. Efficacy of ivermectin in a patient population concomitantly infected with intestinal helminths and ectoparasites. Arzneimittelforschung 2004; 54(7): 416–21.
10. Walton SF, Dougall A, Pizzutto S, Holt D, Taplin D, Arlian LG, Morgan M, Currie BJ, Kemp DJ. Genetic epidemiology of *Sarcoptes scabiei* (Acari: Sarcoptidae) in northern Australia. Int. J. Parasitol. 2004; 34(7): 839–49.
11. Sandhu K, Gupta S, Kumar B, Dhandha R, Udigiri NK, Minz M. The pattern of mucocutaneous infections and infestations in renal transplant recipients. J. Dermatol. 2003; 30(8): 590–5.
12. Brinkmeier T, Herbst R, Frosch P. Reactive perforating collagenosis associated with scabies in a diabetic. J. Eur. Acad. Dermatol. Venereol. 2004; 18(5): 588–90.
13. Schaller M, Sander CA, Plewig G. Demodex abscesses: clinical and therapeutic challenges. J. Am. Acad. Dermatol. 2003; 49(5 Suppl): S272–4.
14. Carr ME. Hand–foot syndrome in a patient with multiple fire ant stings. South. Med. J. 2004; 97(7): 707–9.
15. McGain F, Winkel KD. Ant sting mortality in Australia. Toxicon 2002; 40(8): 1095–100.
16. Lombardi A, Vandelli R, Cere E, Di Pasquale G. Silent acute myocardial infarction following a wasp sting. Ital. Heart J. 2003; 4(9): 638–41.
17. Mullins RJ. Anaphylaxis: risk factors for recurrence. Clin. Exp. Allergy. 2003; 33(8): 1033–40.
18. Oude Elberink JN, De Monchy JG, Van Der Heide S, Guyatt GH, Dubois AE. Venom immunotherapy improves health-related quality of life in patients allergic to yellow jacket venom. J. Allergy Clin. Immunol. 2002; 110(1): 174–82.
19. Yoshida N, Fukuda T. Efficacy and safety of rush immunotherapy in patients with Hymenoptera allergy in Japan. Asian Pac. J. Allergy Immunol. 2003; 21(2): 89–94.
20. Kocer U, Ozer Tiftikcioglu Y, Mete Aksoy H, Karaaslan O. Skin and soft tissue necrosis following hymenoptera sting. J. Cutan. Med. Surg. 2003; 7(2): 133–5.
21. Bentur Y, Taitelman U, Aloufy A. Evaluation of scorpion stings: the poison center perspective. Vet. Hum. Toxicol. 2003; 45(2): 108–11.
22. Isbister GK, Warner G. Acute myocardial injury caused by Sydney funnel-web spider (*Atrax robustus*) envenoming. Anaesth. Intensive Care 2003; 31(6): 672–4.
23. Kriz B, Benes C, Danielova V, Daniel M. Socio-economic conditions and other anthropogenic factors influencing tick-borne encephalitis incidence in the Czech Republic. Int. J. Med. Microbiol. 2004; 293(Suppl 37): 63–8.

24. Nowakowski J, Nadelman RB, Sell R, McKenna D, Cavaliere LF, Holmgren D, Gaidici A, Wormser GP. Long-term follow-up of patients with culture-confirmed Lyme disease. Am. J. Med. 2003; 115(2): 91–6.
25. Centers for Disease Control and Prevention (CDC). Knowledge, attitudes, and behaviors about West Nile virus—Connecticut, 2002. MMWR 2003; 52(37): 886–8.
26. Holtz TH, Kachur SP, MacArthur JR, Roberts JM, Barber AM, Steketee RW, Parise ME. Malaria surveillance—United States, 1998. MMWR CDC Surveill. Summ. 2001; 50(5): 1–20.
27. Verma SB. Necrotizing fascitis induced by mosquito bite. J. Eur. Acad. Dermatol. Venereol. 2003; 17(5): 591–3.
28. Cepeda LT, Pieretti M, Chapman SF, Horenstein MG. CD30-positive atypical lymphoid cells in common non-neoplastic cutaneous infiltrates rich in neutrophils and eosinophils. Am. J. Surg. Pathol. 2003; 27(7): 912–8.

Chapter 17

Psychoneurodermatologic Disorders

Erica Liverant

A psychodermatologic disorder is a disease that involves an interaction between the mind and the skin. The skin holds a powerful position as an organ of communication and plays an important interaction with one's social environment [1]. Between 20 and 40% of patients seeking treatment from dermatologists have some type of psychological or psychiatric problem causing or influencing the skin lesions [1]. The majority of these patients often lack insight into the cause of their skin disease and will refuse treatment by any mental health professional. Thus, it becomes the role of the dermatologist to be able to recognize these patients. The dermatologist must be able to recognize and diagnose these psychocutaneous diseases and understand the basic treatments that are available.

The majority of psychocutaneous diseases fall into three categories: psychophysiologic disorders, primary psychiatric disorders, and secondary psychiatric disorders. Psychophysiologic diseases involve skin problems that react to emotional states but which themselves are not considered to be of psychiatric origin. Atopic dermatitis and psoriaris are examples of psychophysiologic disorders. Primary psychiatric disorders are considered when the primary illness is psychological and the patient then presents with self-induced cutaneous inflictions. The diseases that are described as primary psychiatric include delusions of parasotosis, factitial dermatitis, and neurotic excoriations. Secondary psychiatric disorders involve disfiguring skin disorders which result in severe psychological distress. Secondary psychiatric diseases include acne and vitiligo. These categories are not mutually exclusive with some disorders may falling into more than one subgroup.

The treatment of these disorders requires evaluating both the cutaneous and social issues underlying the problem. Only after addressing all aspects of the psychodermatologic disorder can the patient be successfully treated. Even with a primary psychiatric illness, the dermatologist must address the skin infection in order to avoid any complicating infections. And vice versa, the dermatologist must also be able to tackle the psychological factors involved in order to successfully treat the patient. The examples mentioned will be discussed in detail with regard to their diagnosis, pharmacological treatment, and psychological treatment in the following.

R.A. Norman (ed.), *Diagnosis of Aging Skin Diseases,*
© Springer-Verlag London Limited 2008

Psychophysiologic Disease

The skin has serious psychological implications, playing an important role as an organ of communication. A wide variety of authors have supported the opinion that stressful life events can precipitate the onset and recurrence of many skin diseases or exert a negative influence on their course. The role of stress is of particular relevance in patients affected by chronic skin conditions, such as psoriasis, atopic dermatitis, and chronic urticaria. The psychophysiologic diseases are those that not only have a dermatopathologic basis but are also influenced by emotional factors. These disorders are recognized as having a psychosomatic component primarily because emotional stress has been observed to exacerbate or affect the course of these disorders [2].

Psoriasis, which affects 1.5–2% of the population in western countries, is a hereditary disorder of the skin with several clinical expressions. Psoriasis vulgaris, the most frequent type, occurs as salmon pink papules and plaques, sharply marginated with marked silvery white scale [3]. Psychosocial factors have been implicated in the onset and exacerbation of psoriasis in 40–80% of patients [4]. Patients with psoriasis were more likely to report that stress predated the onset and exacerbation of their condition than were patients with urticaria, acne, alopecia, or nonatopic eczema [5]. Many psoriasis sufferers have indicated that the disease has had at least "somewhat" of a negative psychosocial impact on them [6]. These patients often express feelings of helplessness, embarrassment, anger, or frustration when asked about their disease [6]. Many psoriasis patients become depressed, and the degree of depressive psychopathology directly correlates with pruritis severity [7].

Psychiatric aspects of treatment. Psychosocial issues appear to be closely linked to the psoriasis sufferer. Assessing the daily difficulties faced by the patient is important, especially in those patients with stress-reactive psoriasis because the psoriasis-related stress may exacerbate the skin lesions [8]. Individual or group psychotherapy, behavioral approaches, and biofeedback have resulted in the improvement of skin lesions and the psychological component of psoriasis patients [9, 10]. In addition, hypnosis significantly improved psoriasis patients' mental states [11]. Treatment of depressive symptoms with antidepressant drug therapy may demonstrate to be helpful in the treatment of pruritis [12]. Because of the antihistaminic and antipruritic properties of the tricyclic antidepressant medication, they have proven useful in dermatology clinics for the treatment of psoriasis. Doxepin (Sinequan), imipramine (Tofranil), and clomipramine (Anafranil) have all been used to treat the pruritis and depressive symptoms. Because doxepin has the greatest antihistaminic and antipruritic effects, it is one of the most widely prescribed antidepressants in dermatology.

Atopic dermatitis is a chronic relapsing skin disorder which begins in infancy and is characterized by severe pruritis and eczematous papulovesicular lesions, which lead to repeated rubbing and scratching of the skin [3]. Over time, the skin becomes thickened with accentuation of skin markings, which is known as lichenification. Inadequate tactile stimulation and a rejecting mother figure have been implicated in childhood atopic dermatitis [13]. In some instances, the maternal rejection is a reaction to the child's dermatitis; in other words, when the skin lesions appear the mother tends to reject the child [14]. The disturbed mother–child relationship then aggravates the skin lesions. Patients with atopic dermatitis tend to be more irritable, resentful, guilt ridden, and hostile compared to those without eczema [15]. In a recent study of atopic dermatitis patients, a direct correlation was found between the severity of the pruritis and the degree of depression [12].

Psychiatric aspects of treatment. Children with intractable atopic dermatitis tend to have dysfunctional family relationships. In order to successfully treat these patients, the dermatologist needs to assess the family dynamics in addition to the standard medical treatments. A variety of techniques, including a psychosocial evaluation, parental guidance, and aggressive medical therapy, have all been used by dermatologists. The parents need to recognize that their interaction with the child is dysfunctional in nature and that this interaction is exacerbating the dermatitis. The dermatologist must be empathetic and understanding towards the parents in order for them to accept the negative feelings they are subconsciously hiding towards the child. With this insight, the parents can then set limits with the child and improve the child's eczema along with the family relationships. If depression is severe in a patient with marked pruritis, antidepressant medications may prove helpful [16]. Doxepin, a tricyclic antidepressant, can be used for the pruritis in atopic dermatitis as well as in psoriasis.

Alopecia areata is characterized by one or more hairless well-defined patches on the scalp or beard region without any signs of inflammation. In the majority of cases, the lesions tend to heal spontaneously, but in some patients they can lead to total alopecia. The alopecia evolves from the turnover of the hair follicles from the anagen to catagen phase. The cause of this turnover is unknown, but stress and emotional factors have been implicated in exacerbating alopecia areata. Psychosomatic factors have been important in 22–29% of children and in 27% of adults with alopecia areata [17]. Mental stress within the preceding months of alopecia is frequently reported by the patient [17]. The prevalence rates of psychiatric disorders associated with alopecia areata are higher than those without AA [18].

Psychiatric aspects of treatment. Alopecia areata is a difficult disease for the dermatologist to treat because of the frequent exacerbations and remissions. Recognizing the psychological and social impact of hair loss is critical when caring for alopecia areata patients. Thus, evaluating various psychosocial therapies aimed to treat the lesions is difficult. Psychotherapy has been shown to help the patient's mental state, but may not help with the skin lesions [19]. Self-help and support groups can also help the patient cope with the psychosocial impact of the disease. If drug therapy is warranted, imipramine (Tofranil) used for 6 months has been shown to cause hair regrowth in alopecia areata patients along with improving mild depressive symptoms [20].

Urticaria are wheals caused by localized edema, and these lesions are typically associated with severe itching sensations. Urticaria is characterized as chronic if the symptoms last beyond 6 weeks, often times persisting for many months. Psychogenic factors are thought to precipitate urticaria in 35–65% of cases [21].

Increased mental tension, fatigue, catastrophic events, and stressful life situations are all associated with the onset of symptoms [22].

Psychiatric aspects of treatment. The primary goal of treatment for these patients is the relief of the pruritis. Tricyclic antidepressants, such as doxepin, have been effective in the treatment of chronic urticaria [16]. The efficacy of this class of drugs is related to the potent antihistaminic and anticholinergic properties, and not necessarily to its antidepressant effects. However, recent studies have proven that a greater percentage of patients with chronic urticaria treated with doxepin reported total clearing of pruritis and urticarial lesions versus an antihistamine alone [23]. Once the patient has been free of all symptoms for over a month, the drug can usually be withdrawn gradually. Adjunctive therapies which have been helpful in treating these patients include hypnosis with relaxation, individual and group psychotherapy, and stress management [24].

Lichen planus is an inflammatory keratotic disease that can affect the skin, oral mucosa, or both. Oral lichen planus can have multiple clinical appearances, the most common of which include reticular, papular, plaque-like, atropic, erosive, and bullous. A number of factors relating to emotional stability have been associated with the development of oral lichen planus [25]. Recent studies have confirmed that anxiety may aggravate the clinical manifestations of the disease and patients with lichen planus suffer more anxiety and depression than controls [25]. Patients can often recall a major life stressor, which is considered a major factor in the development and progression, within a few weeks of the appearance of the oral lesions [26]. The stress was most often related to work, relationship problems, and death and illness [26]. It has been hypothesized that these patients are unable to deal effectively with traumatic life events and need help in order to cope with their disease and the underlying psychological issues.

Psychiatric aspects of treatment. A careful history of patients who present with oral lichen planus must be taken, as certain drugs can exacerbate the disease. The elimination of alcohol and tobacco should be encouraged, which may be a factor in some cases [27]. Excess alcohol consumption can lead to feelings of sadness and, by discouraging the usage of it, the patient's depression might also improve. Any anxiety or depression should be addressed, and ways to improve coping mechanisms should be suggested. The dermatologist may want to consider the benefits of stress management and bereavement counseling in these patients. If ineffective, a low-dose antidepressant or anxiolytic may be used; however, if there continues to be no improvement psychologically, the patient should be considered for counseling.

Primary Psychiatric Disease

Cutaneous symptoms are a feature of a wide range of psychiatric disorders. Primary psychiatric disorders are those that are primarily psychiatric in nature, their cause being related to psychopathologic causes in the absence of a primary dermatologic origin. In order to diagnose a psychocutaneous disease of a primary psychiatric origin, organic causes must be excluded. Delusions of parasitosis, dermatitis artefacta, neurotic excoriations, body dysmorphic disorder, and trichotillomania compose the major categories of this group of psychocutaneous diseases. All of the above diagnoses are defined as having an underlying psychological disorder.

Delusions of parasitosis is a disabling psychiatric disorder seen primarily by dermatologists who make the diagnosis. These patients suffer from a strong belief that they are infested with parasites. The belief is so fixed that the patient may pick small pieces of debris from the skin and bring them to the dermatologist to be examined, insisting that there are parasites in the sample. The samples of alleged parasites presented to the dermatologist are often referred to as the "matchbox sign." Cutaneous findings may include excoriations, prurigo nodularis, and ulcerations. A wide variety of psychiatric disorders are associated with delusions of parasitosis, including anxiety, phobias, hypochondriasis, delusional disorder, bipolar disorders, depression, obsessional states, or schizophrenia [28].

Psychiatric aspects of treatment. Because of the complexity of the underlying psychiatric component, treating these patients is difficult. Most of these patients resist suggestions to seek psychiatric help, and thus the dermatologist becomes an important component in treatment. The first steps should be directed at excluding a true infestation, such as scabies, or any other organic cause. A careful and thorough skin evaluation is critical in convincing the patient nonverbally that the complaint is being taken seriously [29]. It is advised not to confront the patient with the possibility of a psychogenic origin of the complaint until a therapeutic alliance is established [29]. Trust must be established first. It is also important to not inadvertently make any statements that might reinforce the patient's delusions. If the patient continues to have no insight into his/her disease and his/her belief in infestation is unshakeable, the patient is considered to have a true delusional disorder and the possibility of introducing a therapeutic trial of pimozide can be sought. Pimozide (Orap) is an antipsychotic medication approved for the treatment of Tourette's syndrome and is also proclaimed as the superior neuroleptic medicine for delusions of parasitosis [28]. The physician should present pimozide to the patient gradually with the idea that the medicine will help the patient decrease his/her agitation and mental preoccupation. Once the patient is successfully started on pimozide, a therapeutic endpoint needs to be defined. It is recommended to taper the medicine once the patient experiences significant decrease in the level of agitation and mental preoccupation. If the dermatologist continues to have little success with the patient, a psychiatric referral should ultimately be made.

Dermatitis artefacta is a disease in which the patient creates skin lesions in order to satisfy an unconscious need to be taken care of. The patient may be aware that he/she is creating the lesions but will typically deny any part in the process when questioned. The lesions are often bizarre looking with sharp, geometric, angulated borders and surrounded by normal looking skin. They are often located on body parts that are easy to reach with the hands. The lesions can present as erythema, edema, blisters, ulcers, purpura, and nodules. Consistent, however, is the hollow history provided by the patient. The patient will be unable to give an exact description of how the lesion started or spread. Also consistent with these patients is the underlying immature personality, with the disease being an appeal for help [30]. In a minority of patients, the lesions may be seen as a transient maladaptive response to a stressor or the result of a dissociative personality disorder [31]. The majority of patients, however, suffer from a borderline personality disorder.

Psychiatric aspects of treatment. Treating these patients is often difficult for the dermatologist. A supportive and empathetic approach is recommended, avoiding direct confrontation with how the lesions evolved. Medical treatment often involves the use of occlusive dressings, emollients, and bland ointments to replace the desire to destroy the skin. The patient should be encouraged to return to the clinic often, whether or not lesions are present, at least once a week, in order to permit a relationship to develop. Once a therapeutic relationship is established, a more insight-oriented approach should be used [30, 32]. The dermatologist's understanding and acceptance may in some cases permit allusion to the true cause or to an eventual psychiatric referral [31]. Antidepressant medication has been effective in times of exacerbation, and occasionally pimozide (Orap) can be taken if the condition remains.

Neurotic excoriations are lesions produced by the patient as a result of repetitive self-excoriation, which may be initiated by an itch, a disturbing sensation in the skin, or a desire to excoriate an irregularity in the skin [33, 34].This initiates and perpetuates the "itch–scratch" cycle, which in some patients becomes a compulsive ritual [33]. The lesions do not stand out as being bizarre or unusual in appearance as do the lesions of dermatitis artefacta. They are typically a few millimeters in diameter, weeping, crusted, or scarred with postinflammatory hypopigmentation or hyperpigmentation [22]. Psychiatrically, the mild cases may be a response to stress in someone with obsessive-compulsive personality traits [31]. In more severe cases, a psychiatric exam will generally reveal an obsessive-compulsive disorder [31]. Picking that results in neurotic excoriations in some patients may be an expression of a generalized anxiety disorder or depression.

Psychiatric aspects of treatment. After excluding other causes of pruritis, the dermatologist should take an empathetic and supportive approach to these patients. It is often observed that the psychiatric interview alone can initiate improvement in some patients [33]. It is important to establish a therapeutic alliance first. Frequent short visits should be scheduled for supervision and support. The patient should first be offered diversion strategies when the urge to scratch occurs. An attempt should be made to identify any stressors that precipitate the onset of excoriating. Various psychiatric treatments which have been effective include behavior modification, cognitive psychotherapy, and psychodynamic psychotherapy [31]. Because of the compulsiveness of the disease and the recognition that serotonin pathways are involved, selective serotonin reuptake inhibitors have been effective in improving the ritualistic behaviors in a majority of patients. Anxiolytics are also helpful when anxiety is a major component. If these interventions do not help, the dermatologist should then consider a psychiatric referral for these patients.

Trichotillomania is defined as a nonscarring alopecia resulting from a compulsion to pluck out one's own hair [35]. The peak onset is in childhood with a female to male ratio of 5:1. The sites involved are the frontal region of the scalp, eyebrows, eyelashes, and the beard. The areas of hair loss are typically linear or bizarrely shaped. Hairs are broken and show differences in length over the area of alopecia. The patients will typically deny having any part in the process. Underlying psychopathology include obsessive-compulsive disorder, depression, and anxiety [36]. Depressive symptoms and an overconcern about body weight have been reported in a significant number of adolescents with this symptom [37].

Psychiatric aspects of treatment. The patients often deny or rationalize the hair-pulling behavior, making it difficult for the dermatologist to treat these patients successfully. In children, one should address the diagnosis openly, and referral to a child psychiatrist or behavioral therapist should be encouraged [38]. Mothers must be educated about the uncontrollable nature of the compulsion and cautioned against the counterproductive effect of forbidding the activity or responding angrily [39].Treatment utilizing behavioral therapy such as thought stopping, aversive conditioning, simple self-monitoring, hypnosis, and relaxation training have all been reported to be effective [40]. Pharmacotherapy with clomipramine (Anafranil), fluoxetine (Prozac), or venlafaxine (Effexor) may be helpful for obsessive-compulsive disorder [38]. If pruritis is a prominent feature, doxepin (Sinequan) may also be useful [39].

Body dysmorphic disorder is a preoccupation with an imagined defect in appearance, often out of proportion to the physical finding. The individual's concern about the symptom is excessive, and this preoccupation results in significant emotional distress. Complaints commonly involve imagined or slight flaws of the face or head, such as spots, large pores, acne, wrinkles, or scars [22]. Vascular markings, scars, paleness, excessive hairiness are also commonly encountered as complaints. The patients often adopt obsessional, repetitive behavior and may spend most of their day checking their perceived imperfections. Their behaviors prevent them from functioning as normal beings, causing significant social and occupational suffering. The underlying psychopathology of these patients includes obsessive-compulsive disorder, depression, bipolar disease, borderline personality disorder, and schizophrenia.

Psychiatric aspects of treatment. The management of this group of patients is often difficult and challenging for the dermatologist. Body dysmorphic disorder can be divided into those patients who are truly deluded (psychotic) and those who have some insight into their behaviors. The truly deluded patients are often angry, which may be turned in on themselves or directed at the physician. Direct confrontation should be avoided because of this anger; rather, a supportive and empathetic approach is advised. In time, patients with body dysmorphic disorder come to trust the doctor who looks after them. Previous trials have indicated that selective serotonin receptor inhibitors (SSRIs) are valuable in many patients with body dysmorphic disorder. The effective dosage of the SSRI medication is often higher than the dosage conventionally used to treat depression; however, not all patients will respond to treatment with SSRIs. Successful treatment with exposure therapy, audiovisual confrontation, and systematic desensitization have been reported in the literature [41]. Encouraging the patient to avoid ritualistic behaviors and exposing the patient to the most feared social situations have also proven useful [41]. Supportive psychotherapy can be helpful in those patients who are not truly deluded. All of these techniques were more effective when combined with SSRIs.

Cutaneous dysesthesia syndrome is a disorder characterized by chronic cutaneous symptoms without any objective findings. Patients complain of burning, stinging, or itching, which is often exacerbated by psychological stress. Examples of chronic cutaneous dysesthesia include the burning mouth syndrome or glossodynia, vulvodynia, scrotodynia, and atypical facial pain. There are two main categories of patients suffering from this disorder: the first consists of patients with an organic etiology and the second consists of patients whose dysesthesia is considered to be of psychogenic origin. The psychological factors that have been associated with this disorder include anxiety, depression, hypochondrial reactions, conversion reactions, tics, masochistic behavior, and cancerophobia [42]. Dysthymic disorder, somatization disorder, generalized anxiety disorder have all been diagnosed in patients with chronic cutaneous dysesthesia.

Psychiatric aspects of treatment. When confronted with a patient complaining of pain in a specific area, local and systemic diseases should be ruled out first. Among those patients who have an underlying anxiety disorder or depression, it is suggested to treat the psychiatric disorder regardless of whether there is a direct connection between the psychiatric findings and their subjective complaints [43]. It is hypothesized that patients who are depressed or anxious perceive the itch and pain sensation in an exaggerated manner, and by treating the mental condition, the physical aspect will be relieved as well [43]. Although there may be no direct connection between the psychological component and the perceived sensations, the dermatologist has a justification to treat the underlying psychopathologies in the hope that at least the perception of the discomfort may be lessened [43]. For those patients who do not have an underlying psychopathology, certain psychotropic medications can be used for their analgesic and antipruritic effects. Several studies have documented the efficacy of low-dose tricyclic antidepressants for treating the sensations of pain, burning, and tingling [44]. Antidepressants may have some analgesic properties and the drug may relieve the depression associated with or caused by chronic sensations and thus improve the symptoms [44]. If the dermatologist suspects that the sensations the patient is describing are hallucinatory, a therapeutic trial of pimozide (Orap) may be justified [43]. Pimozide must be given cautiously and under good supervision. If after 3 months there is no improvement in the symptoms with pimozide, the medication should be stopped and the physician should refer the patient to a psychiatrist.

Secondary Psychiatric Disease

Psychiatric symptoms may appear in patients with primary skin disease in reaction to their cutaneous disfigurement or perceived social stigma. The psychological component is a serious consequence of the skin lesions and can lead to treatment resistance. Emotionally, this can leave the patient with marked impairment in social functioning. Two important dermatologic diseases which can cause severe psychological distress include acne vulgaris and vitiligo.

Acne vulgaris is a common skin disease which occurs because of an inflammation of the pilosebaceous units of certain body areas. It occurs most frequently in adolescence and manifests itself as comedones, papulopustules, or nodules and cysts [3]. Some people have only a few blemishes, whereas others are afflicted with severe, scarring cystic acne. The disease's major complications include physical scarring and psychosocial effects, which may persist long after the active lesions have disappeared [31]. These patients often become anxious, depressed, angry, and humiliated because of the acne. The feelings may lead to social withdrawal and social phobia, poor school performance, irritability, and family conflict [45]. There is an increased risk of depression and suicide in those patients with severe acne. For teenagers who are more vulnerable to the negative psychological effects of acne, even a mild case may be distressing. Acne can and does significantly impact on the patient's psychosocial well-being. Acne patients often have problems with self-esteem, self-confidence, body image, embarrassment, social withdrawal, depression, anger, frustration, difficult family relationships [46].

Psychiatric aspects of treatment. In addition to the standard topical and systemic therapies used to treat acne, the psychological issues that result from the disfigurement need to be discussed. The emotions of acne patients are often neglected which may result in a lack of compliance and discontent with treatment [31]. The physician should not merely regard acne as a "cosmetic problem"; the psychosocial aspects should be addressed as well. A recent study suggested the use of a skin disorder questionnaire to identify those patients who are particularly distressed by their disease, in order to initiate appropriate psychological management [31]. The authors of the study concluded that individually evaluating each questionnaire might give the physician clues about which therapies are considered more promising by the patient, thus increasing his/her compliance [31]. Physicians should encourage their acne patients to become active in educating themselves about the disease, which will increase their self-esteem [45]. By becoming more educated about the disease, these patients are more likely to achieve emotional distance from it [45]. Patients who are more educated also have better coping mechanisms and show less subjective impairment by the acne.

Hull et al. [47] treated patients with minimal facial acne but with severe symptoms of dysmorphobobia and/or depression related to their acne with isotretinoin (Accutane) for 16 weeks and found remarkable improvement in all patients' mental states. They concluded that although this medicine is indicated for those with therapy-resistant nodulocystic acne, it can be another option for those patients with severe depression and anxiety in response to their acne [47].

Vitiligo is a common acquired disorder characterized by patches of depigmentation of the skin. Vitiligo is characterized by complete or partial pigment loss on skin areas that increase in size over time. The patches can be local or generalized. Vitiligo can affect all races, skin types, ethnicities, and present in any age group. The disease is most disfiguring in those of a darker racial and ethnic group because of the contrast between depigmented and normal skin color. Although vitiligo is neither painful nor physically limiting, it can have a severe negative psychosocial impact on the patient's functioning. The cosmetic disfigurement is in itself a very difficult and stigmatizing condition. In a society obsessed with appearances, patients are often embarrassed and traumatized [48]. Patients with this disorder experience low self-esteem, job discrimination, and social phobias. Recent studies document that at least two-thirds of patients with vitiligo significantly underachieve their potential due to the psychological difficulties resulting from the disfigurement [49]. Patients also report feelings of depression and rejection by those around them.

Psychiatric aspects of treatment. Vitiligo remains a therapeutically challenging disease to treat. It is one of the most psychologically devastating diseases in dermatology. The treatment of vitiligo requires both dermatologic and psychological interventions. In addition to the standard medical treatment for vitiligo, it is also important to individually assess the effects of the disorder from the patient's point of view. Effective management depends on recognizing the emotional factors that are involved and attempting to cover or blend in the defect. The patient should be informed about the option for cosmetic camouflage and can be referred to a camouflage expert for advice [49]. Camouflage therapists are trained to help patients achieve a healthy self-image, accept their appearance, and be less self-conscious around others [49]. Cognitive-behavioral therapy has also proven to be beneficial in terms of coping and living with vitiligo [50]. Those patients who continue to be emotionally stressed after these interventions should be referred for more intense counseling.

The crossover between psychiatry and dermatology is broad and multifactorial [51–54]. Interactions at all levels, whether it be the physical signs or the social impact of a disfiguring skin disease, are clinically relevant and need to be addressed [55–58]. Psychosomatic dermatologic patients should first be treated by the dermatologist, unless a serious psychiatric illness is present. A variety of psychotropic medications can be used to treat psychocutaneous disorders, which the dermatologist should become familiar with. If a therapeutic trial of medication and various psychological approaches continue to be ineffective, the dermatologist should then think about referral to a psychiatrist.

References

1. Panconesi E, Hautmann G. Psychophysiology of stress in dermatology. Dermatol. Clin. 1996; 14(3): 399–420.
2. Koblenzer CS. Psychosomatic concepts in dermatology. Arch. Dermatol. 1983; 119: 501–12.
3. Fitzpatrick TB, Johnson RA, Wolff K. Color Atlas and Synopsis of Clinical Dermatology. New York: McGraw-Hill, 2001, pp. 50–60.
4. Gupta MA, Gupta AK, Haberman HF. Psoriasis and psychiatry: an update. Gen. Hosp. Psychiatry 1987; 9: 157–66.
5. Arnetz BB, et al. Stress and psoriasis. Psychoendocrine and metabolic reactions in psoriatic patients during standardized stressor exposure. Psychosom. Med. 1985; 47: 528–41.
6. Koo J. Population-based epidemiologic study of psoriasis with emphasis on quality of life assessment. Dermatol. Clin. 1996: 14(3): 485–96.

7. Gupta MA, Gupta AK, Kirkby S, et al. Pruritis in psoriasis: a prospective study of some psychiatric and dermatologic correlates. Arch. Dermatol. 1988; 124: 1052–7.
8. Gupta MA, Gupta AK, Kirkby S, et al. A psychocutaneous profile of psoriasis patients who are stress reactors: a study of 17 patients. Gen. Hosp. Psychiatry 1989; 11: 166–73.
9. Ginsburg IH. Coping with psoriasis: a guide for counseling patients. Cutis 1996; 57: 323–30.
10. Ginsburg IH. Psychological and psychophysiological aspects of psoriasis. Dermatol. Clin. 1995; 13: 793–99.
11. Tausk F, Whitmore SE. A pilot study of hypnosis in the treatment of patients with psoriasis. Psychother. Psychosom. 1991; 68: 221–9.
12. Gupta MA, et al. Depression modulates pruritis perception: a study of pruritis in psoriasis, atopic dermatitis, and chronic idiopathic urticaria. Psychosom. Med. 1994; 56: 36–40.
13. Ullman KC, Moore RW, Redi M. Atopic eczema: a clinical psychiatric study. J. Asthma Res. 1977; 14: 91–9.
14. Kirshbaum BA. Eczema and Emotions. Kalamazoo, MI: Upjohn Company, 1982, pp. 35–55.
15. Jordan JM, Whitlock FA. Emotions and the skin: the conditioning of scratch responses in cases of atopic dermatitis. Br. J. Dermatol. 1972; 86: 574–85.
16. Gupta MA, Gupta AK, Ellis CN. Antidepressant drugs in dermatology. Arch. Dermatol. 1987; 123: 647–52.
17. Muller SA, Winkelman RK. Alopecia areata: an evaluation of 736 patients. Arch. Dermatol. 1963; 88: 290–7.
18. Koo JY, et al. Alopecia areata and increased prevalence of psychiatric disorders. Int. J. Dermatol. 1994; 33: 849–50.
19. MacAlpine I. Is alopecia areata psychosomatic? A psychiatric study. Br. J. Dermatol. 1958; 70: 117–31.
20. Perini G, et al. Imipramine in alopecia areata: a double blind, placebo-controlled study. Psychother. Psychosom. 1994; 61: 195–8.
21. Warin RP, Champion RH. Urticaria. Philadelphia: WB Saunders, 1974.
22. Gupta MA, Gupta AK. Psychodermatology: an update. J. Am. Acad. Dermatol. 1996; 124(6): 1030–46.
23. Greene SL, Reed CE, Schroeter AL. Double blind crossover study comparing doxepin with diphenhydramine for the treatment of chronic urticaria. J. Am. Acad. Dermatol. 1985; 12: 669–75.
24. Shertzer CL, Lookingbill DP. Effects of relaxation therapy and hypnotizability in chronic urticaria. Arch. Dermatol. 1987; 123: 913–6.
25. Garcia-Pola Vallejo MJ, Huerta G, Cerero R. Anxiety and depression as risk factors for oral lichen planus. Dermatology 2001; 203: 303–7.
26. Burkhart NW, et al. Assessing the characteristics of patients with oral lichen planus. J. Am. Acad. Dermatol. 1996; 127: 648–60.
27. Conklin RJ, Blasberg B. Oral lichen planus. Dermatol. Clin. 1987; 5(4): 663–72.
28. Zanol K, Slaughter J, Hall R. An approach to the treatment of psychogenic parasitosis. Int. J. Dermatol. 1998; 37: 56–63.
29. Koo J, Gambla C. Psychopharmacology for dermatologic patients. Dermatol. Clin. 1996; 14(3): 500–22.
30. Fabisch W. Psychiatric aspects of dermatitis artefacta. Br. J. Dermatol. l980; 102: 29–34.
31. Niemeier V, et al. Coping with acne vulgaris. Dermatology 1996: 196: 108–15.
32. Fabisch W. What is dermatitis artefacta? Int. J. Dermatol. 1981; 20: 427–8.
33. Freunsgaard K. Neurotic excoriations: a controlled psychiatric examination. Acta Psychiatr. Scand. 1984; 69(S): 1–52.
34. Seitz PFD. Psychocutaneous aspects of persistent pruritis and excessive excoriation. Arch. Dermatol. Syphiligr. 1951; 64: 136–41.
35. Obermayer ME. Psychocutaneous medicine. Springfield, IL: Charles C. Thomas, 1955.
36. Oguchi T, Miura S. Trichotillomania: its psychopathological aspect. Compr. Psychiatry 1977; 18: 177–82.

37. Greenberg R, Sarner CA. Trichotillomania: symptom and syndrome. Arch. Gen. Psychiatry 1965; 12: 482–9.
38. Odom RB, James WD, Berger TG. Psychodermatology. Andrews Diseases of the Skin. Philadelphia: WB Saunders, 2000, pp. 59–63.
39. Koblenzer CS. Cutaneous manifestations of psychiatric disease that commonly present to the dermatologist. *Int. J. Psychiatry Med.* 1992; 22(1): 47–63.
40. Gupta MA, Gupta AK, Haberman HF. The self-inflicted dermatoses: a critical review. Gen. Hosp. Psychiatry 1987; 9: 45–52.
41. Cotterill JA. Body dysmorphic disorder. Dermatol. Clin. 1996; 14(3): 457–7.
42. Trikkas G, et al. Glossodynia. Personality characteristics and psychopathology. Psychother. Psychosom. 1996; 65: 158–62.
43. Koo J, Gambla C. Cutaneous sensory disorder. Dermatol. Clin. 1996; 14(3): 497–502.
44. Hoss D, Segal S. Scalp dysesthesia. Arch. Dermatol. 1998; 134: 327–30.
45. Ginsburg IH. The psychosocial impact of skin disease. Dermatol. Clin. 1996; 14(3): 473–84.
46. Koo J. The psychosocial impact of acne: patients' perceptions. J. Am. Acad. Dermatol. 1995; 32: S26–30.
47. Hull SM, Cunliffe WJ, Hughes BR. Treatment of the depressed and dysmorphobic acne patient. Clin. Exp. Dermatol. 1991; 16: 210–1.
48. Grimes PE. White patches and bruised souls: advances in the pathogenesis and treatment of vitiligo. J. Am. Acad. Dermatol. 2004; 51(1): S5–6.
49. Mason PJ. Vitiligo. The psychosocial effects. Medsurg. Nurs. 1997; 6: 216–22.
50. Papadopoulos L, Bor R, Legg C. Coping with the disfiguring effects of vitiligo: a preliminary investigation into the effects of cognitive-behavioral therapy. Br. J. Med. Psychol. 1999; 72: 385–96.
51. Rook A, Wilkinson DS. Psychocutaneous disorders. Textbook of Dermatology. Oxford: Blackwell, 1979, pp. 2023–35.
52. Medansky RS, Handler RM. Dermatopsychosomatics. Classification, physiology, and therapeutic approaches. J. Am. Acad. Dermatol. 1981; 5: 125–36.
53. Gupta MA, Voorhees JJ. Psychosomatic dermatology: is it relevant? Arch. Dermatol. 1990; 126: 90–3.
54. Jowett S, Ryan T. Skin disease and handicap: an analysis of the impact of skin conditions. Soc. Sci. Med. 1985; 20: 425–9.
55. Ostlere LS, Hardy D, Denton C, et al. Boxing glove hand: an unusual presentation of dermatitis artefacta. J. Am. Acad. Dermatol. 1993; 28: 120–2.
56. Perry HO, Brunsting LA. Pemphigus foliaceus. Arch. Dermatol. 1965; 91: 10–23.
57. Gupta MA, Gupta AK, Haberman HF. Dermatologic signs in anorexia nervosa and bulimia nervosa. Arch. Dermatol. 1987; 123: 1386–90.
58. Koblenzer CS, Bostrom P. Chronic cutaneous dysesthesia syndrome: a psychotic phenomenon or a depressive symptom? J. Am. Acad. Dermatol. 1994; 30: 370–4.

Chapter 18

Common Vascular Disorders in the Elderly

Athena Theodosatos

Vascular changes that occur with aging are associated with a range of disorders. These vascular disorders affect millions of people in the United States annually, with the majority of patients being over the age of 50 [1]. As the population ages, physicians are faced with an increasing number of patients with these disorders, which include, but are not limited to, venous ulcers, arterial ulcers, diabetic ulcers, varicose ulcers, and varicose veins [2]. Some diseases that can lead to vascular disorders include: erosive pustular dermatosis and squamous cell cancer [3]. Proper education on risk factors and prevention measures associated with the formation of various ulcers can decrease the development of these disorders and complications seen when appropriate treatment is not prescribed [2, 3].

Introduction

Venous insufficiency is the most common cause of leg ulcers, followed by mixed venous and arterial disease [1]. Compression therapy allows previously incompetent valves to regain competency, increasing blood flow in the right direction, and reducing the risk of ulcer development. The financial, social, and psychological costs associated with leg ulcers are increasing at a rapid rate [1, 2]. This chapter reviews commonly encountered vascular disorders and describes some of the structural and functional changes that occur in our vascular system during the process of aging.

Structural and Functional Changes

With age, arterial compliance decreases and arterial wall stiffness increases [4]. This finding helps explain why many elderly individuals develop an increase in systolic blood pressure, often leading to the development of hypertension. As blood vessels increase in diameter and thickness they are able to compensate for decreases in blood flow, but other changes also occur, such as blood leakage from the vessels causing vascular insufficiency and edema [4]. Collagen and smooth muscle cells accumulate in the subendothelial space causing the surrounding area to thicken and

R.A. Norman (ed.), *Diagnosis of Aging Skin Diseases,*
© Springer-Verlag London Limited 2008

compromise tissue perfusion leading to the development of pain, skin color changes, and eventually ulceration [4]. Aging is also associated with a decrease in relaxation of the endothelium [4]. Endothelial cells normally produce relaxing factors, such as nitric oxide and prostacyclin, but these compounds are reduced as we age [4]. The decrease in these factors along with other compound changes also contributes to the development of vascular disorders.

Venous Ulcers

Leg ulcers are becoming a severe problem in the United States, with about 600,000 new cases per year [5]. Recent literature reports that 81% of patients with venous stasis ulcers experience decreased mobility, and 57% report that their mobility is severely limited [6]. Also, 68% were reported to have a negative emotional impact on their lives as a result of the ulcers [6]. The etiologic causes are usually linked to venous or arterial insufficiencies [5, 6]. Venous insufficiency is a dysfunction of the venous system that causes high venous pressure in the legs. It develops when there is incompetence of the venous valves leading to an increase in pressure in the superficial venous system [4]. Normally, blood flows from the superficial system to the deep, which lowers pressure and allows continued competency of the venous valves [2–6]. Eventually, the increased pressure causes the veins to elongate and dilate which prevents proper circulation [2–6]. Characteristics of venous insufficiency ulcers on the skin include: reddish-brown color, shallow depth, irregular margins, and minimal pain [2–6]. Sometimes, clinical findings from a physical exam are not conclusive and other studies such as ultrasound testing for venous reflux may be necessary. The majority of leg ulcers develop from high venous pressure in the legs. Other causes of venous insufficiency include outflow obstruction and thrombosis [2–6]. Burn scars and chronic infections are some of the other predisposing factors for their development. Case reports have shown that venous leg ulcers are more common in women and the rate increases with advancing age [6]. Even though venous ulcers are rarely fatal, they frequently result in repeated hospitalizations costing a great deal of money, and an increased morbidity [2–6]. Long-term treatment success may be achieved, and quality of life may be improved by determining the exact cause of the ulcer and providing the appropriate treatment for the patient. Standard venous ulcer treatment involves elevation of the leg, compression therapy, and topical therapy to absorb the exudate and maintain a moist wound environment [7]. Sometimes it may be necessary to surgically debride the ulcerated tissue. The removal of the necrotic tissue will allow granulation and epithelialization to occur and it will also decrease the chances of bacterial infection [7]. Compression with the Unna boot or with elastic bandages is another mode for decreasing pressure in areas where there are distended veins [7]. It is important to apply the bandages while the patient is supine and when their foot is dorsiflexed [7]. Although there are many noninvasive ways to treat ulcers successfully, sometimes minimally invasive vein surgery may be necessary to increase recovery time and decrease other complications associated with wound infections and limited mobility [7, 8]. Examples of these surgeries include: mechanical ablation of enlarged veins and endoscopic incompetent vein ligation [7, 8]. These procedures are considered to have minimal postoperative pain and the majority of patients are able to return to their daily activities within a couple of days [8]. Some of the complications that can develop when treatment is delayed include: gait changes, leg pain, and infection [7, 8]. Gait changes can be prevented with mild to moderate exercise of the calf muscles [7, 8]. If an infection is suspected, tissue sampling and curettage of the base of the ulcer should be performed [8]. Broad-spectrum antibiotics can be prescribed until the specific organism is identified [8]. Generally, oral antibiotics are given but if the infection persists, parenteral antibiotics may be needed. General prevention measures aim at keeping the lower extremities clean and dry, controlling glucose levels, not standing for long periods of time, and wearing support stockings when necessary [6–8]. Proper understanding of how various ulcers present will help healthcare practitioners identify and treat the ulcers earlier.

Arterial insufficiency causes only about 5–10% of leg ulcers. The causes of arterial insufficiency include atherosclerosis and vasculitis [1]. These causes are common in people with medical conditions such as, hypertension, diabetes, and other circulatory diseases [1–3]. Arterial ulcer lesions occur more frequently over bony prominences and they gradually increase in size [3]. Leg ulcers caused by arterial insufficiencies are much more painful than those caused by venous insufficiency, and elevation of the ulcerated leg tends to make the symptoms worse [1–3].

Erosive pustular dermatosis of the leg is a rare disorder that can affect the lower limbs of elderly patients that present with chronic venous insufficiency or stasis dermatitis [3]. Clinical features of the disease include pustule formation and moist eroded lesions on the leg [3].

Squamous cell carcinomas are also known to cause leg ulcers, especially in the elderly patients with poor general health [3, 7]. Ulcers that are unresponsive to therapy for 3 months or more are highly suspicious of malignancy [3, 6, 7, 9]. A simple biopsy can also be performed in office to determine if the ulcer is malignant [3, 6–9]. Regular physical exams are necessary to determine if any changes are occurring that may lead to ulcer formation.

Diabetic Foot Ulcers

Over 16 million people are estimated to be in the United States with diabetes and approximately 15% of those diabetics develop foot ulcers at some time in their life [10]. Ulcers are chronic wounds that need aggressive treatment in order to heal properly. Diabetic ulcers are currently the most common cause of nontraumatic lower extremity amputations in the United States [10, 11]. There are many components involved in the development of diabetic ulcers. The most common risk factors for ulcer formation include: peripheral neuropathy, foot deformities, and peripheral arterial occlusive disease [10, 11]. Diabetic nerve damage affects the motor, sensory, and autonomic pathways, causing muscle weakness, atrophy, loss of sensation, and loss of skin integrity, which can lead to microbial infections [10–12]. Foot deformities can develop from calluses, ingrown toenails, and poor fitting footwear [10–12]. Arterial occlusion usually involves the tibial and peroneal arteries and it can be exacerbated by smoking, hypertension, and hyperlipidemia [10–12].

Diabetic patients exhibit impaired wound healing and increased susceptibility to infection; therefore early intervention is critical to successful treatment of the ulcers [13]. Persistent ulcers suggest underlying infection and require cultures and broad-spectrum antibiotics until the cultures are identified [12, 13]. Ulcerated feet are one of the leading causes of hospitalization in diabetic patients; therefore it is important to thoroughly evaluate the feet of diabetic patients at every office visit [12]. The physical exam should focus on any changes in the skin and special attention should be given to the lower extremities. If an ulcer is noted on exam its characteristics should be described by size, depth, appearance, and location [12]. There are several classification systems for diabetic foot ulcers, but the Wagner Ulcer Classification System, modified by Brodsky, is the most widely used [10]. This system classifies the ulcer based on depth and the presence and extent of ischemia. The stage of the ulcer is indicative of prognosis and it indicates what mode of treatment may be necessary. Diabetic ulcers are best managed and treated by a multidisciplinary team [13]. These teams or programs should focus on prevention, education, regular foot exams, and early aggressive treatment to prevent complications. One of the main goals of treatment is to obtain wound closure [12, 13]. The various modes of treatment should be employed in a systematic manner. For example, once an ulcer has been detected, the affected foot should be elevated to relieve pressure and footwear should be replaced with pressure relieving footwear. Sometimes crutches or a wheelchair may be needed and other times removable walking braces are used [12–14]. The next step should be debridement, because nonviable, infected tissues do not allow for new tissue to form and they exacerbate the ulcer allowing them to extend further [12–14]. The wound should be kept moist to enhance epidermal migration across the wound. If the ulcer shows signs of local or systemic infection, antibiotics should be prescribed and bacterial cultures should be obtained [12–14]. Topical antibiotics are generally used for the superficial infections, although they are not always effective if used alone. Underlying ischemia must also be treated for successful results [14]. Minor trauma from stress to the foot and increased shoe pressure are pathways leading to ulceration [14]. One way to decrease the increased pressure involves the use of total contrast casting [12, 14]. This type of cast molds to the foot and redistributes weight away from the ulcer sites. The problem with this type of treatment is that daily wound inspection is not possible and if the cast is not properly applied, the ulcers will worsen [12, 14]. One way to gauge effective treatment is to measure the wound length and width at least once a week and document it, instead of using subjective statements, such as "the wound looks like it's getting better [13, 15]." The best approach in multidisciplinary teams is prevention along with patient education. Patient education on good foot hygiene and proper footwear help prevent new ulcers from developing. Regular foot care exams are especially important, since the majority of elderly patients rely on healthcare professionals for routine foot care [3]. Diabetic foot ulcers account for billions of dollars in medical expenditures each year therefore, early recognition of risk factors is important, along with routine foot exams [11, 12].

Varicose Ulcers

Varicose ulcers develop when veins in the legs dilate causing problems with valve function [16]. The valves either cease to function or they partially close, allowing backflow of blood to pool in the lower extremities [16]. Varicose ulcers usually develop on the outer areas of the lower extremities, particularly the ankle area [17]. The ulcers can swell and develop a scaly, pruritic area around the border but they are noted to have minimal pain. These ulcers tend to last for several months to several years [16, 17]. The etiology of the varicose ulcer was first recognized and described by John Homans in 1917 [16]. He recognized the significance of the perforator veins of the leg, playing a major part in the postphlebitic syndrome and ulcer formation. During his time imaging studies were not yet available. As a result, Homan diagnosed varicose veins by using techniques such as the Trendelenburg test, which enabled observation of rapid refill through the surface vessels [16]. He also used the constriction test, which blocked proximal veins. Distal filling time was measured to determine incompetence of the perforator veins [16]. Homan also described the various categories of advance venous disease and many of his points are still accepted today [16]. Treatment of the varicose ulcers may involve excision of the simple varicose veins down to the ulcer [15–17]. Complicated cases may need a more radical procedure, like complete groin dissection of the saphenous vein and stripping in the thigh to get down to the ulcer, so it can be excised [15–17].

Varicose Veins

Varicose veins are a common problem in many individuals. The challenge of correcting the problem is being able to conservatively treat the veins in a cosmetically acceptable manner versus preventing recurrence and complications [18]. Clinical presentation varies from person to person, with ranges causing no pain or mild localized pain to widespread symptoms affecting the entire leg causing fatigue, aching, and swelling. Varicose veins are either associated with primary valve degeneration from superficial venous insufficiency or secondary varicose veins can develop from chronic deep venous insufficiency [18]. Complications, such as phlebitis or bleeding can occur if there is trauma or prolonged standing. In order to properly treat a patient, one must take a precise history and physical exam. Sometimes a patient may describe musculoskeletal symptoms with their varicose veins; if this occurs, treatment will not be very effective if both problems are not addressed and treated [18]. Important risk factors for developing these unsightly veins include: increased age, female gender, multiple pregnancies, and positive family history.

Conservative management should be considered for elderly patients that may not tolerate invasive treatment measures [16, 18]. First-line conservative management involves compression stockings, which are inexpensive and risk free. Successful management involves addressing the etiology of the underlying venous hypertension causing the varicosities [16, 18]. Chronic venous insufficiency is treated well with surgical stripping of the saphenous vein [17]. One drawback to the stripping procedure is the ability to damage the saphenous nerve during the stripping procedure. Other methods of invasive treatment involve minimally invasive techniques, which involve dissection of the saphenofemoral junction, laser therapy, and stab avulsion of the symptomatic varicose vein [17, 18].

Conclusion

Vascular disorders are increasing at a rapid rate, especially in the elderly population [6]. Costs involved with treatment are enormous; they not only involve financial costs but also affect social and psychological factors [5,6]. The changes that occur in our vascular system as we age contribute to the development of a variety of disorders commonly seen in healthcare facilities everyday [2]. With proper education of the risk factors and prevention methods associated with many of the common vascular disorders, we can effectively decrease the amount of ulcers and other vascular problems seen in many elderly individuals [2–6].

References

1. Rojas AI, Bello YM, Phillips TJ. Leg ulcers: diagnostic approach and management. 2001; 10: 129–42.
2. Paquette D, Falanga V. Leg Ulcers. Clin. Geriatr. Med. 2002; 18: 1.
3. Theodosat A. Skin diseases of the lower extremities in the elderly. Dermatol. Clin. North Am. 2004; 22: 13–21.
4. Ciocon J, Nemade S, Galindo D. Common and challenging vascular disorders in the elderly. Clin. Geriatr. 1999; 7: 3.
5. De Sanctis JT. Percutaneous interventions for lower extremity peripheral vascular disease. Am. Fam. Phys. 2001; 64: 12.
6. Margolis DJ, Bilker W, et al. Venous leg ulcer: incidence and prevalence in the elderly. J. Am. Acad. Dermatol. 2002; 46: 3.
7. Brem H, Kirsner RS, Falanga V. Protocol for the successful treatment of venous ulcers. Am. J. Surg. 2004; 188: 1.
8. Elias SM, Frasier KL. Minimally invasive vein surgery: its role in treatment of venous stasis ulceration. Am. J. Surg. 2004; 188: 1.
9. Hill DP, Poore S, Wilson J, et al. Initial healing rates of venous ulcers: are they useful as predictors of healing? Am. J. Surg. 2004; 188: 1.
10. Pinzur MS, et al. Diabetic foot. Available: www.emedicine.com. Accessed 7/13/2005.
11. Armstrong DG, Lavery LA. Diabetic foot ulcers: prevention, diagnosis and classification. Am. Fam. Phys. 1998; 57: 6.
12. Frykberg RG. Diabetic foot ulcers: pathogenesis and management. 2002; 66: 9.

13. Gottrup F. A specialized wound-healing center concept: importance of a multidisciplinary department structure and surgical treatment facilities in the treatment of chronic wounds. Am. J. Surg. 2004; 187: 5.
14. Brem H, Sheehan P, Boulton AJ. Protocol for treatment of diabetic foot ulcers. Am. J. Surg. 2004; 187: 5.
15. Mostow EN. Wound healing: a multidisciplinary approach for dermatologists 2003; 21: 2.
16. Kistner RL. Etiology and treatment of varicose ulcers of the leg. J. Am. Coll. Surg. 2005; 200: 5.
17. Valencia IC, Falabella D, et al. Chronic venous insufficiency and venous leg ulceration. J. Am. Acad. Dermatol. 2001; 44: 401–21.
18. Teruya TH, Ballard JL. New approaches for the treatment of varicose veins. Surg. Clin. North Am. 2004; 84: 5.

Chapter 19

Pressure Ulcers

Cynthia A. Fleck

Pressure ulcers are one of the largest dilemmas facing long-term care providers and clinicians who care for geriatric patients. Two-thirds of pressure sores occur in patients older than 70 years of age [1]. Pressure ulcer prevalence is estimated to be around 15% in acute care, up to 28% in long-term care and up to 29% in home care [2]. Pressure ulcers account for $2.2–3.6 billion/year in expenditures [3], can cost up to $70,000 to treat [4] and kill 60,000 people in the US every year [5]. Patients inclined to pressure ulcers are at higher risk of morbidity and mortality with infection, osteomyelitis and sepsis being the most common major complications.

The term *pressure ulcer* is somewhat of a misnomer since pressure is only part of the problem. Other terms such as bedsore, pressure sore or decubitus ulcer are often used interchangeably in the medical community. Decubitus comes from the Latin *decumbere*, meaning "to lie down." Hence, "decubitus" does not adequately describe the breakdown or ulceration that can occur from other positions such as sitting, which can cause ischial tuberosity (sitting bones) ulcers. Pressure ulcers are any lesions caused by unrelieved pressure resulting in damage of underlying tissue (National Pressure Ulcer Advisory Panel, available at http://www.npuap.org).

Pressure ulcers have affected us for ages. Yet, dealing with the general management of pressure ulcers has only just begun to gain notoriety among national and worldwide healthcare concerns. In spite of present attention and development in the areas of medicine, surgery, nursing care, physical therapy and self-care education, pressure ulcers continue to be a major source of morbidity and mortality. This is especially true for our elders and for those with impaired sensation and prolonged immobility [6].

It is theorized that pressure ulcers are caused by localized pressure or shear forces that lead to ischemia and cell death, thus causing skin and tissue breakdown. Pressure is equal to force, divided by area. So the greater the surface area of the load, the less the pressure exerted. For instance, a sitting individual is at higher risk of developing a pressure ulcer than a person who is lying supine. Kosiak proved that tissue compression and ischemia can lead to tissue destruction and pressure ulcer formation. He also showed that the amount of pressure and the duration of the pressure are inversely proportional [7]. For instance, low amounts of pressure over longer periods of time can be just as detrimental as high pressure for shorter times.

R.A. Norman (ed.), *Diagnosis of Aging Skin Diseases,*
© Springer-Verlag London Limited 2008

Pathophysiology

Many factors contribute to the development of pressure ulcers, but pressure leading to ischemia and necrosis is the final shared path. Pressure is exerted on the skin, soft tissue, muscle, underlying tissue and bone by the weight of an individual against the contacting surface. These pressures often are in excess of capillary-filling pressure, thought to be approximately 32 mmHg [8] although this number is rather random, given the wide variations of weight, age and other issues and that these early studies were performed on young college-aged men. Tissues are capable of withstanding enormous pressures when brief in duration, but prolonged exposure to pressures just slightly above capillary-filling pressure initiates a series of events potentially leading to tissue necrosis and ulceration. The provocative event is compression or deformation of the tissues (due to shear forces) against an external object such as a mattress, shoe, wheelchair, bed rail or other surfaces.

Shear forces and friction aggravate the effects of pressure and are important components of the mechanism of injury. Many sores that we term "pressure ulcers" are actually shear-induced ulcers. In addition, maceration may occur in the incontinent patient, predisposing the skin to injury by decreasing its tensile strength. Pressure, shear and friction cause microcirculatory occlusion resulting in ischemia, which leads to inflammation and tissue anoxia. Tissue anoxia can then lead to cell death, necrosis and ulceration. Irreversible changes may occur during as little as 2 h of uninterrupted pressure depending on the individual's risk and co-morbidities [9]. Reswick and Rogers [10] suggested the routine of turning patients every two hours which continues to be a foundation of preventing pressure ulcers.

Healthy individuals with normal sensation, mobility and mental faculty usually do not succumb to pressure ulcers. Feedback, both conscious and unconscious, from the areas of compression leads us to change our position. We constantly make micro-movements to compensate. This shifts the pressure from one area to another prior to any irreversible ischemic damage to the tissues. Weight shifting for insensate or those individuals with poor mobility should take place every 15 min in the seated person and at least every 2 h in the recumbent individual [11].

Individuals with decreased mobility or sensation or those who are unable to avoid long periods of uninterrupted pressure are at increased risk for developing necrosis and ulceration. This group of patients typically includes the elderly, the neurologically impaired, the chronically ill, those with altered mental status, those with decreased sensation and/or paralysis and patients hospitalized or institutionalized with acute or chronic illness.

Causes

Although prolonged, uninterrupted pressure is the main cause of pressure ulcers, impaired mobility is probably the most common reason patients are exposed to unrelieved pressure. This is common in those who are neurologically impaired, heavily sedated or anesthetized, restrained, demented or those suffering traumatic injury such as a pelvic or femur fracture. These patients are incapable of assuming the responsibility of altering their position to relieve pressure. Moreover, this immobility, if prolonged, leads to muscle and soft tissue atrophy, decreasing the bulk over which bony prominences are supported, further increasing the risk of developing a pressure ulcer.

History

When initially evaluating a patient with pressure ulceration, it is important to note the following information from the history:

- Overall physical and mental health

  - Concurrent diseases and/or disabilities

- Prior hospitalizations, operations or wounds
- Diet

  - Recent weight changes
  - Food avoidances

- Bowel and bladder habits

  - Continence status

- Presence of spasticity or flexion contractures
- Medications and allergies
- Tobacco, alcohol and recreational drug use
- Place of residence
- Any paralysis or breeches in sensation
- Support surface used in bed or while sitting
- Level of independence, mobility and ability to comprehend and cooperate with care
- Underlying social and financial support structure
- Presence of specific cultural, religious or ethnic issues
- Presence of advanced directives, power of attorney or specific preferences regarding care
- Presence of signs or symptoms related to the current ulceration

  - Pain
  - Fever
  - Exudate
  - Odor

- History of the present ulcer

  - Length of time the ulcer has been present
  - Treatments attempted in the past

Where Do Pressure Ulcers Occur?

Generally, pressure ulcers occur over bony prominences like the heels, sacrum, ischial tuberosities (sitting bones) or the greater trochanters (hip bones). In adults, many are concentrated in and around the pelvis due to its bony structure and posture issues, both sitting and reclining. Heels present a big challenge since pressure, coupled with other co-morbid states such as arterial disease and/or diabetes mellitus, can further complicate treatment and increase risk. The frail elderly [12] and the very young [13] are at greater risk for development of pressure ulcers.

Risk Assessment

A risk assessment tool is helpful to identify risk factors and alert the clinical team of increased pressure ulcer risk. The Braden Scale for predicting pressure ulcer risk and the Norton Scale are two of the most common risk assessment tools [14]. Both are valid and reliable.

BRADEN SCALE FOR PREDICTING PRESSURE SORE RISK

Patient's Name _____ Evaluator* _____

SENSORY PERCEPTION ability to respond meaningfully to pressure-related discomfort	**1. Completely Limited** Unresponsive (does not moan, flinch, or grasp) to painful stimuli, due to diminished level of con-sciousness or sedation. OR limited ability to feel pain over most of body	**2. Very Limited** Responds only to painful stimuli. Cannot communicate discomfort except by moaning or restlessness OR has a sensory impairment which limits the ability to feel pain or discomfort over ½ of body.	**3. Slightly Limited** Responds to verbal commands, but cannot always communicate discomfort or the need to be turned. OR has some sensory impairment which limits ability to feel pain or discomfort in 1 or 2 extremities.	**4. No Impairment** Responds to verbal commands. Has no sensory deficit which would limit ability to feel or voice pain or discomfort..			
MOISTURE degree to which skin is exposed to moisture	**1. Constantly Moist** Skin is kept moist almost constantly by perspiration, urine, etc. Dampness is detected every time patient is moved or turned.	**2. Very Moist** Skin is often, but not always moist. Linen must be changed at least once a shift.	**3. Occasionally Moist:** Skin is occasionally moist, requiring an extra linen change approximately once a day.	**4. Rarely Moist** Skin is usually dry, linen only requires changing at routine intervals.			
ACTIVITY degree of physical activity	**1. Bedfast** Confined to bed.	**2. Chairfast** Ability to walk severely limited or non-existent. Cannot bear own weight and/or must be assisted into chair or wheelchair.	**3. Walks Occasionally** Walks occasionally during day, but for very short distances, with or without assistance. Spends majority of each shift in bed or chair	**4. Walks Frequently** Walks outside room at least twice a day and inside room at least once every two hours during waking hours			
MOBILITY ability to change and control body position	**1. Completely Immobile** Does not make even slight changes in body or extremity position without assistance	**2. Very Limited** Makes occasional slight changes in body or extremity position but unable to make frequent or significant changes independently.	**3. Slightly Limited** Makes frequent though slight changes in body or extremity position independently.	**4. No Limitation** Makes major and frequent changes in position without assistance.			
NUTRITION usual food intake pattern	**1. Very Poor** Never eats a complete meal. Rarely eats more than ⅓ of any food offered. Eats 2 servings or less of protein (meat or dairy products) per day. Takes fluids poorly. Does not take a liquid dietary supplement OR is NPO and/or maintained on clear liquids or IV's for more than 5 days.	**2. Probably Inadequate** Rarely eats a complete meal and generally eats only about ½ of any food offered. Protein intake includes only 3 servings of meat or dairy products per day. Occasionally will take a dietary supplement. OR receives less than optimum amount of liquid diet or tube feeding	**3. Adequate** Eats over half of most meals. Eats a total of 4 servings of protein (meat, dairy products per day. Occasionally will refuse a meal, but will usually take a supplement when offered OR is on a tube feeding or TPN regimen which probably meets most of nutritional needs	**4. Excellent** Eats most of every meal. Never refuses a meal. Usually eats a total of 4 or more servings of meat and dairy products. Occasionally eats between meals. Does not require supplementation.			
FRICTION & SHEAR	**1. Problem** Requires moderate to maximum assistance in moving. Complete lifting without sliding against sheets is impossible. Frequently slides down in bed or chair, requiring frequent repositioning with maximum assistance. Spasticity, contractures or agitation leads to almost constant friction	**2. Potential Problem** Moves feebly or requires minimum assistance. During a move skin probably slides to some extent against sheets, chair, restraints or other devices. Maintains relatively good position in chair or bed most of the time but occasionally slides down.	**3. No Apparent Problem** Moves in bed and in chair independently and has sufficient muscle strength to lift up completely during move. Maintains good position in bed or chair.				
				Total Score			

Fig. 19.1 The Braden Scale. © Barbara Braden and Nancy Bergstrom, 1988. reprinted with permission

Using the Braden Scale, healthcare professionals can assess six broad categories, which include sensory perception, moisture, activity, mobility, nutrition, friction and shear. A score of 18 or below indicates a risk for developing a pressure ulcer (Fig. 19.1).

As an alternative, the Norton Scale assesses physical condition, mental state, activity, mobility and incontinence. A score of 16 or below indicates risk for ulceration.

Table 19.1 The Braden Scale suggested protocol

*At risk (15–18)**	*Manage moisture*
Frequent turning	Use commercial moisture barrier
Maximal remobilization	Use absorbant pads or diapers that
Protect heels	wick and hold moisture
Manage moisture, nutrition and friction and shear	Address cause if possible
Pressure-reduction support surface if bed- or chair-bound	Offer bedpan/urinal and glass of
* If other major risk factors are present	water in conjunction with turning
(advanced age, fever, poor dietary intake of protein,	schedules
diastolic pressure below 60, hemodynamic instability),	
advance to next level of risk	
*Moderate risk (13–14)**	*Manage nutrition*
Turning schedule	Increase protein intake
Use foam wedges for 30E lateral positioning	Increase calorie intake to spare
Pressure-reduction support surface	proteins
Maximal remobilization	Supplement with multi-vitamin
Protect heels	(should have vit A, C and E)
Manage moisture, nutrition and friction and shear	Act quickly to alleviate deficits
* If other major risk factors present,	Consult dietitian
advance to next level of risk	
High risk (10–12)	*Manage friction and shear*
Increase frequency of turning	Elevate hob no more than 30E
Supplement with small shifts	Use trapeze when indicated
Pressure-reduction support surface	Use lift sheet to move patient
Use foam wedges for 30E lateral positioning	Protect elbows and heels if being
Maximal remobilization	exposed to friction
Protect heels	
Manage moisture, nutrition	
and friction and shear	
Very high risk (9 or below)	*Other general care issues*
All of the above	No massage of reddened bony
+	prominences
Use pressure-relieving surface if	No donut-type devices
patient has intractable pain or severe pain exacerbated by	Maintain good hydration
turning or additional risk factors	Avoid drying the skin
*Low air loss beds do not substitute for turning schedules	

Barbara Braden, 2001, reprinted with permission

Use of the Braden Scale should also include a plan of action based on the patient's risk assessment score. A suggested protocol is given in Table 19.1.

It is generally accepted that risk for pressure ulcer formation is both intrinsic and extrinsic. The intrinsic factors include age, nutrition, disease process, drug therapy, lack of sensation, immobility, bed rest, smoking, radiation, obesity, infection, low blood pressure, incontinence, dehydration, edema and so on. Extrinsic risk factors include pressure, shear, friction, moisture and heat.

Assessment

Assessment includes all of the same criteria that we equate with any and all chronic wounds. When evaluating the pressure ulcers, however, it is important to determine the greatest or lowest level of tissue destruction or the ulcer's stage. A number of systems have been developed over the years for classification or "staging" of wounds involving the skin and underlying structures. The staging system currently recommended by Agency for Healthcare Policy and Research (AHCPR) and Wound Ostomy and Continence Nursing Society (WOCN) (and accepted by Medicare/CMS) is a four-stage system based on the tissue layers involved. This system was derived from previous staging systems proposed by Shea [15], the International Association for Enterostomal Therapy [16] and the National Pressure Ulcer Advisory Panel [17]; WOCN Society Position Statements Staging Pressure Ulcers, 1996, available at http://www.wocn.org/publications/posstate/staging.html).

See Fig. 19.2 for skin strata and a comparison of various pressure ulcer stages.

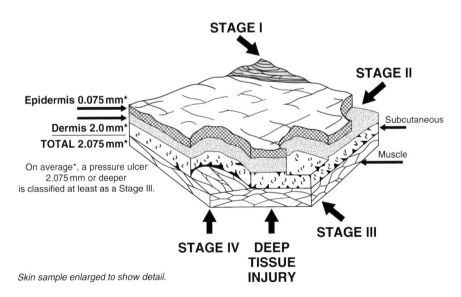

Fig. 19.2 Skin strata and comparison of various pressure ulcer stages

Table 19.2 NPUAP pressure ulcer staging system

Stage I	Intact skin with non-blanchable redness of a localized area usually over a bony prominence. Darkly pigmented skin may not have visible blanching; its color may differ from the surrounding area *Further description:* The area may be painful, firm, soft, warmer or cooler as compared to adjacent tissue. Stage I may be difficult to detect in individuals with dark skin tones. May indicate "at risk" persons (a heralding sign of risk)
Stage II	Partial thickness loss of dermis presenting as a shallow open ulcer with a red pink wound bed, without slough. May also present as an intact or open/ruptured serum-filled blister *Further description:* Presents as a shiny or dry shallow ulcer without slough or bruising.* This stage should not be used to describe skin tears, tape burns, perineal dermatitis, maceration or excoriation *Bruising indicates suspected deep tissue injury
Stage III	Full-thickness tissue loss. Subcutaneous fat may be visible but bone, tendon and muscle are not exposed. Slough may be present but does not obscure the depth of tissue loss. May include undermining and tunneling *Further description:* The depth of a stage III pressure ulcer varies by anatomical location. The bridge of the nose, ear, occiput and malleolus do not have subcutaneous tissue and stage III ulcers can be shallow. In contrast, areas of significant adiposity can develop extremely deep stage III pressure ulcers Bone/tendon is not visible or directly palpable
Stage IV	Full-thickness tissue loss with exposed bone, tendon or muscle. Slough or eschar may be present on some parts of the wound bed. Often include undermining and tunneling *Further description:* The depth of a stage IV pressure ulcer varies by anatomical location. The bridge of the nose, ear, occiput and malleolus do not have subcutaneous tissue and these ulcers can be shallow. Stage IV ulcers can extend into muscle and/or supporting structures (e.g., fascia, tendon or joint capsule) making osteomyelitis possible. Exposed bone/tendon is visible or directly palpable
Unstageable	Full-thickness tissue loss in which the base of the ulcer is covered by slough (yellow, tan, gray, green or brown) and/or eschar (tan, brown or black) in the wound bed *Further description:* Until enough slough and/or eschar is removed to expose the base of the wound, the true depth, and therefore stage, cannot be determined. Stable (dry, adherent, intact without erythema or fluctuance) eschar on the heels serves as "the body's natural (biological) cover" and should not be removed
Suspected deep tissue injury	Purple or maroon localized area of discolored intact skin or blood-filled blister due to damage of underlying soft tissue from pressure and/or shear. The area may be preceded by tissue that is painful, firm, mushy, boggy, warmer or cooler as compared to adjacent tissue *Further description:* Deep tissue injury may be difficult to detect in individuals with dark skin tones. Evolution may include a thin blister over a dark wound bed. The wound may further evolve and become covered by thin eschar. Evolution may be rapid exposing additional layers of tissue even with optimal treatment

The National Pressure Ulcer Advisory Panel has redefined the definition of a pressure ulcer and the stages of pressure ulcers, including the original four stages and adding two stages on deep tissue injury and unstageable pressure ulcers (Table 19.2). This work is the culmination of over 5 years of work beginning with the identification of deep tissue injury in 2001. For more information, go to the NPUAP's website at http://www.npuap.org.

Pressure Ulcer Definition

A pressure ulcer is localized injury to the skin and/or underlying tissue usually over a bony prominence, as a result of pressure or pressure in combination with shear and/or friction.

A number of contributing or confounding factors are also associated with pressure ulcers; the significance of these factors is yet to be elucidated.

Do not confuse deep purple areas or dark necrotic tissue to be a stage I pressure ulcer (Fig. 19.3 and (Fig. 19.4). These areas are usually indicative of deeper, full-thickness damage to the muscle underlying the tissue and not superficial damage of a stage I. The proposed theory is that suspected "deep tissue injury" (DTI) occurs near the bone or from the "outside in" from a myosubcutaneous infarct [18]. Later,

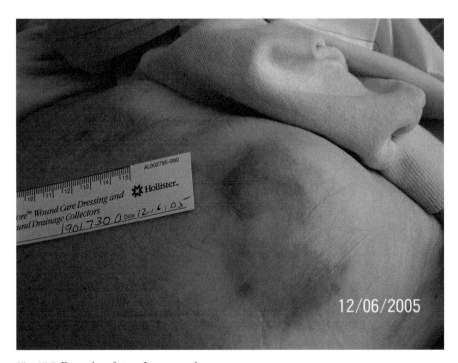

Fig. 19.3 Examples of stage I pressure ulcers

Fig. 19.4 Examples of stage I pressure ulcers

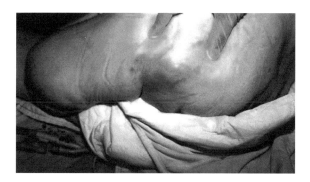

damage is seen superficially when the tissue dies or necroses and reaches the outer layers of skin and then the skin opens [19].

Deep tissue injury due to pressure exists as a form of pressure ulcer and is not well captured by the current staging system. Several pressure ulcer staging systems are frequently cited but none defines pressure-related injury under intact skin [20]. The National Pressure Ulcer Advisory Panel (NPUAP) recommended using the terms "pressure-related deep tissue injury under intact skin" or "deep tissue injury under intact skin" for describing these lesions. Since their February 2007 Consensus Meeting and NPUAP Biennial Conference [21], the definition has been updated to reflect [22] accuracy, clarity, succinctness, utility and discrimination.

The lesions are unique forms of "dangerous" pressure ulcers that should be differentiated from superficial stage I damage since they can deteriorate very quickly. They should not be confused with a bruise, contusion, hematoma or gangrene [23] (Fig. 19.5).

In addition, dermatologic manifestations such as incontinent perineal dermatitis, candidiasis or tinea, maceration or denudation should not be classified as a "pressure ulcer." Describe skin conditions as what you see. These are not pressure-related assaults (Figs. 19.6–19.12).

Assessment of all wounds, no matter their etiology, should include the location, size (length, width and depth), the wound bed (color and type of tissue), any devitalized material, the peri wound or surrounding skin, the exudates or drainage type, amount, color, consistency and odor, the wound margins and any turning under of the wound's edge (undermining), tunneling as well as assessment of pain and possible cause. The comprehensive assessment should then be documented on the medical record and be re-evaluated periodically. As the wound changes, so too should the plan of care.

Pressure ulcers can also be painful, regardless of the stage. Dallam and her associates reported that 59% of persons with pressure ulcers experienced pain and only 2% of these patients that reported their pain received pharmacological treatments [24]. Furthermore, the American Geriatric Society Panel of Persistent Pain in Older Persons found that up to 80% of nursing home residents with pressure ulcer have significant pain that is under treated [25].

Fig. 19.5 Example of suspected deep tissue injury that eventually opened up to full-thickness tissue loss

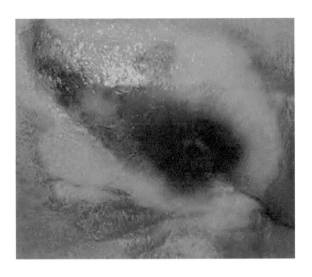

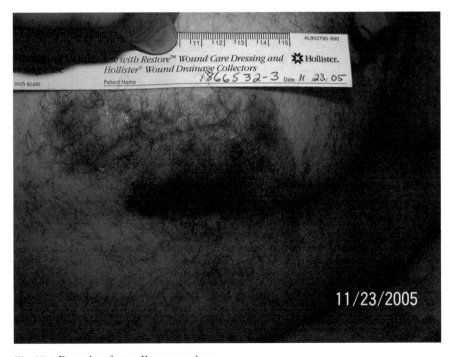

Fig. 19.6 Examples of stage II pressure ulcers

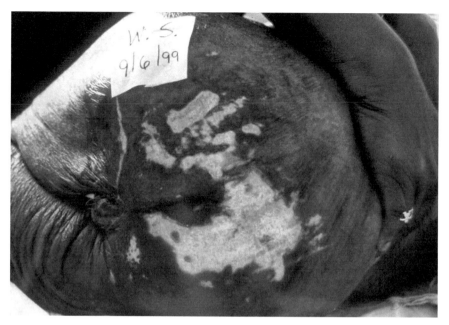

Fig. 19.7 Examples of stage II pressure ulcers

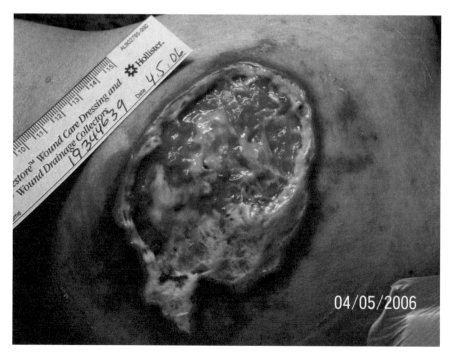

Fig. 19.8 Examples of stage III pressure ulcers

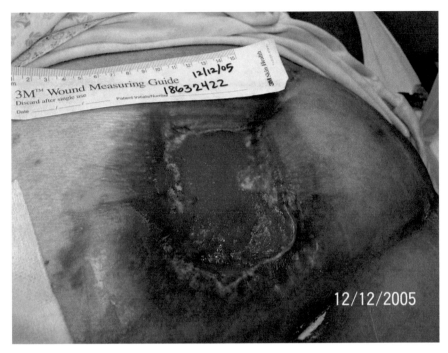

Fig. 19.9 Examples of stage III pressure ulcers

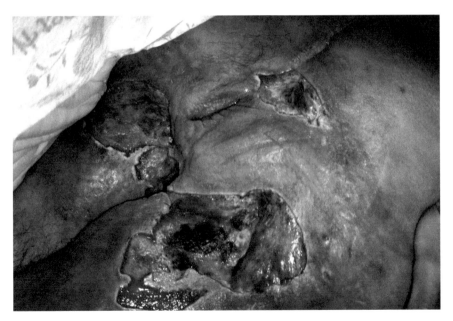

Fig. 19.10 Examples of stage IV ulcers

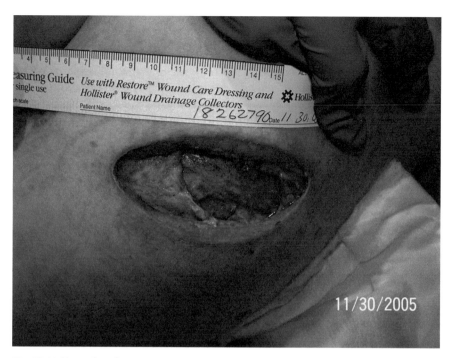

Fig. 19.11 Examples of stage IV ulcers

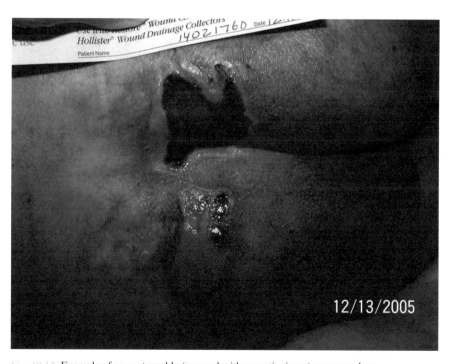

Fig. 19.12 Example of an unstageable (covered with necrotic tissue) pressure ulcer

Caveats

Keep in mind that only a full-thickness wound (stage III and IV pressure ulcers) can develop devitalized material such as slough and/or eschar. These wounds heal by granulation, contraction and, finally, epithelialization. Since the various strata are not replaced (i.e., muscle, fascia, subcutaneous), a wound does not "reverse" stage as it heals or closes [26]. For example, a stage III pressure ulcer is always a stage III pressure ulcer, even as it granulates, contracts and epithelializes to closure. A stage III does not become a stage II and a stage I for instance. It could be described in terms of percentage of healing as the wound's size decreases. A helpful way to quantify healing is demonstrated by the P.U.S.H. Tool available at http://www.npuap.org.

Even after a wound has granulated and epithelialized to closure, the tissue continues to "remodel" and gain strength for up to 2 years. Furthermore, the healed tissue will never regain its entire tensile straight it once had. At best it will regain 70–80% its original strength [27].

Kennedy observed and described pressure ulcers that some people get as a result of the dying process [28]. Kennedy terminal ulcers (KTU) are considered a predictor of imminent death within 14–21 days. They are often shaped like a pear, usually appear on the sacrum, are often dark yellow but can also be black or red, have irregular borders, suddenly appear and can start as a blister or stage II pressure ulcer and quickly progress to a stage III or IV.

Skin Tears

Although skin tears are not considered "pressure ulcers," it is important to mention these traumatic sores as they tend to occur to some of the same individuals as pressure ulcers. As the skin ages, the basement membrane (junction between the epidermis and the dermis) flattens, making it "loose," thus more prone to traumatic injury and unintentional separation, in essence, a skin tear. The anatomy of aging skin makes skin tears nearly inevitable in the elderly. In addition, harsh soaps and surfactant cleansers as well as non-nutritional moisturizers and protectants containing hydrocarbons such as petroleum and mineral oil, which do not contribute to lipid replacement, further add to the skin's vulnerability. Choosing a skin care regime that replaces soap and harsh surfactant cleansers (detergent type) with pH-balanced mild cleansers and phospholipids cleansers can decrease the incidence of skin tears, additionally providing overall cost savings and comfort [29] (Fig. 19.13).

Heel Pressure Ulcers

The heel presents a problematic source of pressure due to its bony prominence, especially in the recumbent individual. Care should be taken to mobilize the immobile, providing good skin care and off-loading with pressure relief equipment, to

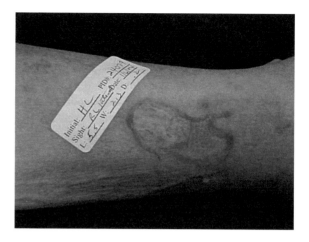

Fig. 19.13 Example of a skin tear on the posterior arm

the vulnerable heel area. Unlike pressure ulcers on other areas of the body, if the heel ulcer is dry, black and intact, it should be left alone, without debridement. This is considered best practice if there is a chance of compromised blood flow and if there is no edema, redness or drainage, in other words, a "stable" heel eschar [30] (Fig. 19.14).

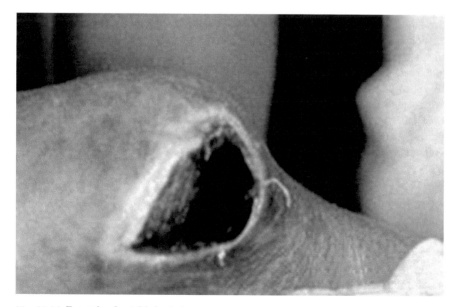

Fig. 19.14 Example of a stable heel ulcer

Healing

Pressure ulcers do not heal by regeneration, rather granulation tissue fills in the tissue void, the wound surface contracts and the wound seals off by epithelialization. Muscle, fascia, subcutaneous and underlying tissue such as bone that is destroyed will be replaced by scar tissue. The individual is therefore at higher risk for developing another pressure ulcer in the same area. Prevention measures should commence immediately after healing takes place to reduce the chance of reoccurrence. Simple strategies such as continuing the use of a prevention support surface and/or pressure-relieving cushion or device, providing good skin care, off-loading problem areas, mobilizing the immobile and utilizing preventative dressings can avert future pressure ulcers.

Treatment Strategies

Treatment of pressure ulcers includes supporting the host medically, surgically and nutritionally if necessary, mobilizing the immobile, relieving pressure with recumbent and seated support surfaces and preparing the wound bed, consisting of cleaning, debriding, management of any bioburden, providing moist wound dressings and protecting the peri wound skin as well as possible adjunctive therapies.

Prevention Basics

Pressure ulcer prevention encompasses alleviating the possible causative factors. If we consider that lack of viable blood flow to the tissue is the main cause of pressure ulcers we can further classify that damage into pressure, shear, friction, moisture and heat, and thus better support the host. We can also prevent pressure ulcers by managing the following negative effects. These prevention recommendations are adapted from the 1992 Agency for Healthcare Policy and Research (AHCPR, now the Agency for Healthcare Policy and Research (AHRQ)) clinical practice guidelines [31] and the Wound Ostomy and Continence Nursed Association's 2003 Guidelines for Prevention and Management of Pressure Ulcers [32].

Pressure

- Pressure can be lessened by establishing a patient turning schedule that can be documented. The standard of care for turning and repositioning is every 2 h in the recumbent individual and every 15 min in the seated person.
- Use the 30° lateral position in a supine patient instead of placing a patient side lying at 90°. This dramatically decreases the peak pressure caused by the greater trochanter.

- Implement an appropriate pressure-redistribution support surface to both the seated and recumbent surfaces that the patient's body contacts at the first sign of risk.
- Avoid the use of invalid rings, "donuts," rubber rings or any technology that has a cut-out area for cushioning a seated client since this can actually increase pressures, especially over bony prominences.
- Limit the time that the patient spends on the commode or bedpan.
- Off-load the heels with a pillow, heel protection device or wedge.

Shear

- Limit the elevation of the head of the bed to 30° or less.
- Use draw sheets to turn and reposition patients.
- Use the bed's side rails and consider adding a trapeze to the bed frame to optimize mobility and decrease shear forces.
- Never perform massage over bony prominences that have been compressed. This can cause tissue damage, although there is conflicting information in the literature [33].

Miscellaneous

- Apply high-quality moisturizers to the skin to increase the water content and thus pliability and strength. Apply moisturizers anytime water comes in contact with the skin, especially after the bath or shower. Look for products that allow the skin to breath while decreasing excessive transepidermal water loss (e-TEWL).
- Use a skin prepping solution or sealant before using tape on a patient's skin.
- Teach the patient and care givers to visually inspect the skin daily for early detection.
- Encourage proper hydration and nutrition.
- Institute an active or passive range-of-motion routine.
- Calculate a risk assessment score on every patient to identify those at high risk for development of pressure ulcers (see "Risk Assessment," Braden Scale).
- Apply transparent dressings or skin sealants to protect the epidermis.

Moisture

- Protect the skin from body fluids and drainage by absorption.
- Decrease baths and address a patient's need for skin cleansing individually and by body region.
- Use moisturizing, soap-free cleansers with a neutral or slightly acidic pH.
- Apply barrier creams that remain in contact with the skin despite cleaning to offer

protection from incontinence episodes. Good examples of ingredients include zinc oxide, dimethicone and other high-quality silicones. Products containing petrolatum-based protectants should be avoided since they protect for a very short time and do not remain in contact with the skin.

- Institute a bowel and bladder program that is customized to each resident and can be documented.
- Consider the use of some of the newer high-tech polymer-based incontinent products (briefs, pad, etc.) and customize to each resident's needs.

Seated dependent

- Avoid uninterrupted sitting.
- Teach the patient to perform a weight shift (stand up with assist, push up, bend at the waist or shift from side to side) every 15 min.
- If the patient is not able to perform an independent weight shift, they should be repositioned or put back to bed once per hour.
- Utilize a high-quality pressure-redistribution cushion (high-density foam, air or viscous gel) for all seated-dependent individuals.

Current Controversy

The latest debate with pressure ulcers is whether or not they are unavoidable. Are they secondary only to poor care or are some ulcers simply inescapable? According to the CMS Guidance to Surveyors (available at http://www.cms.hhs.gov/manuals/pm_trans/R4SOM.pdf) an *avoidable* pressure ulcer is one that the resident developed while under a facility's care and the facility did not do one of the following:

- *Evaluate* the resident's clinical condition and pressure ulcer risk assessment.
- *Define* and implement interventions that are consistent with resident needs, resident goals and recognize standards of practice.
- *Monitor* and evaluate the impact of the interventions or revise them as appropriate.

Unavoidable pressure ulcers are those that the resident develops even though the facility:

- *Evaluated* the resident's clinical condition and pressure ulcer risk factors
- *Defined* and implemented interventions that are consistent with resident needs, goals and recognized standards of practice
- *Monitored* and evaluated the impact of the interventions
- *Revised* the approaches as appropriate

It is imperative to document any and all non-modifiable risk factors that a resident may have and why they may lead to the development of a pressure ulcer, for instance, refusal or inability to eat in addition to the refusal of a feeding tube.

Pressure ulcers will continue to be a big area for debate and litigation until we as healthcare providers recognize that the body's largest organ, the skin, can and will fail, just as any other major organ.

Helpful Websites

- American Medical Directors Association (AMDA): www.amda.com
- Wound, Ostomy and Continence Nurses Society (WOCN): www.wocn.org
- National Pressure Ulcer Advisory Panel (NPUAP): www.npuap.org
- Braden Scale: www.bradenscale.com
- Norton Scale: www.coa.kumc.edu
- Guideline clearing house: www.guidelines.gov
- Paralyzed Veterans of America (PVA): www.pva.org
- Agency for Healthcare Policy and Research (now the Agency for Healthcare Research and Quality), AHCPR Guidelines for Prevention and Management of Pressure Ulcers and Treatment of Pressure Ulcer Guidelines: www.ahrq.gov
- Advancing the Practice: www.advancingthepractice.org
- Association for the Advancement of Wound Care (AAWC): www.aawconline.org
- American Academy of Wound Management (AAWM): www.aawm.org

References

1. Revis DR. Decubitus Ulcers, October 2005, eMedicine at http://www.emedicine.com.
2. Cuddigan J, et al., eds. Pressure Ulcers in America: Prevalence, Incidence and Implications for the Future. Reston, VA: National Pressure Ulcer Advisory Panel (NPUAP), 2001.
3. Beckrich K, Aronovitch S. Hospital acquired pressure ulcers: a comparison of costs in medical vs. surgical patients. Nurs. Econ. 1999; 17(5): 263–71.
4. Young ZF, Evans A, Davis J. Nosocomial pressure ulcer prevention: a successful project. J. Nurs. Adm. 2003; 33: 380–3.
5. Allman RM. Pressure ulcers among the elderly. N. Engl. J. Med. 1989; 320(13): 850–3.
6. Abrussezze RS. Early assessment and prevention of pressure ulcers. In: Lee BY, ed. Chronic Ulcers of the Skin. New York: McGraw-Hill, 1985, pp. 1–9.
7. Kosiak M. Etiology and pathology of ischemic ulcers. Arch. Phys. Med. Rehabil. 1959; 40(2): 62.
8. Landis EM. Micro-injection studies of capillary blood pressure in human skin. Heart 1930; 15: 209–28.
9. Fleck C. Pressure ulcer prevention: getting back to basics. Adv. Provid. Post-Acute Care 2000; 63–4.
10. Reswick JB, Rogers JE. Experience at Rancho Los Amigos Hospital with devices and techniques to prevent pressure sores. In Kenedi RM, Cowden JM, Scales JT, eds. Bedsore Biomechanics. London: University Park Press, 1976, p. 3003.
11. Fleck, C. Reducing the pressure: methods for effective wound care management. Contin. Care 2002.

12. Thomson JS, Brooks RG. The economics of preventing and treating pressure ulcers; a pilot study. J. Wound Care 1999; 8(6):312–6.
13. Quigley SM, Curley MA. Skin integrity in the pediatric population: preventing and managing pressure ulcers. J. Soc. Pediatr. Nurs. 1996; 1: 7–18.
14. Bergstrom N, Braden B, Laguzza A, Holman A. The Braden Scale for predicting pressure sore risk. Nurs. Res. 1987; 36(4): 205–10.
15. Shea JD. Pressure sores: classification and management. Clin. Orthop. Relat. Res. 1975; 112: 89–100.
16. IAET, 1988.
17. NPUAP, 1989 Consensus Conference.
18. Salcido R. Myosubcutaneous infarct: deep tissue injury. Adv. Skin Wound Care 2007; 20(5): 248–50.
19. Maklebust J, Sieggreen M. Pressure Ulcers: Guidelines for Prevention and Management, 3rd ed. Philadelphia, PA: Lippincott Williams and Wilkins, 2001.
20. Ankrom AM, Bennett RG, Sprigle, S, et al. Pressure-related deep tissue injury under intact skin and the current pressure ulcer staging system. Adv. Skin Wound Care 2005; 18(1): 35–42.
21. NPUAP Biennial Conference: Charting the Course for Pressure Ulcer Prevention & Treatment, San Antonio, TX, 9–10 February 2007.
22. Press Release—Pressure Ulcer Stages Revised by NPUAP, National Pressure Ulcer Advisory Panel, Washington, DC, February 2007.
23. Black JM. Moving toward consensus on deep tissue injury and pressure ulcer staging. Adv. Skin Wound Care 2005; 415–2.
24. Dallam L, Smyth C, Jackson BS, et al. Pressure ulcer pain: assessment and quantification. J. Wound Ostomy Continence Nurs. 1995; 22: 211–8.
25. AGS Panel on Persistent Pain in Older Persons. The management of persistent pain in older persons. American Geriatrics Society. J. Am. Geriatr. Soc. 2002; 50: S205–24.
26. NPUAP position on reverse staging of pressure ulcers. NPUAP Rep. 1995; 4(2).
27. Bryant RA, ed. Acute and Chronic Wounds: Nursing Management, 2nd ed. St. Louis: Mosby-Yearbook, 2000.
28. Kennedy KLE. The Kennedy Terminal Ulcer, available at http://www.kennedyterminalulcer.com/.
29. Groom M. Decreasing the incidence of skin tears in the extended care setting with the use of a new line of advanced skin care products containing olivamine. Symposium on Advances in Skin and Wound Care, San Diego, CA, April 2005.
30. Bergstrom N, Bennett MA, Carlson CE, et al. Treatment of pressure ulcers. Clinical Practice Guide, No. 15, AHCPR Publication No. 95-0653. Rockville, MD: US Department of Health and Human Services, Agency for Health Care Policy and Research, December 1994.
31. AHCPR. Panel for the Prediction and Prevention of Pressure Ulcers in Adults: Pressure ulcers in adults: prediction and prevention. Clinical Practice Guidelines, No. 3, AHCPR Publication No. 92-0047. Rockville, MD: US Department of Health and Human Services, Agency for Health Care Policy and Research, Public Health Service, May 1992.
32. Ratliff C, Bryant D. Guideline for prevention and management of pressure ulcers. WOCN Clinical Practice Guideline Series, No. 2. Wound, Ostomy and Continence Nurses Society. Available at http://www.wocn.org.
33. Duimel-Peeters I, et al. The effects of massage as a method to prevent pressure ulcers: A review of the literature. Ostomy/Wound Manag. 2005; 51(4): 70–80.

Chapter 20

Cutaneous Manifestations of Diabetes

Arun Chakrabarty, Robert A. Norman, and Tania J. Phillips

Diabetes mellitus is a heterogenous group of metabolic disorders characterized by elevated serum glucose levels resulting from defects in insulin production, insulin action, or a combination. Complications include retinopathy, nephropathy, and neuropathy. The two main types of diabetes are Type1 insulin-dependent diabetes mellitus characterized by the destruction of insulin-producing beta cells of the pancreas creating the absolute need for exogenous insulin and Type2 non-insulin-dependent mellitus associated with an older age, obesity, physical inactivity, and family history. Type2 diabetes is increasingly being diagnosed in children and adolescents. Diabetes has been implicated as the single largest cause of end-stage renal disease, the main reason for non-traumatic amputation, and an independent risk factor for cardiovascular disease [1]. Nearly one-third of diabetic patients have some type of dermatologic manifestation. With time, the skin of all diabetic patients is affected in some form or another. Cutaneous signs of diabetes mellitus are extremely valuable to the clinician. For example, diabetic bullae, diabetic dermopathy, necrobiosis lipoidica diabeticorum, and the scleroderma-like syndrome of waxy skin with limited joint mobility can alert the physician to the diagnosis of diabetes [2,3]. Eruptive xanthomas reflect the status of glucose and lipid metabolism. This review will focus on the clinical features, the pathogenesis, and treatment strategies of the cutaneous manifestations of diabetes.

Necrobiosis Lipoidica Diabeticorum (Fig. 20.1)

Necrobiosis lipoidica diabeticorum is a degenerative disease of collagen in the dermis and subcutaneous fat with an atrophic epidermis and granulomatous dermis. The initial lesions of NLD are well-circumscribed erythematous plaques with a depressed, waxy telangiectatic center [4,5]. In early lesions, a neutrophilic vasculitis is evident. With the passage of time, granulomatous lesions evolve into a sclerotic stage of the reticular dermis and subcutaneous fat [6–8]. One-third of lesions may progress to ulcers if predisposed to any trauma. The vast majority of lesions occur on the pretibial region of the lower extremities. When NLD occurs in regions other than the legs, there is less of an association with diabetes. NLD affects females more than males and only 3–7% of diabetics ever develop the lesions [4,9].

R.A. Norman (ed.), *Diagnosis of Aging Skin Diseases,*
© Springer-Verlag London Limited 2008

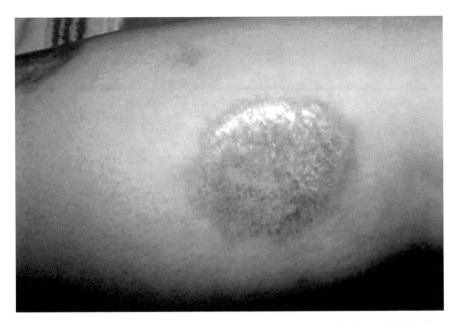

Fig. 20.1 Necrobiosis lipoidica diabeticorum of the lower extremity; well-circumscribed erythematous plaque of the lower extremity, with a waxy telangiectatic center. Courtesy of Dr Daniel Loo, MD

The etiology of NLD has not been clearly defined. Most popular theories suggest that a microangiopathic basis with neuropathy leads to the degradation of collagen [4, 10]. Few studies have found a correlation between NLD and the microvascular effects of diabetic retinopathy and nephropathy [4, 10, 11]. An immunologic role, such as the release of cytokines from inflammatory cells, may lead to the destruction of the collagenous matrix.

At present, there is no standard therapy for necrobiosis lipoidica. The majority of the literature on the management of necrobiosis lipoidica refers to anecdotal reports. The main modalities of treatment options include non-steroidal anti-inflammatory agents, intra-lesional, systemic, or topical corticosteroids, and even laser surgery [3, 4, 7]. A randomized double-blind Swedish trial of aspirin and dipyridamole combination versus a placebo did not reveal any significant benefit [12].

Acanthosis Nigricans (Fig. 20.2)

Acanthosis nigricans is a disorder characterized by a velvety light brown-to-black hyperpigmented, cutaneous thickening usually on the back, the sides of the neck, the axillae, and flexural surfaces. Lesions of acanthosis nigricans show marked

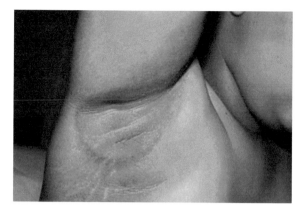

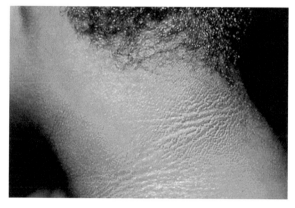

Fig. 20.2 (**a**) Acanthosis nigricans in the axillary region of diabetic patient; there is hyperpigmentation and skin thickness. Courtesy of Dr Daniel Loo, MD. (**b**) Acanthosis nigricans in the posterior aspect of neck; hyperpigmented velvety appearing plaques. Courtesy of Dr Daniel Loo, MD

hyperkeratosis and papillomatosis with mild acanthosis and hyperpigmentation [4]. The first cutaneous sign is hyperpigmentation followed by intensified hypertrophy of the epidermis.

The exact mechanism of acanthosis nigricans is unknown. There are eight types of acanthosis nigricans, the most common type being "obesity-associated acanthosis nigricans [13]." Malignancy has also been associated with acanthosis nigricans. The first major breakthrough association of acanthosis nigricans with insulin resistance came from a study by Kahn in 1976 [14]. Insulin resistance contributes a significant role in non-insulin-dependent diabetes and in a number of syndromes [14–16]. Insulin resistance may be caused by pre-receptor defects (autoantibodies against the insulin receptor), receptor resistance (genetic or functional defects in the insulin receptors), and/or post-receptor abnormalities (genetic or functional defects leading to inability to activate the receptor tyrosine kinase) [17–22]. There have been suggestions that insulin at high concentrations may stimulate insulin-like growth factor receptors on keratinocytes [23], thereby promoting epidermal cell proliferation.

There is no cure for acanthosis nigricans. The principal management should be targeted at the underlying problem [13,16]. Overweight individuals have considerable improvement with weight reduction. In patients with malignancy, elimination of the tumor may decrease the prominence of acanthosis nigricans.

Diabetic Dermopathy (Fig. 20.3)

Diabetic dermopathy, also known as shin spots, is considered the most common cutaneous finding in diabetes. According to one study, 40% of diabetic patients in an Israeli hospital had diabetic dermopathy, which was statistically significant in patients over the age of 50 [24]. Diabetic dermopathy appears as round to oval atrophic hyperpigmented lesions on the pretibial areas of the lower extremities. The lesions are usually bilateral and have an asymmetrical distribution. Histologically, lesions show edema of the papillary dermis, thickened superficial blood vessels, extravasation of erythrocytes, and a mild lymphocytic infiltrate [7, 25, 26]. The extravasated erythrocytes leave hemosiderin deposits, which provide the brownish hyperpigmentation. The lesions of diabetic dermopathy resolve spontaneously, leaving scars behind [2].

Diabetic Thick Skin

Physicians have noticed that patients with diabetes mellitus tend to have thicker skin than those without. This has been confirmed using ultrasound [27]. Diabetic thick skin has been separated into three main categories: (a) scleroderma-like changes of the hand associated with stiff joints and limited mobility; (b) measurable skin thickness which is clinically insignificant; and (c) scleredema diabeticorum. Thickening of the dorsum of the hands may occur in a third of patients with diabetes [7]. Other signs of increased skin thickening include pebbled or rough skin, known as Huntley's papules, over the inter-phalangeal joints, particularly the knuckles. Waxy skin

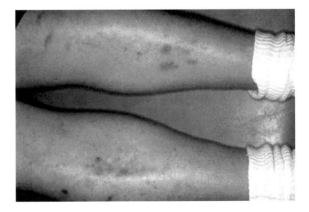

Fig. 20.3 Diabetic dermopathy of the pretibial regions; common cutaneous marker of diabetes; atrophic circumscribed hyperpigmented patches. Courtesy of Dr Daniel Loo, MD

and stiff joints have been correlated with increasing age and duration of diabetes, more so for Type1 DM, rather than the glycemic value [4, 28]. The term scleredema describes a clinical picture of thickening of the skin and non-pitting induration of which there are two types. The first, scleredema of Buschke, can occur at any age and usually subsequent to a viral or streptococcal infection. The posterior neck and upper part of the back are frequently affected. Scleredema diabeticorum has the same distribution as scleredema of Buschke but the skin thickening extends to the upper extremities, including the hands.

Histologically, large disorganized collagen bundles in a thickened dermis are separated by clear spaces with small amounts of acid mucopolysaccharides. Diabetic scleredema may be difficult to distinguish clinically from scleroderma. Hanna and Friesen reveal that diabetic thick skin has distinct light and electron microscopic features from those seen in scleroderma [29]. Unlike scleroderma, diabetic thick skin seldom had collagen fibers below 60 nm and bimodality of fibers was not observed [29]. Some studies have mentioned an increased synthesis of type 3 collagen (small fibers) in scleroderma, resulting in a bimodal distribution of collagen size [29–32]. Another study mentioned an increase in hyaluronic acid in diabetic scleredema while a predominance of dermatan sulfate in scleroderma [29, 33]. The pathogenesis of diabetic thick skin has not been clearly defined. Potential explanations include the hydration of collagen secondary to polyol accumulation [4, 34] and non-enzymatic glycosylation of collagen [4, 35]. There is no treatment for this condition although strict glycemic controlmay be beneficial [36].

Diabetic Bullae (Fig. 20.4)

Diabetic bullae are usually confined to the hands and feet. The blisters occur spontaneously and most are non-scarring. Patients tend to have adequate circulation in the affected extremity but have signs of diabetic peripheral neuropathy. There are three types of diabetic bullae. The most common type is sterile, fluid-containing

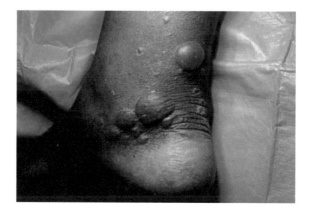

Fig. 20.4 Diabetic bullae of the posterior heel; fluid-containing bullae usually sterile and usually confined to the hands and feet; they tend to heal without scarring. Courtesy of Dr Daniel Loo, MD

and heals without scarring. Histology shows intra-epidermal cleavage without acantholysis [7]. The second type is hemorrhagic and heals with scarring. Histology depicts cleavage below the dermoepidermal junction with destruction of anchoring fibrils [7, 37]. The third type involves mostly multiple non-scarring bullae on sun-exposed, tanned skin. Histology reveals cleavage at the lamina lucida [37, 38]. One study mentioned an association with long-term Type2 DM [39] with peripheral neuropathy and another study mentioned a connection with chronic Type1 DM [4]. The pathogenesis of these lesions has not been clearly elaborated. Therapy of diabetic bullae is focused upon preventing infection.

Yellow Skin

Yellow nails and skin associated with diabetes is a benign condition with no known significance. The pathological cause of yellow skin remains controversial. The change may be due to either elevated levels of carotene or non-enzymatic glycosylation of dermal collagen [4]. One glycosylation end product, 2-(2-furoyl)-4 [5]-(2-furanyl)-1H-imidazole, has a yellow hue, which could provide the characteristic color of yellow skin [3, 16]. The yellow color is best appreciated at the distal hallux of the nails and palms and soles. There is no current treatment for this condition.

Diabetic Ulcers (Fig. 20.5)

Diabetic patients form the single largest group of non-traumatic amputations in the United States [40]. For the majority of diabetic patients, the initial condition that leads eventually to amputation begins with a skin ulcer. Diabetic foot ulcers are separated into two categories: ischemic and neuropathic ulcers [40]. Peripheral neuropathy plays a central role in nearly four-fifths of diabetic patients. The most common neuropathy is a mixed distal motor and sensory neuropathy [4, 41]. In the

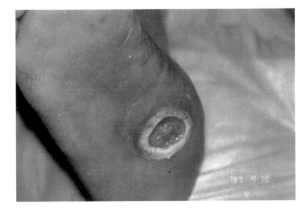

Fig. 20.5 Diabetic neuropathic ulcer of the plantar surface of the foot; peripheral neuropathy leading to loss of sensation is an early warning sign. Courtesy of Dr Tania J. Phillips, MD

majority of cases, ulceration occurs as a consequence of the loss of protective sensation. The combination of motor and sensory neuropathy along with mechanical factors plays a role in the pathogenesis of neuropathic ulcers [4,42]. Clinical signs of paresthesias with loss of temperature and pain sensation along with disturbances in sweating are prevalent in neuropathic diabetic ulcers. The pathogenesis of ischemic ulcers involves diabetic atherosclerotic disease. The ischemic patient will present with disproportionately excruciating pain associated with a superficial ulcer while the neuropathic patient is unaware of a large, deep ulcer. The ischemic patients will often elicit a history of intermittent claudication, foot pain on leg elevation, and pain on exertion relieved with resting [40].

Prevention of foot ulcers is critical. Clinicians should routinely examine the feet of diabetic patients. A nylon monofilament test provides an early method for the loss of peripheral sensation and identifies patients at risk for ulceration. Education in foot care, proper footwear, avoidance of burns and trauma, and close medical follow-up are steps needed for the prevention of diabetic ulcers [40]. Glycemic control will diminish the progression of peripheral neuropathy, a key factor in the development of ulcers. Smoking cessation must be emphasized. Patient compliance along with physician intervention are the mainstays of the prevention strategy of diabetic ulcers.

Treatment of diabetic ulcers becomes necessary once preventive measures have failed. Many diabetic ulcers fail to heal because patients continue to put weight on their affected lower extremity. Approximately, 90% of ulcers can be treated by relieving weight from the ulcerated area, treatment of infections with systemic antibiotics, and arterial perfusion restoration [43]. A common mistake is the use of wet to dry dressings on a clean ulcer bed [40]. The removal of the dry dressing interrupts the healing process of re-epithelialization. Dressings which maintain a moist wound environment are preferred. New adjunctive therapies such as Becaplermin (recombinant platelet-derived growth factor) show modest benefit in improving granulation tissue and wound repair [44]. The role of growth factors and cytokines in the process of wound healing is an area of ongoing investigation. Bioengineered skin equivalents, such as Apligraf^{TM} and Dermagraft^{TM}, promote more rapid healing [45]. These innovative therapies are not a substitute for basic management of diabetic ulcers, such as adequate off-loading, treatment of infections, and debridement [40, 44]. The decision to perform vascular surgery depends on the severity of the vascular impairment, the surgical risks, and rehabilitation potential. The therapeutic goal of the treatment of diabetic ulcers is the eventual healing and avoidance of amputation, thereby improving function and quality of life.

Diabetic Cutaneous Infections

Well-controlled diabetic patients are no more susceptible to infections than the normal population [3]. Patients with uncontrolled diabetes mellitus and ketosis are more predisposed to severe systemic and cutaneous bacterial infections [3, 4]. Bacterial infections of the skin, usually caused by *Staphylococcus aureus* and beta-hemolytic streptococci, include impetigo, erysipelas, cellulitis, and necrotizing fasciitis [4,46]. Obese patients with diabetes mellitus have a higher predisposition to erythrasma, caused by *Corynebacterium minutissimum* [4,46]. Systemic antibiotic therapy and surgical debridement are indicated for severe infections, particularly for necrotizing fasciitis. *Candida* is one organism correlated with increased serum glucose levels and an early indicator of undiagnosed diabetes mellitus [3, 4, 47]. Commonly affected areas involve the nail folds and the web spaces of the fingers and toes. Normalization of blood glucose, topical, and systemic antifungals are the main modalities of treatment. Patients with diabetes mellitus are also at risk for rhinocerebral mucormycosis, an extensive life-threatening infection beginning in the nasal passages and spreading into the orbit and cerebrum [4, 48]. Treatment consists of debridement and intravenous fungal therapy, such as amphotericin B. Malignant external otitis caused by *Pseudomonas aeruginosa* is a rare but serious infection in elderly diabetics. Initially, there is a purulent discharge and severe pain of the external auditory meatus, which then progresses to a cellulitis and then to a meningitis [4,7,48]. Treatment involves surgical debridement and intravenous antipseudomonal antibiotics. Patients with malignant otitis externa have a high mortality [49].

Perforating Dermatosis

The majority of patients with adult-onset acquired perforating dermatosis have kidney failure associated with diabetes [50]. Itching and scratching accompany this entity, also known as Kyrle's disease or reactive perforating collagenosis. The lesions are located primarily on the extensor surfaces of the lower extremities but can occur on the face and trunk. The lesions are described as a few millimeters in diameter, papular, often with a keratotic plug. Another feature consists of the elimination of collagen and elastin throughout the affected epidermis. Histologic examination of these lesions reveals a hyperplastic epidermis surrounding a plug of degenerated material, which has elements of leukocytes, collagen, and nuclear debris [3,4,51]. Acquired perforating dermatosis is difficult to treat. Retinoic acid has shown some benefit along with topical anti-histamines to alleviate the pruritus [52]. A Chinese study showed a reduction of pruritus with the use of transcutaneous electrical nerve stimulation [53]. A German article mentioned two patients being successfully treated with allopurinol [54].

Eruptive Xanthomas

Eruptive xanthomatosis in the context of diabetes mellitus is accompanied by hyperlipidemic and hyperglycemic states. The lesions are described as waxy, yellow papules surrounded by an erythematous rim and usually occur on the extensor surfaces and popliteal region. Histologic samples depict lipid-laden histiocytes and a mixed lymphoneutrophilic infiltrate in the dermis. The main treatment option is strict control of the hyperlipidemic and hyperglycemic condition associated with the diabetes mellitus [55].

Other Dermatoses

There is some evidence of higher incidence of vitiligo in diabetic patients [56]. Patients with vitiligo have a family history of autoimmune diseases such as Addison's disease, Hashimoto's thyroiditis, pernicious anemia. Vitiligo has a higher incidence among adult diabetics and therefore, it is recommended to evaluate for diabetes among late-onset vitiligo [57]. One-fourth of porphyria cutanea tarda patients have diabetes [56]. Diabetes generally precedes the onset of porphyria, a possible result of the non-enzymatic glycosylation of the heme pathway [56–58]. Granuloma annulare is a chronic, asymptomatic dermatosis with a predilection for the dorsum of the hands, feet, and elbow. The lesions may be difficult to distinguish from necrobiosis lipoidica diabeticorum and are self-limited. The generalized form may have an association with diabetes mellitus [59]. Nearly one-half of diabetic patients with psoriasis develop psoriasis before diabetes but the association between diabetes and psoriasis has not been clearly defined [56]. Similarly, the association between diabetes and lichen planus, Kaposi's sarcoma, and skin tags remain controversial [56].

References

1. Nathan M. Long-term complications of diabetes mellitus. N. Engl. J. Med. 1993; 305: 1676–85.
2. Jelinek JE. Cutaneous manifestations of diabetes mellitus. Int. J. Dermatol. 1994; 33: 605–17.
3. Norman A. Dermal Manifestations of Diabetes. New York: Geriatric Dermatology Text, 2001, pp. 143–54.
4. Perez I, Kohn R. Cutaneous manifestations of diabetes. J. Am. Acad. Dermatol. 1994; 30: 519–31.
5. Meurer M, Szeimies RM. Diabetes mellitus and skin diseases. Curr. Probl. 1991; 20: 11–23.
6. Braverman IM. Skin Signs of Systemic Disease. Philadelphia, PA: WB Saunders Text, 1981, 654–64.
7. Huntley AC. Cutaneous manifestations of diabetes mellitus. Dermatol. Clin. 1989; 7: 531–46.
8. Huntley AC. The cutaneous manifestations of diabetes mellitus. J. Am. Acad. Dermatol. 1982; 7: 427–55.
9. Muller SA. Dermatologic disorders associated with diabetes mellitus. Mayo Clin. Proc. 1966; 41: 689–703.
10. Sibbald RG, Schachter RK. The skin and diabetes mellitus. Int. J. Dermatol. 1984; 23: 567–84.
11. Boulton AJM, Cutfield RG, Abouganem D, et al. Necrobiosis lipoidica diabeticorum: a clinicopathologic study. J. Am. Acad. Dermatol. 1988; 18: 530–7.
12. Stratham B, Finlay AY, Marks R. A randomized double-blind comparison of aspirin and dipyridamole combination versus a placebo in the treatment of necrobiosis lipoidica. Acta Derm. Venereol. (Stockh) 1981; 61: 270–1.
13. Schwartz A. Acanthosis nigricans. J. Am. Acad. Dermatol. 1994; 31: 1–19.
14. Kahn CR, Flier JS, Bar RS, et al. The syndromes of insulin resistance and acanthosis nigricans: insulin-receptor disorders in man. N. Engl. J. Med. 1976; 294: 739–45.
15. Reaven GM. Role of insulin resistance in human disease. Diabetes 1988; 37: 1595–607.

16. Electronic Textbook of Dermatology. http://www.telemedicine.org/stamford.

17. Tsushima T, Omori Y, Murakami H, et al. Demonstration of heterogeneity of autoantibodies to insulin receptors in type B insulin resistance by isoelectric focusing. Diabetes 1989; 38: 1090–6.

18. Moller DE, Cohen O, Yamaguchi Y, et al. Prevalence of mutations in the insulin receptor gene in subjects with features of the type A syndrome of insulin resistance. Diabetes 1994; 43: 247–55.

19. Moller DE, Flier JS. Insulin resistance-mechanisms, syndromes, and implications. N. Engl. J. Med. 1991; 325: 938–48.

20. Rendon MI, Cruz PD Jr, Sonthheimer RD, et al. Acanthosis nigricans: a cutaneous marker of tissue resistance to insulin. J. Am. Acad. Dermatol. 1989; 21: 461–9.

21. Taylor SI. Lilly lecture: molecular mechanisms of insulin resistance. Lessons from patients with mutations in the insulin-receptor gene. Diabetes 1992; 41: 1473–90.

22. Cama A, Sierra MDDL, Ottini L, et al. A mutation in the tyrosine kinase domain of the insulin receptor associated with insulin resistance in an obese woman. J. Clin. Endocrinol. Metabol. 1991; 73: 894–901.

23. Cruz PD Jr, Hud JA Jr. Excess insulin binding to insulin like growth factor receptors: proposed mechanism for acanthosis nigricans. J. Invest. Dermatol. 1992; 98(Suppl): 82S–5S.

24. Shemer A, Bergman R, Linn S, et al. Diabetic dermopathy and internal complications in diabetes mellitus. Int. J. Dermatol. 1998; 37(2): 113–5.

25. Bauer M, Levan NE. Diabetic dermangiopathy: a spectrum including pretibial pigmented patches and necrobiosis lipoidica diabeticorum. Br. J. Dermatol. 1970; 83: 528–35.

26. Binkley GW, Giraldo B, Stoughton RB. Diabetic dermopathy: a clinical study. Cutis 1967; 3: 955–8.

27. Huntley AC, Walter RM. Quantitative evaluation of skin thickness in diabetes mellitus: relationship to disease parameters. J. Med. 1990; 21: 257–64.

28. Brik R, Berant M, Verdi P. The scleroderma-like syndrome of insulin-dependent diabetes mellitus. Diabetes Metab. Rev. 1991; 7: 121–8.

29. Hanna W, Friesen D, Bombardier C, et al. Pathologic features of diabetic thick skin. J. Am. Acad. Dermatol. 1987; 16: 546–53.

30. Fleischmajer R, Damiano V, Nedwich A. Alteration of subcutaneous tissue in systemic scleroderma. Arch. Dermatol. 1972; 105: 59–66.

31. Hayes RL, Rodnan GP. The ultrastructure of skin in progressive systemic sclerosis (scleroderma). I. Dermal collage fibers. Am. J. Pathol. 1971; 63: 433–42.

32. Fleischmajer R, Gay S, Perlish JS, et al. Immunoelectron microscopy of type III collagen in normal and scleroderma skin. J. Invest. Dermatol. 1980; 75: 189–91.

33. Fleischmajer R, Perlish JS. Glycosaminoglycans in scleroderma and scleredema. J. Invest. Dermatol. 1972; 58: 129–32.

34. Eaton PR. The collagen hydration hypothesis: a new paradigm for the secondary complications of diabetes mellitus. J. Chronic Dis. 1986; 39: 753–66.

35. Buckingham BA, Uitto J, Sandborg C, et al. Scleredema-like changes in insulin dependent diabetes mellitus: clinical and biochemical studies. Diabetes Care 1984; 7: 163–9.

36. Lieberman LS, Rosenblum AL, Riley WJ, et al. Reduced skin thickness with pump administration of insulin. N. Engl. J. Med. 1980; 303: 940–1.

37. Bernstein JE, Medenica M, Soltani K, et al. Bullous eruption of diabetes mellitus. Arch. Dermatol. 1979; 115: 324–5.

38. Toonstra J. Bullous diabeticorum. J. Am. Acad. Dermatol. 1985; 13: 799–805.

39. Sibald GR, et al. Skin and diabetes. Endocrinol. Metab. Clin. North Am. 1996; 25: 463–72.

40. Miller F III. Management of diabetic foot ulcers. J. Cutan. Med. Surg. 1998; 3(Suppl. 1): 13–17.

41. Bleich HL, Boro ES. Diabetic polyneuropathy: the importance of insulin deficiency, hyperglycemia and alterations in myoinositol metabolism in its pathogenesis. N. Engl. J. Med. 1976; 295: 1416–20.

42. Grunfeld C. Diabetic foot ulcers: etiology, treatment, and prevention. Adv. Intern. Med. 1991; 37: 103–32.
43. Caputo M, Cavanagh P, Ulbrecht J, et al. Assessment and management of foot disease in patients with diabetes. N. Engl. J. Med. 1994; 331: 854–60.
44. Cavanagh P, Buse J, Frykberg R, et al. Consensus development conference on diabetic foot wound care. Diabetes Care 1999; 22: 1354–60.
45. Veves A, Falanga V, Armstrong DG, et al. Graftskin, a human skin equivalent, is effective in the management of noninfected neuropathic diabetic foot ulcers: a prospective randomized multicenter clinical trial. Diabetes Care 2001; 24(2): 290–5.
46. Meurer M, Szeimies RM. Diabetes mellitus and skin diseases. Curr Probl 1991; 20: 11–23.
47. Knight L, Fletcher J. Growth of *Candida albicans* in saliva: stimulation by glucose associated with antibiotics, steroids, and diabetes mellitus. J. Infect. Dis. 1971; 123: 371–7.
48. Tierney MR, Baker AS. Infections of the head and neck in diabetes mellitus. Infect. Dis. Clin. North Am. 1995; 9(1): 195–216.
49. Petrozzi JW, Warthan TL. Malignant external otitis. Arch. Dermatol. 1974; 110: 258–60.
50. Rapini RP, Hebert AA, Drucker CR. Acquired perforating dermatosis: evidence for combined transepidermal elimination of both collagen and elastic fibers. Arch. Dermatol. 1989; 125: 1074–8.
51. Zelger B, Hintner H, Aubock J, et al. Acquired perforating dermatosis: transepidermal elimination of DNA material and possible role of leukocytes in pathogenesis. Arch. Dermatol. 1991; 127: 695–700.
52. Berger RS. Reactive perforating collagenosis of renal failure: diabetes responsive to topical retinoic acid. Cutis 1989; 43: 540–2.
53. Chan LY, Tang WY, Lo KK. Treatment of pruritus of reactive perforating collagenosis using transcutaneous electrical nerve stimulation. Eur. J. Dermatol. 2000; 10(1): 59–61.
54. Kruger K, Tebbe B, Krengel S, et al. Acquired reactive perforating dermatosis. Successful treatment with allopurinol in 2 cases. Hautarzt 1999; 50(2): 115–20.
55. Cruz PO, East C, Berstresser PR. Dermal, subcutaneous, and tendon exanthomas: diagnostic markers for specific lipoprotein disorders. J. Am. Acad. Dermatol. 1988; 19: 95–111.
56. Cohen-Sabban E, Cabo H, Woscoff A. Dermatoses most frequently related to diabetes. J. Clin. Dermatol. 1999; 2: 15–22.
57. Burnham TK, Fosnaugh RP. Porphyria, diabetes, and their relationship. Arch. Dermatol. 1961; 83: 55–60.
58. Epstein JH, Tuffanelli DL, Epstein WL. Cutaneous changes in the porphyrias. Arch. Dermatol. 1973; 107: 689–98.
59. Fitzpatrick TB, RA Johnson, Wolff K. Color Atlas and Synopsis of Clinical Dermatology, 4th ed. New York: McGraw-Hill, 2001, 120–2.

Chapter 21

Pain Management in Acute and Chronic Wounds

Cynthia A. Fleck

The American Pain Society (APS) defines pain as "an unpleasant sensory and emotional experience associated with actual or potential tissue damage, or described in terms of such damage" (APS. Available at: http://www.ampainsoc.org/advocacy/). It may seem obvious that tissue damage associated with wounds and the resultant pain, go hand in hand; however, many current wound care practices are outdated and do not take this into consideration. Unfortunately, there are no definitive diagnostic tests to measure pain or, more specifically, wound pain; there is only our patient's perception. The APS considers pain to be the "fifth vital sign" (APS. Available at: http://www.ampainsoc.org/advocacy/). According to pain management pioneer Margo McCaffrey, "Pain is whatever the patient indicates it to be" [1].

History

Accounts of pain were recorded by ancient man. Early humans related pain to evil, magic and demons. Relief of pain was believed to be the responsibility of sorcerers, priests and other purveyors of the supernatural. Treatment involved healing rites. With some advancement in knowledge about pain, pressure, heat, water and sun became treatments of choice. The Greeks and Romans were the first to advance a theory of sensation, the idea that the brain and nervous system have a role in producing the perception of pain. But it was not until well into the fifteenth and sixteenth centuries that evidence began to accumulate in support of these theories. It was then that the Renaissance-era artist and scientist Leonardo Da Vinci and his contemporaries came to believe that the brain was the central organ responsible for sensation. Da Vinci also developed the idea that the spinal cord transmitted sensations to the brain.

In the seventeenth and eighteenth centuries, the study of the body and the senses continued to be a source of wonder for the world's philosophers. In 1664, the French philosopher René Descartes described what to this day is still called a "pain pathway." Descartes illustrated how particles of fire, in contact with the foot, travel to the brain, and he compared pain sensation to the ringing of a bell.

R.A. Norman (ed.), *Diagnosis of Aging Skin Diseases,*
© Springer-Verlag London Limited 2008

In the nineteenth century, pain came to dwell under the domain of science, paving the way for advances in pain therapy. Physician-scientists discovered that opium, morphine, codeine and cocaine could be used to treat pain. These drugs led to the development of aspirin—to this day, the most commonly used pain reliever. Before long, anesthesia—both general and regional—was refined and applied during surgery.

In the last 10 years, research has focused on healing as the major outcome of wound treatment, with very little attention paid to other patient-centered outcomes, such as pain. However, with the development of quality-of-life assessment in patients with chronic wounds, pain has been identified as a major issue.

The Basics of Pain

The current understanding of wound pain is primarily drawn from the literature relating to other conditions and the physiology of acute and chronic pain. A quick review will be helpful in comprehending wound-specific pain. There are two major types of pain: *nociceptive* and *neuropathic*.

Nociceptive pain involves the ordinary processing of stimuli that damages normal tissues or has the potential to do so if prolonged. It results from mechanical or thermal excitation or trauma to peripheral receptors called nociceptors. In this way pain becomes a "conscious" perception. This type of pain is usually responsive to non-opioid and/or opioid drugs.

Nociceptive pain can be categorized into *somatic* and *visceral* pain. Somatic pain arises from bone, joint, muscle, skin or connective tissue. It is generally aching or throbbing in quality and is well localized. Visceral pain arises from visceral organs, such as the gastrointestinal (GI) tract and pancreas. Visceral pain tends to be vague and poorly localized and may radiate to unexpected locations.

Neuropathic pain is described as burning, "pins and needles," electrical, shooting or lightning-like pain. It results from either injury to or malfunction of the central or peripheral nervous system. Nerves can be affected this way by either compression or infiltration by such factors as infections, scar tissue or tumors. Neuropathic pain responds poorly to opioids and analgesic treatment and may persist for years.

Neuropathic pain may be subdivided into *central* and *peripheral* pain. Centrally generated pain involves injury to either the peripheral or central nervous system. Phantom limb pain and diabetic neuropathy are examples of centrally generated neuropathic pain. Peripherally generated pain is pain that is felt along the distribution of many peripheral nerves or is associated with a known peripheral nerve. An example is trigeminal neuralgia.

Pain can be further broken down into *chronic* or *persistent* and *acute* pain. Acute pain is an episode of pain that can be short or long lasting and represents some type of direct injury. It can be recurring or an exacerbation, occurring periodically over an extended period. Examples include burns, lacerations or a bee sting.

Chronic pain is defined as pain that has lasted 3–6 months or longer, often continuing long after an injury has healed. Often, normal treatment methods will fail and the pain may continue for the remainder of the patient's life. Examples include headache, abdominal pain, low back pain and the pain of fibromyalgia. An example of acute pain in a chronic situation is sickle cell crisis.

Another classification important to this discussion is *procedural* and *non-procedural* pain. Procedural pain is straightforward and something our patients experience perhaps every day. There are many causes. Reasons specific to the wound care client include biopsy, wound and burn debridement, incision and drainage and, perhaps most commonly, dressing changes.

Despite efforts to improve pain control in institutions, many barriers remain. Some of the most bothersome are those that result in the under-treatment of pain during procedures. Traditional clinical practice has largely ignored the pain related to procedures, and clinicians have continued to rationalize this on the basis of out-dated information about methods of pain control. Patients fail to request pain relief because of their own misconceptions and faulty assumptions. It is important to relay to the patient that pain is not a part of the healing process and that it is okay and even necessary to request pain and anxiety relief.

Establishing goals of procedural pain management are one of the first steps in creating standardized pain management plans and protocols. The primary goal is for the patient to experience adequate pain relief during the procedure. Other goals include minimizing anxiety and fear related to the procedure; cooperation during the procedure; and a prompt, safe recovery from the effects of the procedure. Therefore, informed consent and patient/family teaching are imperative.

Non-procedural pain results from conditions or syndromes, such as cancer, human immunodeficiency virus (HIV), trauma, chronic diabetes and, in the wound care patient, infection and inflammation. A perfect example of non-procedural wound pain is an infected foot with cellulites. Infection and inflammation are both causes of non-procedural wound pain.

Risk

All patients with wounds are at risk of experiencing pain. In fact, all wounds should be considered painful unless the patient tells you otherwise. Several groups of individuals are most vulnerable for under-treatment of pain: the elderly, infants and children, cognitively impaired patients and those patients with communication or language barriers. Whether because of their generation or their inability to communicate effectively, we must look for non-verbal cues to indicate that patients are in pain. Acting out, holding or rubbing a specific body part, yelling or moaning, avoiding dressing changes, withdrawal and constant sleeping can indicate that the patient is in pain.

Assessment

All patients with wounds should be assessed for pain—no exceptions. The Department of Veterans Affairs considers pain assessment "the fifth vital sign" and collects

Fig. 21.1 Pain measurement
scales

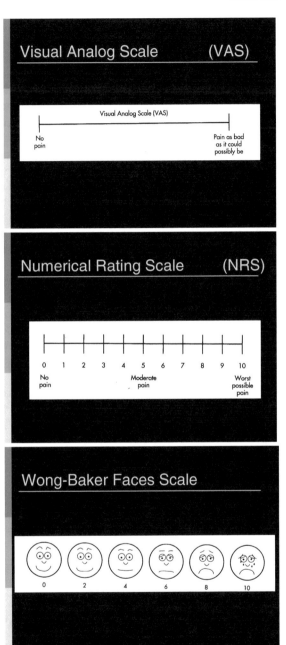

pain data with each vital sign measurement [2]. An easy pneumonic to remember the components of wound pain is the letters P-Q-R-S-T [3]. Pain assessment should cover:

- **P**alliative/**p**roactive factors: The question "What makes the pain better or worse?" is helpful.
- **Q**uality of pain: Ask "What kind of pain are you experiencing?" and "How would you describe it: sore, burning, or throbbing?"
- **R**egion and **r**adiation of pain: Eliciting questions, including "Where is the pain right now?" and "Does it radiate?" can help pinpoint the pain.
- **S**everity of pain: Use one of the many quantitative scales, such as the Visual Analog Scale, the Numerical Rating Scale or the Wong–Baker Faces Scale, to assess the severity of the patient's pain. The Verbal Rating Scale (VRS) is one the simplest scales to use and consists of no more than four words (none, mild, moderate and severe) [1].
- **T**emporal aspects of pain: Questions, such as, "When does the pain stop and start?" and "Is it better or worse any particular time of day or night?" can help.

Be aware of non-verbal cues, such as restlessness, guarding the area or wound, grimacing, sweating, muscle tightness, squinting, dilated pupils and either constant sleep or inability to sleep, as indicators of pain. Caregivers may overlook infants and patients who are elderly, deaf, non-verbal or cognitively impaired. Make sure their pain is assessed.

Providing scales to quantitatively and consistently measure pain is useful. The Visual Analog Scale, Numerical Rating Scales and Wong-Baker Faces are helpful and generally understood and accepted [1], see Fig. 21.1.

Asking the patient to keep a diary with dates, times and triggers can be useful. Documentation is imperative. Pain assessment should be documented at regular intervals. All treatments and interventions, even something as simple as administration of acetaminophen, need to be evaluated and documented.

Pain Management Strategies

Pain management strategies include medications, devices and adjunctive treatments. The key to effective pain relief is quite simple: stay on top of it. Balanced analgesia is considered ideal. Balanced analgesia uses combined analgesic regimens, reducing the likelihood of significant side effects from a single agent or method. The oral and intravenous (IV) routes are always preferred for ongoing pain management. But this is not to say that an intramuscular (IM) injection is never recommended, as it is for certain medications and vaccines, for example.

At times preemptive analgesia is needed to prevent noxious stimuli before surgery, during painful procedures and whenever pain management is expected to be difficult. To maintain a pain rating that is acceptable to the patient, around-the-clock (ATC) dosing is often used. To prevent recurrence of pain, ATC dosing is indicated whenever pain is predicted to be present for more than 12 out of 24 h. The patient's requirement for analgesia must be assessed accurately prior to wound care and/or dressing changes. If there is wound pain, or antecedent pain from other pathologies, the patient's current analgesic regime should be reviewed by a pain specialist. In the meantime, basic principles of good pain management techniques must be applied. The World Health Organization (WHO) developed an analgesic ladder that is a useful guideline for titrating the strength and dose of analgesia to the level of pain [4]. Table 21.1 describes and summarizes the WHO Analgesic Ladder.

Medication choices include non-opioids and opioids:

Non-opioids:

- Aspirin (ASA)
- Acetaminophen: use of it carries the risk of hepatotoxicity in excessive doses
- Non-steroidal anti-inflammatory drugs (NSAIDS), which carry the risk of GI bleeding and renal insufficiency

Adjuvants:

- Gabapentin is an adjuvant medication useful for neuropathic pain. It enhances the action of opioids [5] with very few adverse effects. It can be used orally or topically. However, there are no studies examining its direct effects or absorption when directly applied to wounds.
- Tricyclic antidepressants are also good adjuvants, though they are less effective than gabapentin and their side effects include dry mouth, sedation and urinary retention.

Opioids: The main fear with opioid use is addiction, although when used carefully in those with moderate to severe pain, this rarely occurs. Opioids may also cause confusion in the elderly. The risk of constipation is so high with these drugs, it is important to proactively initiate the use of stool softeners and/or laxatives.

Table 21.1 WHO Analgesic Ladder

	Pain	Treatment
1	Pain persisting or increasing	Nonopioid ± adjuvant
2	Pain persisting or increasing	Opioid for mild to moderate pain ± nonopioid ± adjuvant
3	Freedom from cancer pain	Opioid for moderate to severe pain ± nonopioid ± adjuvant

Adjunctive Pain Management

Adjunctive and device strategies are other methods of relieving and controlling pain. They can be used alone or in conjunction with pharmacologic intervention and include:

- *Heat and cold*. Heat and cold have been used for centuries. Heat vasodilates and increases blood flow. Heat is usually preferred to cold for pressure ulcers, superficial boils and hematoma resolution. Cold vasoconstricts and decreases inflammation and edema and is preferred for acute trauma, swelling and headache pain. Heat should not be used in the case of severe peripheral vascular disease as the metabolic rate of the limb may be raised beyond the ability of the arterial system to provide oxygen to the area.
- *Transcutaneous electrical nerve stimulation* (TENS). TENS use was widespread in the 1980s for post-operative pain. Today, it is rarely seen but it can offer an adjunct to traditional pain management, especially as a method of reducing the opioid dose required for satisfactory pain relief.
- *Electrical stimulation* (e-stim). E-stim involves the application of an electrical current at various wavelengths to help reduce edema and pain while promoting tissue regeneration and collagen production. TENS and e-stim use different types of electrical current.
- *Ultrasound*. Long used for pain management, ultrasound has now also proven beneficial to at least a low degree for wound healing [6, 7]. Settings should be 3 MHz for dermal wounds, 1 MHz for deeper wounds, and 0.3 watts/square cm, 20% duty cycle.
- *Acupuncture*. This method has been long used in the East, though it is still very poorly accepted in the West.
- *Dressings with lidocaine or morphine*. These dressings, compounded into a hydrogel by a pharmacist and ordered by a physician, are useful for painful wounds and are gaining acceptance in the wound care community. Gabapentin has also been used topically but should only be used on the peri-wound area until its absorption has not been studied through open wounds.
- *Moisture-retentive dressings*. Moisture-retentive wound care dressings like hydrocolloids, sheet and amorphous hydrogels, contact layers, soft silicones, cellulose and polyacrylate dressings have shown to decrease wound and peri-wound pain and pain associated with dressing changes.
- *Therapeutic support surfaces*. Therapeutic support surfaces take pressure off the body's frame, conform to the body's contours, equalize soft tissue pressure, diminish ischemia, promote healthy blood flow and skin microclimate and decrease discomfort and pain.
- *Monochromatic infrared energy* (MIRE). MIRE has been shown to be independently useful for pain management as well as for wound care. The United States Food and Drug Administration has approved MIRE for pain management and wound healing.

Wound Pain

There is an increasing acknowledgment that pain is a major issue for patients suffering from many different wound types. Ineffective wound pain management results in delayed healing, lack of compliance and prolonged care. Greater attention should be paid to wound product evaluations and surveys where characteristics such as pain, maceration, trauma and comfort are observed [8]. From a sensory dimension, information about how the wound "hurts" and what it feels like is uncovered. Following the initial tissue damage, the inflammatory response sensitizes the pain receptors in the skin. This helps the individual locate the extent and site of the wound so that it can be protected. When evaluating non-verbal and/or cognitively impaired individuals, start by performing a physical exam for evidence of purulent discharge, bone involvement, tenderness, erythema or induration. Many cognitively impaired patients can respond to a simple pain scale like the FACES if only they are asked [1].

In the acute wound, the pain subsides with healing. In chronic wounds, however, the impact of the prolonged inflammatory response can cause the patient to have an increased sensitivity in the wound (primary hyperalgesia) and surrounding skin (secondary hyperalgesia). If further painful or noxious stimuli are added to the equation as the result of repeated manipulation, such as during dressing changes, this acts as a "wind-up" mechanism, which locks the patient into a cycle where any sensory stimulus will register as pain (this is known as allodynia) [8].

Since wounds consistently involve damage to nerves, some patients may experience altered sensations as a result of the changes in how the nerves respond (neuropathic pain). Even the lightest sensation, such as a change in temperature or air blowing on the wound, can produce an exaggerated response from the central nervous system, causing the individual excruciating pain (allodynia). Wound healing complications, such as maceration, infection and ischemia, may further contribute to the pain response.

The European Wound Management Association (EWMA) published a position statement on pain during wound dressing change [8]. The key findings of this report are shown in Table 21.2.

Wound pain can serve as an indicator of inadequate wound management, an untreated underlying cause and/or an infection. Such pain frequently happens during dressing change or debridement; because of exudate pressure; around wound edges; in the infected wound; with the application of antiseptics; and during certain wound cleansing procedures [8]. Be sure to consider not only pain-free wound dressings but also advanced dressings to decrease the frequency of dressing changes.

Professionals often define and understand a patient's wound pain based on clinical assumptions. For example, it is frequently accepted that arterial ulcers are more painful than venous ulcers and that small ulcers are less painful than large ulcers. The relationship, however, between the intensity of pain a patient experiences and the type or size of the injury is highly variable and is not an accurate predictor of pain [8]. Between 60 and 80% of patients with chronic wounds experience some degree of pain, and 50% of patients with pressure ulcers have pain, particularly those

Table 21.2 Key findings of EWMA Position Statement

EWMA Position Statement

- □ Dressing removal is considered to be the time of most pain
- □ Dried out dressing and adherent products are most likely to cause pain and trauma at dressing changes
- □ Products designed to be nontraumatic are most frequently used to prevent tissue trauma
- □ Gauze is most likely to cause pain
- □ Newer products, such as hydrogels, alginates, soft silicones and polyacrylates are the least likely to cause pain
- □ Use of valid pain assessment tools is considered a low priority in assessment with greater reliance on body language and nonverbal cues

with stages 3 and 4 pressure ulcers [9]. The degree of pain has also been correlated to the stage of the pressure ulcer, thus contradicting the common wisdom that stage 4 pressure ulcers are painless [10].

Szor and Bourguignon have reported that 87.5% of patients reported pain at dressing change and 84.4% of patients with wounds reported pain at rest. Of those patients reporting pain during dressing changes, 18% described their pain as "horrible" or "excruciating." Forty-two percent of patients reported their pain as continuous, occurring both at rest and at dressing change. Only 6% of the patients had been prescribed analgesics to address their pain [10].

Wound Pain Essentials

Assume that every wound is painful and every patient who has a wound is in pain. Patients frequently experience pain during dressing changes (e.g., from dried dressings, strong adhesives, debridement and the pressure of exudate), around wound edges and in infected or inflamed wounds. Wound pain can serve as an important indicator of inadequate wound management, untreated underlying cause and/or infection.

Moist wound healing has been demonstrated to result in faster healing, less scarring and less pain. The pain reduction is attributed to the bathing of nerve endings in fluid, preventing dehydration of the nerve receptors [11].

In summary, the following pain relief strategies are intuitive but sometimes forgotten.

Strategies for pain relief at dressing change include:

- Handling all wounds gently. Flush, do not rub, when cleaning.
- Avoiding unnecessary stimulus to the wound, such as drafts from an open window, fan or vent, and prodding or poking.
- Protecting wound edges with barrier co-polymer, cream or a hydrocolloid wafer cut to fit around the wound.
- Allowing patients to change their own dressing if possible.
- Allowing patients to call "time out" verbally or by some non-verbal cue like raising their hand.
- Encouraging slow, rhythmic breathing and other relaxation techniques.
- Letting patients know that there are "no points for bravery" and that blood flow can actually be decreased during episodes of pain.
- Medicating prior to dressing change and debridement. Topical EMLA (eutectic mixture of local anesthesia) cream (AstraZeneca Pharmaceuticals, Wayne, Pennsylvania) or Lidoderm® (Endo Pharmaceuticals, Chadds Ford, Pennsylvania) cream (2.5% lidocaine and 2.5% prilocaine) is a useful anesthetic that is safe and easy to use. It should be applied approximately 1–2 h before the procedure, depending on the area to be treated and the extent of treatment.
- Using dressings least likely to adhere and cause pain like hydrogels, hydrofibers, alginates, soft silicones, cellulose and polyacrylates. Dressings that can dry out, such as gauze and others, can cause tremendous pain, especially when removed.
- Avoid using gauze. It is a key factor in the development of painful wounds [8]. Novel alternatives like the polyacrylate dressings provide moist wound healing and fast, efficient debriding without pain.
- Choosing high-tech dressings that are appropriate for a particular wound and can remain in situ for longer periods of time to reduce the need for frequent dressing changes.
- Select dressings with absorbency that matches exudate levels.

Wound Pain and Types

Wound pain usually relates to the etiology or treatment of the wound. Etiology issues that can cause pain include inflammation, edema, ischemia, claudication, infection (cellulitis and osteomyelitis), venous hypertension and malignancy. Treatment concerns consist of dressing adherence, debridement, cleansing and manipulation of the wound bed and peri-wound skin.

When first addressing wound pain, it is necessary to understand the etiology of the wound, treat the cause and remove the noxious stimuli. Let us review various wound types, the potential causes of pain and the treatment recommendations.

Pressure ulcer pain is often due to ischemia from pressure and shear leading to discomfort caused by inflammation. Langemo and associates found that half of all patients with pressure ulcers have pain, particularly those with stage 3 and stage 4 ulcers [9]. Treatment is aimed at the cause: assessing risk for every potential client, providing appropriate pressure redistribution (support surfaces, both mattresses and cushions), supporting the host holistically, maximizing nutrition, mobilizing the immobile, treating bioburden and infection and practicing appropriate preventative care. Pain that interferes with movement and/or affects mood may contribute to immobility and to the potential for developing a pressure ulcer or for delayed wound healing of an already existing ulcer.

Venous ulcer pain is described as dull, aching heaviness that can continue after the ulcer heals. This pain is often secondary to edema and internal pressure. Venous ulcers were historically believed to be painless, but we now know that this is far from true. Seven recent studies determined most venous ulcer patients (63% or more) experienced pain [12]. Addressing the pain involves treating the cause. For known venous insufficiency (with an ABI > 0.8), treatment includes compression, support stockings and leg elevation.

Neuropathy is the most common complication of diabetes. The amount of pain depends on the severity of neuropathy and can interfere with the patient's entire life, including the ability to sleep. The pain is often described as "pins and needles" or burning and itching. New pain can indicate a developing infection. Teach every patient with diabetes to report this important sign. We begin to address neuropathic wound pain by eliminating or controlling the source. Proper control of diabetes, preventative foot care, offloading, and pharmacologic intervention—often with tricyclics and other types of antidepressants—are key.

Arterial ulcer pain is frequently associated with peripheral vascular disease and intermittent claudication, which can occur at night, when the patient's legs are elevated at periods of rest or as a result of activity or exercise. It is usually described as burning, cramping or aching. Treating the source of the arterial ulcer pain consists of teaching the patient to dangle his or her legs with an unrelieved pain episode and, if medically necessary, bypass grafting or balloon angioplasty to revascularize the ischemic area.

Edema, swelling and inflammation can cause or contribute to the pain experience. Infection and inflammation alone can be painful. Superficial infection may cause local pain or discomfort due to the release of mediators by the bacteria and the host. The exudate of chronic wounds has abnormally high concentrations of proteases, particularly matrix metalloproteinases (MMPs) [13]. These increased proteases shift the wound healing balance into a continuing chronic-inflammatory phase. The use of compression bandages, hosiery and binders can offer relief. Also, look to newer dressings, such as activated polyacrylates, which diminish edema at the wound site.

Below are a few caveats to consider:

- Encourage the use of compression bandages, hose and binders to decrease swelling and edema, thereby decreasing pain unless contraindicated by congestive heart failure or peripheral vascular disease.
- Use newer dressings like polyacrylates to help further diminish edema at the wound site and the peri-wound area.
- For known chronic venous insufficiency (CVI) with an ankle brachial pressure index (ABI) > 0.8, apply appropriate compression stockings or four-layer com-

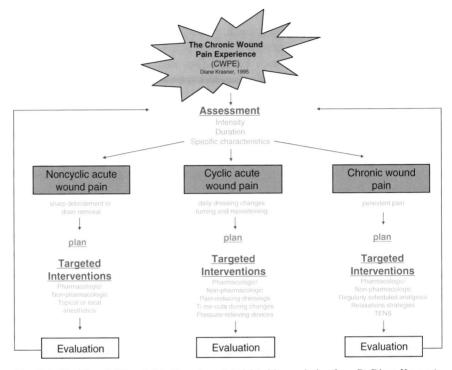

Fig. 21.2 The Chronic Wound Pain Experience Model (with permission from Dr Diane Krasner)

pression dressings and make sure that your residents elevate their lower extremities. This in turn decreases edema, which can alleviate discomfort.

The first model for chronic wound pain assessment and treatment was presented by Krasner in 1995 [14]. This useful model highlights the difference between background pain associated with the underlying etiology of the wound and the pain caused by treatment (iatrogenic pain), such as dressing pain. The model is shown in Fig. 21.2.

Dressing and Treatment Strategies

Dressing removal is considered to be the time of most pain [8]. Dried dressing and adherent products are most likely to cause pain and trauma at dressing changes. Products designed to be non-traumatic should be used to prevent tissue trauma. Gauze is most likely to cause pain and should be avoided. Clinicians should avoid wet-to-dry regimens, as well.

Consider novel alternatives, such as polyacrylate debriding. This method of debridement debrides at an average rate of 38% and produces no discomfort [15].

New research shows that activated polyacrylate gel absorbents (TenderWet®, Medline Industries, Inc., Mundelein, IL, USA) debride just as well as collagenase [16]. These methods can also cause substantial pain. Recent literature has also revealed that activated polyacrylate gel absorbents may be effective in reducing wound bioburden by interfering with biofilm as well [17].

One of the most important things to consider in selecting a dressing to diminish pain in the wound is that the chosen dressing must minimize the degree of sensory stimulus to the sensitized wound area. Any dressing that sticks to the wound bed, such as gauze, or dries within the wound bed and is then pulled away sends more sensory information to receptors in the skin than one that is easily rinsed away or slides off the inflamed tissue. Dressings, such as sheet and amorphous hydrogels, hydrofibers, alginates, soft silicones, cellulose dressings, "smart" non-adherent foams and polyacrylates, provide beneficial wound healing environments and also offer a virtually pain-free dressing removal while curtailing the pain experience during wearing time.

Be sure to select dressings with absorbency that matches exudate levels. Choose dressings that can remain in situ for longer periods of time, thus minimizing the chances of wound manipulation and a harmful aggravation of the pain cycle. Contact layers or dressings that remain in close proximity to the wound bed during dressing changes also have proven beneficial in the pain arena. Do not neglect pain management during wound cleansing, either. Appropriate non-cytotoxic wound cleansers used at body temperature ($\sim 100°F$) at 4–15 psi are best to keep discomfort at bay [18]. Avoid cytotoxic solutions, such as povidone iodine or hydrogen peroxide, when cleaning the wound [19] as these can cause discomfort as well as being lethal to fibroblasts and keratinocytes.

Simple measures, such as the use of skin preparations (especially the no-sting varieties), polymers that adhere to the skin to strengthen and prepare it for adhesive application, provide less trauma to sensitive peri-wound skin. Use them whenever you dress a wound. Consider tape alternatives, such as netting, tubular dressings, Velcro wraps and Montgomery straps, to attach dressings. When removing a dressing, make every possible effort to avoid unnecessary manipulation of the wound and prevent further damage to the delicate granulation and healing tissue within the wound bed and peri-wound skin. If the dressing has become dried out, make sure to moisten it with an isotonic solution before removing. Choose dressings that allow less frequent and therefore less painful dressing changes. Also, consider contact layers that stay in place when the dressings are changed, thus staving off potential wound bed pain.

Silver dressings, especially ionic silver hydrogels, could be one of the most ideal pain-free dressings. The dressings provide a broad-spectrum antimicrobial action with no known resistance and maintain moisture balance with pain-free application and removal. They also provide for autolytic, thus pain-free, debridement and display anti-inflammatory actions while eliminating any offensive odors [20]. Another area of concern with regard to the wound care patient and pain is how the dressing is attached. Review the dressing tapes that you and your facility uses. Are they gentle on thin, aging epidermis, holding tight with a low sensitivity adhesive, yet allowing easy removal? Are you and your staff regularly utilizing a co-polymer skin preparation with the application of all adhesives and tapes, providing strength and thus decreasing the chance of a skin tear, which can produce even more pain? Check your protocols and be sure that this important step is not skipped. Do not forget about the state-of-the-art "tapeless" ways of securing a dressing: Montgomery straps, Kling gauze, elastic netting or "grip" elastic support bandages not only provide support to the dressing but further protect from the injury and pain of removal and reapplication of tape.

Pain-Free Tactics

What other pain-relieving tactics can we integrate into our advanced wound caring practice? Dallam and associates showed that pain was significantly lower in patients using support surfaces for pressure reduction [21]. Support surfaces take pressure off the body's frame and soft tissue, promote a healthy microclimate and conform to body contours.

For gentle skin care, use a four-pronged approach: clean, moisturize, protect and nourish the skin of every patient—every time. Consider going soap-free. Newer products without harsh surfactant-type cleansers use phospholipids to clean, leaving the skin healthier and more comfortable. Look for ingredients like methylsulfonyl-methane (MSM), which slows the conduction of pain fibers and helps to reduce inflammation [22].

When utilizing negative pressure wound therapy (NPWT) or vacuum assisted closure (V.A.C.® Therapy, KCI, San Antonio, Texas), if the patient experiences pain, then consider premedicating 30–60 min prior to removal of the dressing. Pain can be dramatically reduced by instilling normal saline onto the dressing and/or by a physician or nurse practitioner's order for lidocaine solution to be injected 30–60 min prior to removal of dressings. Line the wound bed with an amorphous hydrogel or powder with ionic silver—it not only helps relieve pain on initiation and removal but can also cut offensive odor and number of days on negative pressure therapy—or a non-adherent gauze [23]. Also, be sure to apply a skin prep or sealant to the peri-wound skin prior to applying the occlusive drape. Other strategies include keeping exposed tissue moist with normal, saline-soaked gauze or impregnated hydrogel gauze during long dressing changes and NPWT changes. Ensure that adequate personnel participate in the dressing change to minimize the time. More than one clinician is usually necessary to change these complex dressings.

Standards and Evidence

Pain specialists estimate that at least 90% of patients with pain should experience satisfactory pain relief. Yet at least 50% of patients needlessly suffer moderate to severe pain despite two decades of efforts to educate healthcare professionals.

Clinical practice guidelines for pain management have been available since the mid-1980s from organizations such as the American Pain Society and the Agency for Healthcare Research and Quality (AHRQ) (APS. Available at: http://www. ampainsoc.org/advocacy/) [24, 25] but they have not been widely followed.

The Joint Commission on Accreditation of Healthcare Organizations (JCAHO) released revised pain management standards [26]. Among the requirements: pain must be assessed and reassessed regularly; routine and as needed analgesics must be administered; and discharge planning and teaching must include continuing care based on the patient's needs at the time of discharge, including pain management. Additionally, it requires that patients:

- Have the right to appropriate assessment of their pain
- Will be treated for pain or referred for treatment
- Will be taught the importance of effective pain management
- Will be taught that pain management is a part of treatment
- Will be involved in making the care decisions

The Agency for Healthcare Research and Quality (AHRQ) recommends that pressure ulcers be routinely assessed by healthcare workers who should not assume the absence of pain in patients who cannot express or manifest it. Assess all patients for pain related to the pressure ulcer or control the source of pain (e.g., cover wounds, adjust support surfaces, reposition the patient). Provide analgesia as needed and appropriate. Prevent or manage pain associated with debridement as needed [27].

Dallam et al., reported that only 2% of patients with pressure ulcers who reported pain or discomfort received pharmacologic treatments [21].

Krasner found that 42% of patients reported pain as continuous, occurring both at rest and at dressing changes [14]. Only 6% of these patients were prescribed analgesics.

The American Geriatric Society (AGS) Panel on Persistent Pain in Older Persons found that up to 80% of nursing home residents with pressure ulcers have significant pain that is under-treated [28].

The Patient's Perspective

Patient's have many concerns about their wounds. They view pain as the worst aspect of their chronic wound but will often suffer silently, not wanting to be viewed as having a low pain tolerance. The literature demonstrates that patients rank pain control as more important than healing [29]. Pain has been shown to be a primary reason for why individuals fail to attend clinic visits [30]. Patients fail to request pain relief because of their own misconceptions and faulty assumptions.

Many barriers to pain management exist. Myths about the inevitability of pain, fear of addiction, cultural and religious issues and social and socioeconomic factors involved with the patient and the patient's family sometimes block the control of pain. System-related challenges include lack of specialized pain resources, a low priority given to pain management and insufficient reimbursement or expense. Often care providers lack education in pain management or fear that patients will develop dependency to pain medications. Only education will change these unfortunate facts.

Increased cortisol levels lead to immunosuppression and poor wound healing. Delayed healing is associated with emotional stress, higher anxiety and depression [31]. Help your patients relax and cope with stress by referring them to mental health professionals who can offer appropriate therapy and pharmacologic intervention when required. Pain that interferes with movement and/or affects mood may contribute to immobility and to the potential for developing pressure ulcers or for delayed wound healing or non-healing of an already existing ulcer. Therefore, our ultimate goal is to assess, measure, document, manage and evaluate patients' wound pain experience to their satisfaction. McCaffrey suggests that pain is whatever the experiencing person says it is and exists whenever he or she says it does [1]. It is always a subjective experience.

Future Discoveries

What does the future hold? The lidocaine 5-percent patch (Lidoderm® Patch, Endo Pharmaceutical, Chadds Ford, PA) was recently approved by the Food and Drug Administration for local anesthesia of neuropathic pain. Experimental use of lidocaine-infused amorphous hydrogels, compounded for sustained release into painful wounds, is being undertaken. A commercial product available by prescription is Regenecare® Wound Gel with 2% lidocaine (MPM Medical, Inc., Irving, Texas). Bioengineered cellulose (XCell® Cellulose Wound Dressing, Medline Industries, Inc., Mundelein, IL), already proven to be a pain-free dressing choice [32] is currently being studied for its ability to deliver analgesics directly into the wound bed in a time-released fashion. Additionally, exploration of the effects of topical opioids, such as morphine-infused hydrogels, on treatment of painful wounds continues. Another novel topical which offers lidocaine-infused cream and lotion for painful intact skin and peri-wound applications is LidaMantle® Lotion (Lidocaine HCL 3%) and LidaMantle® Cream (Lidocaine HCL 3%) (Doak Dermatologics, Fairfield, NJ). It is also available with hydrocortisone acetate 0.5%, LidaMantle HC.

Providing tailored pain relief to our patients with wounds is common sense. It is one of our primary functions to relieve pain and suffering. It is basic to the human spirit and enjoyment and quality of life. Remember that individual pain responses vary and treatment may require a variety of approaches including sensory, affective, cognitive and sociocultural dimensions.

The bottom line is to be aware of non-verbal cues that your patient is experiencing wound pain. Pain is whatever the patient indicates it to be. Expect that your patient suffering with a wound is automatically suffering from pain, unless she or he tells you differently. To assess how your facility addresses pain, ask yourself the

Table 21.3 Helpful Pain Websites

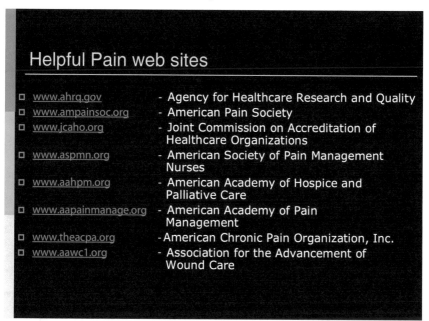

following questions. Do your protocols include the pain management components of wound care? Do you have a pain specialist on your wound care team? Are you using appropriate wound management techniques and dressings to help alleviate pain? Are you offering your patients a pain-free wound care experience? Make sure these goals extend to your wound care practices and you'll be performing twenty-first century care with a gentle hand! Today's clinician can now offer virtually pain-free wound care with state-of-the-art topicals, advanced dressings and treatments (Table 21.3).

References

1. McCaffrey M, Paero C. Pain: Clinical Manual, 2nd ed. St Louis, MO: Mosby, 1999.
2. Department of Veterans Affairs. VA initiates pain management program. Available at: http://www1.va.gov/opa/pressrel/pressrelease.cfm?id = 244.
3. Baranoski S, Ayello EA. Wound Care Essentials Practice Principles. Springhouse, PA: Lippincott Williams and Wilkins, 2004, 225–6.
4. World Health Organization. Cancer Pain Relief,2nd ed. Geneva: WHO, 1996.
5. Gilron I, et al. Morphine, gabapentin or their combination for neuropathic pain. N. Engl. J. Med. 2005; 352(13): 1324–34.
6. Ernst E. Ultrasound for cutaneous wound healing. Phlebology 1995; 10: 2–4.

7. Hashish, II. The effect of ultrasound therapy on post-operative inflammation, PhD Thesis, University of London, 1966.
8. European Wound Management Society Position Document: Pain at Wound Dressing Changes. London, UK: Medical Education Partnership Ltd., 2002, pp. 2, 8. Available at http://www.ewma.org/english/english.htm.
9. Langemo D, Bates-Jensen B, Hanson D. Pressure Ulcers in Individuals at the End of Life: Palliative Care and Hospice, Pressure Ulcers in America: Prevalence, Incidence and Implications for the Future, NPUAP Monograph, 2001, p. 145.
10. Szor JK, Bourguignon C. Description of pressure ulcer pain at rest and at dressing change. J. Wound Ostomy Continence Nurs. 1999; 26: pp. 115–20.
11. Kannon GA, Garrett AB. Moist wound healing with occlusive dressings. A clinical review. Dermatol. Surg. 1995; 21: 583–90.
12. Siobhan R, Eager C, Sibbald RG. Venous leg ulcer pain. Ostomy Wound Manage. 2003; 49(4A suppl): 16–23.
13. Mast BA, Shulz GS. Interaction of cytokines, growth factors and proteases in acute and chronic wounds. Wound Repair Regen. 1996; 4: 411–20.
14. Krasner DL. Caring for the person experiencing chronic wound pain. In Krasner DL, Rodeheaver GT, Sibbald RG, eds. Chronic Wound Care: A Clinical Source Book for Healthcare Professionals, 3rd ed. Wayne, PA: HMP Communications, 2001, pp. 79–89.
15. Paustian C. Debridement rates with activated polyacrylate dressings. Ostomy Wound Manage. 2003; 49(Suppl 1): 2.
16. Konig M, et al. Enzymatic versus autolytic debridement of chronic leg ulcers; a prospective randomized trial. J. Wound Care 2005; 14(7): 320–3.
17. Bruggisser R. Bacterial and fungal absorption properties of a hydrogel dressing with a super absorbent polymer core. J. Wound Care 2005; 14(9): 1–5.
18. van Rijswijk L, Braden BJ. Pressure ulcer patient and wound assessment: an AHCPR clinical practice guideline update. Ostomy Wound Manage. 1999; 45(Suppl 1A): 56S.
19. Rodeheaver GT. Wound cleansing, wound irrigation, wound disinfection. In Krasner DL, Rodeheaver GT, Sibbald RG, eds. Chronic Wound Care: A Clinical Sourcebook for Healthcare Professionals, 3rd ed. Wayne, PA: HMP Communications, 2001, pp. 369–83.
20. Reddy M. Chronic wound pain in older adults. Geriatrics Aging 2004; 7(3): 16.
21. Dallam L, Smyth C, Jackson BS, et al. Pressure ulcer pain: assessment and quantification. J. Wound Ostomy Continence Nurs. 1995; 22: 211–8.
22. Fleck CA, McCord D. The dawn of advanced skin care. Extended Care Prod. News 2004; 95: 32–9.
23. Sibbald RG, Mahoney J. the V.A.C.®Therapy Canadian Consensus Group. A consensus report of the use of vacuum-assisted closure in chronic, difficult-to-heal wounds. Ostomy Wound Manage. 2003; 49(1): 52–66.
24. Acute Pain Management Guideline Panel. Acute Pain Management: Operative or Medical Procedures and Trauma. Rockville, MD: US Department of Health and Human Services, Agency for Health Care Policy and Research, 1992, AHCPR Publication Number 92-0032.
25. Jacox A, Carr DB, Payne R, et al. Clinical Practice Guideline Number 9: Management of Cancer Pain. Rockville, MD: US Department of Health and Human Services, Agency for Health Care Policy and Research, 1994, AHCPR Publication Number 94-0592.
26. Comprehensive Accreditation Manual for Hospitals: The Official Handbook (CAMH). JCAHO, 1999.
27. Acute Pain Management Guideline Panel. Clinical Practice Guideline: Acute Pain Management: Operative or Medical Procedures and Trauma. Rockville, MD: US Department of Health and Human Services, Agency for Health Care Policy and Research, 1992, AHCPR Publication 92-0032.
28. AGS Panel on Persistent Pain in Older Persons. The management of persistent pain in older persons. J. Am. Geriatr. Soc. 2002; 50: 205–24.
29. Eager CA. Survey of best practices in wound care. Presented at the 16th Annual Symposium on Advanced Wound Care in Las Vegas, Nevada, April 28–May 1, 2003.

30. Pieper B, Dinardo E. Reasons for non-attendance for the treatment of venous ulcers in an inner-city clinic. J. Wound Ostomy Continence Nurs. 1998; 25: 180–6.
31. Cole-King A, Harding KG. Psychological factors and delayed health in chronic wounds. Psychosom. Med. 2001; 63: 216–20.
32. Alvarez OM, Patel M, Booker J, Markowitz L. Effectiveness of a bioengineered cellulose dressing for the treatment of chronic venous leg ulcers: results of a single center randomized study involving 24 patients. Wounds 2004; 16(7): 224–33.
33. Alvarez OM, Fernandez-Obregon A, Rogers RS, et al. Chemical debridement of pressure ulcers: a prospective, randomized, comparative trial of collagenase and papain/urea formulations. Wounds 2000; 12(2): 15–25.
34. Dallam LE, Barkauskus C, Ayello EA, Baranoski S. Pain management and wounds. In Baranoski S, Ayello EA, eds. Wound Care Essentials: Practice Principles. Philadelphia, PA: Lippincott Williams and Wilkins, 2004, pp. 217–38.

Chapter 22

The Geriatric Patient: Head to Toe Skin Evaluation

Robert A. Norman

Objectives

Upon completion of this chapter, the reader will be able to

Apply a comprehensive geriatric dermatology history and physical examination.
Differentiate between intrinsic and extrinsic aging.
Describe and recognize the common benign dermatoses: solar lentigines, sebaceous hyperplasia, acrochordons, seborrheic keratoses, Favre-Racouchot, xerosis, seborrheic dermatitis, purpura, cherry hemangiomas, and venous lakes.
Describe the appearance and management of the more common malignant skin neoplasms: actinic keratosis, basal cell carcinoma, squamous cell carcinoma, keratoacanthoma, and malignant melanoma.
Contrast the appearance of bullous pemphigoid, allergic contact dermatitis, herpes zoster, and tinea pedis.
Arrange skin diseases by their color and location and shape to help classify the condition.

This chapter is not intended to include all the possible conditions that can manifest in the geriatric patient, nor does it address every possible differential diagnosis or treatment available for the various conditions. Included here are only the most commonly found conditions among the geriatric population and some of the appropriate treatments. A more comprehensive and detailed list of geriatric conditions can be found in the references listed.

Because there are many cutaneous diseases, a thorough and detailed evaluation of each patient is necessary to gather as much information as possible. As presented in medical programs and books, a thorough history and physical examination includes, but is not limited to, the following points [1]:

The name, age, race, and gender of the patient.
Chief complaint: The reason for the visit. For a dermatologic history and

physical, the questions would involve the existence, location, and history of a skin lesion.

Onset: This would involve when the patient first noticed the lesion, whether it is an acute occurrence or a chronic one.

Progression: This would include the progression of the lesion, whether it is rapid or slow, whether it is contained or widespread.

Impacting factors: Do heat, cold, sun, exercise, travel, drugs, pregnancy, or change of seasons affect the lesion/ailment? If so, how? If not, what does affect the lesion/ailment?

Associated symptoms: Does the area itch, hurt, or burn? Does it have drainage? Is it malodorous? Is the drainage purulent?

Previous occurrence/treatment: Has it happened before? When? If more than once, how many times? How was it treated? Was the medication topical vs oral? How long did the treatment last? What was the result of the treatment?

Summary of information: This is basically a verbal recap of the information during or at the end of the interview to ensure understanding on both sides.

Allergies: To drugs, foods, etc.

Past medical and surgical histories: All previous illnesses and surgeries.

Medications: Dosages, instructions, compliance. Ask patients to bring a list of the medications and dosages with them to each appointment.

Family history: Diabetes, coronary artery disease, hypertension, etc., affecting parents, siblings, grandparents.

Social history: Occupation; use of tobacco, alcohol, or recreational drugs.

Review of systems

Physical examination: Vital signs, appearance, any lesions appreciated.

Type: Flat vs raised vs depressed (these include macules, papules, nodules, scales, crusts, pustules, cysts, blisters, fissures, erosions, ulcers, atrophic lesions, lichenification, vesicles, excoriations, plaques); color of the lesion; consistency—what does the lesion feel like; is it mobile; is it tender.

Shape: Is the lesion round vs oval vs annular vs umbilicated; does it have regular vs irregular borders.

Arrangement: Does the area in question have grouped vs disseminated lesions.

Distribution: Is the lesion isolated vs localized vs generalized; symmetrical vs intertriginous area vs follicular vs random; what kind of pattern does it have; is the pattern characteristic of that type of lesion.

Differential diagnosis.

Diagnostic tests to confirm diagnosis.

Treatment plans [1].

The following is a compilation of descriptions, signs/symptoms, differential diagnoses, and treatment [1–4] of the most common diseases and conditions [3–6] that a practitioner may find in an abbreviated and systematic head to toe evaluation of the geriatric patient, with relevance to the region examined [1, 7].

Scalp

Tinea Capitis

Description: A dermatophytic infection of the hair shaft most commonly caused by *Trichophyton tonsurans* and *Microsporum canis* [5,6]. It normally affects children but should be considered when elderly patients present with scalp conditions refractory to treatment. It affects elderly women more than men [5] (Fig. 22.1).

Signs/symptoms: Elderly patients can present with alopecia, folliculitis, pustules, or crusting [5,6].

Differential diagnosis: Includes seborrheic dermatitis and discoid lupus erythematosus, alopecia areata, folliculitis, and scalp psoriasis [5,6].

Treatment: Head & Shoulders, Selsun Blue, Nizoral A-D. Antifungals, selenium sulfide shampoo left on the scalp for 5 min two to three times weekly [5,6]. Treatment with griseofulvin for tinea of the scalp should continue for 4–8 weeks [3].

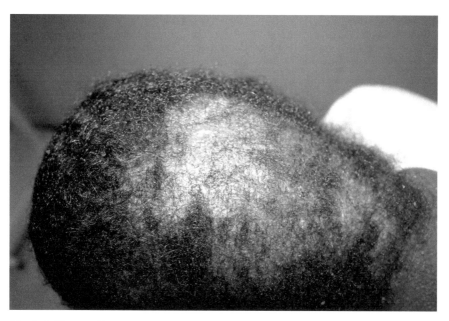

Fig. 22.1 Tinea capitis

Pilar Cyst

Description: Also known as a wen or atheroma [2–4, 7]. It is an easily movable
single nodule or multiple nodules formed by the trichilemmal epithelium of
the hair follicle, resembling epidermoid cysts but with macerated, soft, and
cheesy layers of dry keratin [2, 3].
Differential diagnosis: Epidermoid cyst, steatocystoma, cylindroma [4].
Treatment: Excision, incision, and drainage [2–4, 7].

Alopecia Areata

Description: Patches of hair loss on the scalp [1, 2] (Fig. 22.2).
Signs/symptoms: Usually none, but occasionally redness in area of hair loss,
nail pitting, and dystrophy [1, 2].
Differential diagnosis: Secondary syphilis, tinea capitis, traction alopecia [1,2].
Treatment: Topical and systemic steroids, PUVA, Minoxidil.

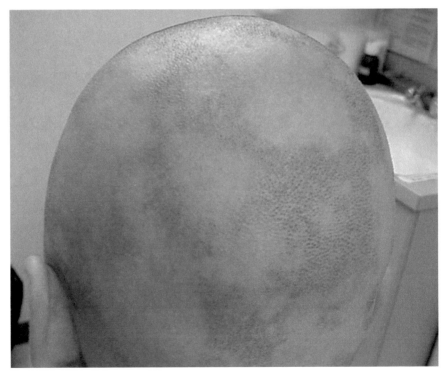

Fig. 22.2 Alopecia areata

Actinic (Solar) Keratosis

Description: Dry, rough, and scaly lesions in sun-exposed areas [1–4].
Signs/symptoms: Usually none, although some may become irritated and cause some discomfort [1–4].
Differential diagnosis: Verruca vulgaris, seborrheic keratosis, squamous cell carcinoma, basal cell carcinoma [1–4].
Treatment: UVB, cryotherapy, retinoids, laser, chemical peels, 5-FU.

Cutaneous Horn

Description: Macular, papular base with horn-like kertatotic growth. The distribution of cutaneous horn usually is in sun-exposed areas, particularly the face, scalp, pinna, nose, forearms, and dorsal hands (Fig. 22.3).
Signs/symptoms: Usually none. Because of their excessive height, they can be traumatized that may result in inflammation at the base with resulting pain. Rapid growth may occur.

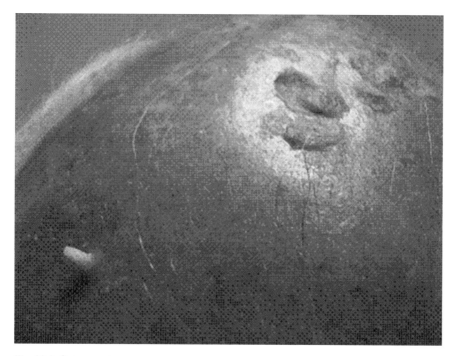

Fig. 22.3 Cutaneous horn

Differential diagnosis: Verruca vulgaris, SCC, actinic keratosis, keratoacanthoma.

Treatment: It is essential to perform a biopsy of the lesion that includes the base of the horn to rule out SCC or actinic keratosis.

Face

Epidermal Inclusion Cyst

Epidermal cysts are very common and are filled with keratin originating from true epidermis, most often from a hair follicle. They arise spontaneously and are prone to rupture. These cysts are most commonly found on the trunk, posterior neck, and post auricular fold. They present as dome-shaped, slightly mobile, cystic nodules ranging from 0.5 to 5.0 cm in size. If they are inflamed, they appear red and boggy and may be tender to palpation. When these lesions are drained, thick cheesy keratin debris along with purulent material can sometimes be expressed. Elective surgical excision is often the treatment of choice and the best results occur when the cyst lining is removed with blunt dissection. Very large cysts may require packing and further treatment [8].

Lentigines (Solar)

Description: Brownish patches that are smooth and are found on sun-exposed areas [1–4].

Signs/symptoms: None [1–4].

Differential diagnosis: Seborrheic keratosis, ephelides, nevi, melanoma [1–4].

Treatment: Chemical peels, bleaching creams, cryotherapy [1, 2, 4].

Rosacea

Description: History of frequent facial flushing and worsened by spicy foods, alcohol consumption, sunlight exposure.

Signs and symptoms: Inflammatory papules and pustules, erythema and telangiectasias, can show thickened and disfigured nose (rhinophyma).

Differential diagnosis: Seborrheic dermatitis, acne ulgaris, lupus erythematosus.

Treatment: Systemic antibiotics used in anti-inflammatory doses, topical retinoids, laser ablation of telangiectasias, dermabrasion.

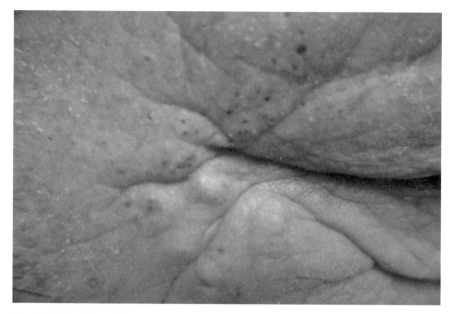

Fig. 22.4 Favre-Racouchot Syndrome

Favre-Racouchot Syndrome

Favre-Racouchot includes a variety of primarily sun-induced skin changes—nodular elastosis with cysts and comedones, and sebaceous hyperplasia. Superficial vascular changes result in erythema and telangiectasias. Irregular melanocyte distribution via alteration in pigmentation may manifest as multiple areas of hyperpigmentation, hypopigmentation, and scattered lentigines (Fig. 22.4).

Seborrheic Dermatitis

Description: Erythematous patches with raised plaques and/or yellow greasy looking scales found in the hairline, on the face, behind the ears, in the beard, on the trunk, and on the genitalia [1, 2, 4] (Fig. 22.5).
Signs/symptoms: Pruritus, redness, and scaling [1, 2, 4].
Differential diagnosis: Psoriasis vulgaris, impetigo, dermatophytosis, candidiasis, pityriasis versicolor [1–4].
Treatment: Topical steroids, UVB, retinoids, topical antifungal agents [1, 2, 4].

Melanoma

Description: Slowly enlarging, irregularly and darkly pigmented, aymmetric macule or nodule [1–4] (Fig. 22.6).

Fig. 22.5 Seborrheic
dermatitis

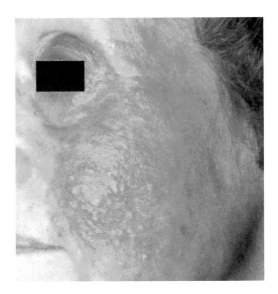

Signs/symptoms: Usually none, although some may become irritated, bleed and
  cause some discomfort [1–4].

Differential diagnosis: Melanocytic nevus, dysplastic nevus, pyogenic granuloma, pigmented seborrheic keratosis, pigmented basal carcinoma [1–3, 6].

Treatment: Surgery is the primary treatment of all stages of melanoma. Treatment of advanced (stage III and higher) melanoma may involve surgical
  removal of the tumors and any affected lymph nodes, followed by systemic
  or local chemotherapy with single or multiple agents.

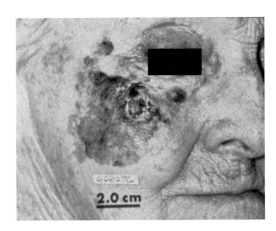

Fig. 22.6 Melanoma

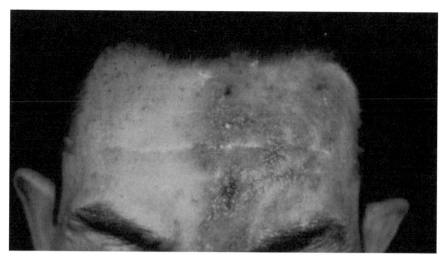

Fig. 22.7 Herpes zoster

Herpes Zoster

Description: Viral infection dormant in a dorsal root ganglion, also known as shingles, reactivated in an immunocompromised adult [2–6]. Then vesicles appear and later form crusts [2]. It is possible for a person who has never been exposed to the virus to catch chickenpox from someone who has an outbreak of shingles [3]. The practitioner should be suspicious of an underlying lymphoma, leukemia, or AIDS [3] (Fig. 22.7).

Signs/symptoms: Pain and/or paresthesias followed by eruption of red plaques that become vesicles, usually along a single dermatome, which later become covered by crusts. The pain may be felt before, during, and after (postherpetic neuralgia) the vesicular eruption [1–4].

Differential diagnosis: Herpes simplex (especially recurrent outbreaks), poison ivy, zoster sine herpete, cellulitis [1–4].

Treatment: Valacyclovir 1 g TID, nerve blocks, topical lidocaine patch or capsaicin cream. TCAs or gabapentin can be considered. The use of prednisone 60 mg × 2–4 weeks, then tapered over 4–6 weeks thereafter to prevent postherpetic neuralgia is still controversial [1, 2].

Venous Lake

Description: Asymptomatic, solitary, sofy, compressible, dark blue to violaceous, 0.2- to 1-cm papule commonly found on sun-exposed surfaces of the vermilion border of the lip, face and ears (Fig. 22.8).

Signs/symptoms: Generally none.

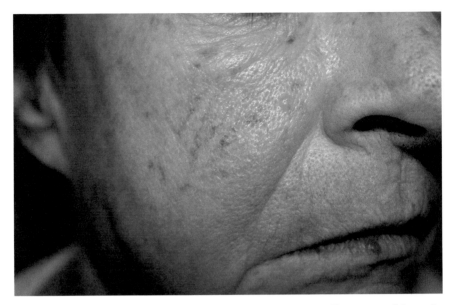

Fig. 22.8 Patient with alcohol abuse and persistent telangiectasias as well as a venous lake on the right lower lip

Differential diagnosis: Melanoma, blue nevus.
Treatment: None needed.

Basal Cell Carcinoma

Description: Most common form of skin cancer. There are five types: nodular/cystic (smooth surface, hard/firm), sclerosing/morpheaform (infiltrating type, whitish patches with irregular borders), ulcerating (crust covered with raised border), superficial (multiple areas usually on trunk, erythematous with thin scales), and pigmented (brown, blue, or black) [1, 2] (Fig. 22.9).

Signs/symptoms: Usually none, but can become irritated.

Differential diagnosis: Keratoacanthoma, psoriasis, seborrheic keratosis, tinea corporis, nodular melanoma [1, 2].

Treatment: Excision (Mohs), cryosurgery/electrosurgery except in danger areas or scalp, radiation in certain circumstances.

Sebaceous Hyperplasia [1, 2]

Clinically, hyperplastic glands look like yellow nodules that may have a central pore. The number of sebaceous glands remains constant as a person ages, but the glands increase in size and become more visible, particularly in chronically sun-exposed

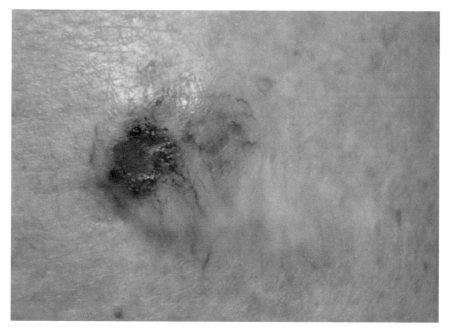

Fig. 22.9 Basal cell carcinoma

skin. Paradoxically, sebum production decreases over time, contributing to the dry skin seen in normally aged as well as photo-aged skin. It is important to distinguish sebaceous hyperplasia from nodular basal cell cancer. In contrast to basal cell cancer, the sebaceous gland is not translucent and does not have telangiectatic blood vessels. Nevertheless, when in doubt, it is always best to perform a biopsy (Fig. 22.10).

Squamous Cell Carcinoma

Description: The second most common non-melanoma skin cancer in the United States. Associated with an increased risk of metastasis, especially in areas of previous radiation, thermal injury, chronic draining sinuses, and chronic ulcers. It has a thick scale, is well defined, may be inflamed at the base [1–5] (Fig. 22.11).

Signs/symptoms: Usually none, although may be prone to bleeding [1].

Differential diagnosis: Actinic keratosis, fibrous papule, hemangioma, keratoacanthoma, wart, angiokeratoma, basal cell carcinoma, sebaceous hyperplasia, seborrheic keratosis, nummular eczema [1–5].

Treatment: Excision (Mohs surgery), electrodesiccation, curettage and cautery, radiation (except radiation-induced SCC), deep cryotherapy [1, 3, 4].

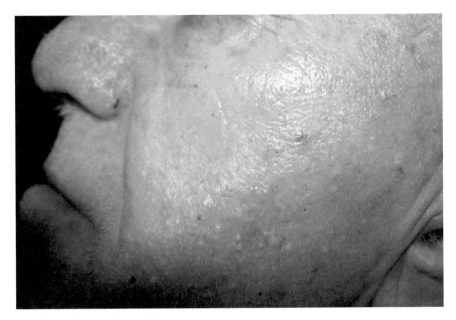

Fig. 22.10 Sebaceous hyperplasia

Photoaging

Description: The damage to the skin caused by intense and chronic exposure to sunlight. It contributes to extrinsic aging and can often make a person look older than his or her chronologic age.

Signs/symptoms: Fine wrinkles, mottling and pigmentation, roughness, redness, comedones.

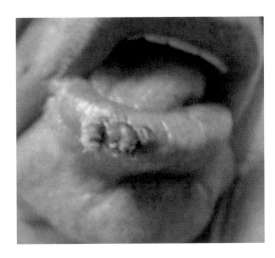

Fig. 22.11 Squamous cell carcinoma

Differential diagnosis: Actinic keratoses, solar lentigines.

Treatment: Sun protection (sunscreen and clothing), skin rejuvenation treatments, tretinoin cream.

Neurodermatitis

Description: Skin conditions that are psychologically related; it is estimated that at least one-third of individuals presenting to a dermatologist have a skin condition due to a psychological factor. Authors use many different names to refer to skin conditions that are psychologically related, including neurodermatitis, psychocutaneous diseases, psychodermatologic disorders, psychosomatic dermatology, and psychocutaneous medicine [1–3]. Neurodermatitis includes delusions of parasitosis, dermatitis artefacta, lichen simplex chronicus, neurotic excoriations, prurigo nodularis, and trichotillomania.

Signs/symptoms: Often intense itching and perception of "bugs in the skin." Multiple excoriations at all different stages of healing, often with clear areas on the central back that cannot be reached by scratching.

Differential diagnosis: scabies, eczema, generalized pruritus, bullous disorders, systemic disease.

Treatment: It includes topical anti-pruritic creams and ointments, oral psychiatric medicines, and counseling.

Neck

Acrochordon

Description: Fleshy or dark-colored benign pedunculated papules or nodules (skin tags) on the neck, axillae, groin, chest, abdomen [1–4] (Fig. 22.12).

Signs/symptoms: Painful when they get tangled in necklaces or clothing [1–4].

Differential diagnosis: Verruca vulgaris, nevi, seborrheic keratosis [1–4].

Treatment: Snip excision, cryotherapy, cautery [1–4].

Lichen Simplex Chronicus

Description: Lichenified, scaly, erythematous plaques found on fingers, elbows, palms, soles [1, 2, 4].

Signs/symptoms: Lion-like facies, pruritus [1, 2].

Differential diagnosis: Mycosis fungoides, dermatophytosis, psoriasis vulgaris, prurigo nodularis, contact dermatitis [1, 2].

Treatment: Topical steroids, tar preparations, antihistamines [1].

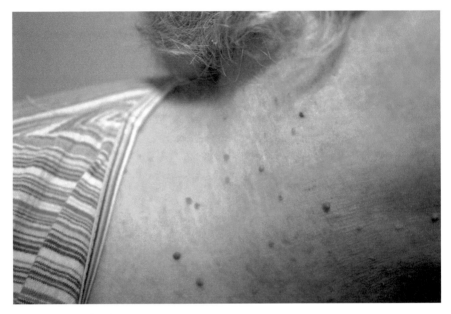

Fig. 22.12 Acrochordons

Trunk

Seborrheic Keratosis

Description: Rough, dark-colored plaques that have a "stuck-on" mole-like appearance [1, 2, 4] (Fig. 22.13).

Signs/symptoms: Usually none, although some may get irritated and cause discomfort [1, 2, 4].

Differential diagnosis: Verruca vulgaris, lichen planus, nevi, melanoma, basal cell carcinoma, lentigines [1–4].

Treatment: None needed. Can perform shave excision, chemical peels, cryotherapy [1, 2, 4].

Allergic Contact Dermatitis

Allergic contact dermatitis is an itchy skin condition caused by an allergic reaction to material in contact with the skin.

Description: The dermatitis is generally confined to the site of contact with the allergen, although severe cases may extend outside the contact area or may become generalized. It occurs hours after contact with the responsible material and will dissipate when the skin is no longer in contact with it.

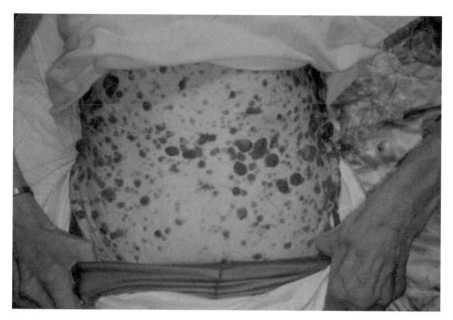

Fig. 22.13 Seborrheic keratosis (front)

An example is a localized irritation underlying a watch strap due to contact allergy to nickel (Fig. 22.14).

Signs/symptoms: Localized itch and irritation, occasional secondary infection.

Differential diagnosis: Contact urticaria, irritant contact dermatitis.

Allergic contact dermatitis is different than contact urticaria, where a rash appears within minutes of exposure and then fades away within minutes to hours, as with the allergic reaction to latex.

Allergic contact dermatitis is also distinct from irritant contact dermatitis, in which a similar skin condition is caused by excessive contact with irritants that include water, soaps, detergents, solvents, acids, alkalis, and friction.

At times a contact allergy arises only after the skin has been exposed to ultraviolet light. Although the allergen may have been in contact with covered areas, the rash is confined to sun exposed areas and is called photocontact dermatitis.

Treatment: Emollient creams, topical steroids, topical or oral antibiotics for secondary infection, oral steroids (short courses for severe cases), tacrolimus ointment, and pimecrolimus cream.

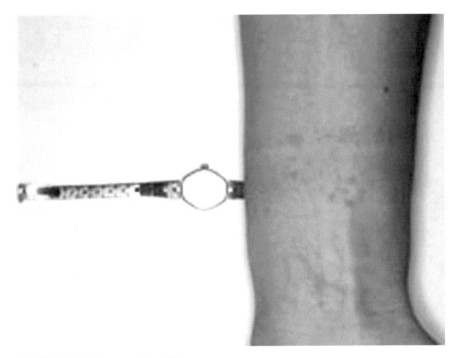

Fig. 22.14 Allergic contact dermatitis

Herpes Zoster

Description: See above (Figs. 22.7 and 22.15).

Lupus

See Fig. 22.16.

Psoriasis Vulgaris

Description: Silver, thick scales on pink-colored plaques on the skin and scalp, and pitting of the nails in psoriatic arthritis. Psoriasis can consist of a localized lesion or it can be widespread, can consist of large irregularly shaped areas or small, round areas [1, 2, 4] (Fig. 22.17).

Signs/symptoms: Pruritus. Psoriatic arthritis can include joint pain. Pustular psoriasis can present with chills, weakness, and fever [1, 2, 4].

Differential diagnosis: Includes, but is not limited to, pityriasis rubra pilaris, seborrheic dermatitis, pityriasis rosea, lichen planus, lichen sclerosis et atrophicus, pityriasis lichenoides, candidiasis, lichen simplex chronicus [1, 2, 4, 6].

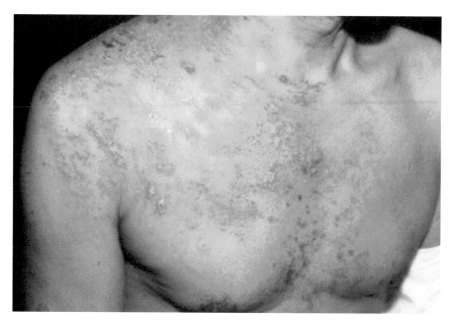

Fig. 22.15 Herpes zoster

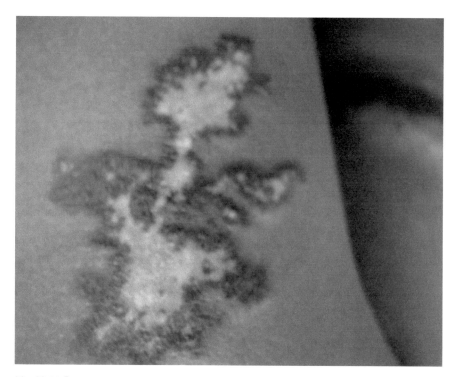

Fig. 22.16 Lupus

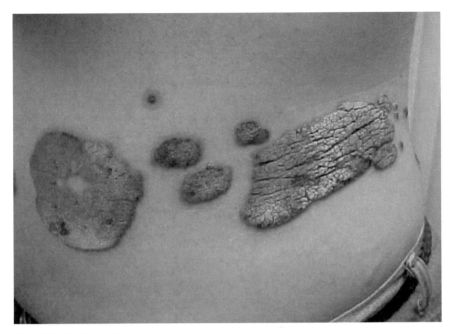

Fig. 22.17 Psoriasis vulgaris

Treatment: Biologic therapy (injectables), retinoids, topical steroids, UVB [1, 2, 4].

Scabies

Description: Transmissible ectoparasite skin infection characterized by superficial burrows, intense pruritus (itching), and secondary infection. The infestation of the skin occurs with the microscopic mite *Sarcoptes scabei*. Infestation is common, found worldwide, and affects people of all races and social classes. Scabies spreads rapidly under crowded conditions where there is frequent skin-to-skin contact between people, such as in hospitals, institutions, child-care facilities, and nursing homes (Fig. 22.18).

Signs/symptoms: Pimple-like irritations, burrows or rash of the skin, the skin folds on the wrist, elbow, or knee, the penis, the breast, or shoulder blades. Intense itching, especially at night and over most of the body.

Differential diagnosis: Lice, eczematous dermatitis, dermatitis herpetiformis, folliculitis, neurodermatitis. Skin scraping will help with diagnosis.

Treatment: Elimite (permethrin), Stromectol (Ivermectin). All clothes, bedding, and towels used by the infested person 2 days before treatment should be washed in hot water and dried in a hot dryer. A second treatment of the body with the same therapy may be necessary 7–10 days later.

Fig. 22.18 Scabies of upper arm and trunk

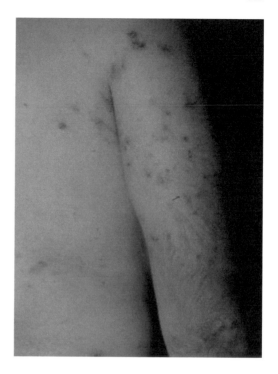

Scratching the rash may break the skin and make secondary infection more likely. For those with severe immunity such as advanced HIV infection, or those being treated with immunosuppressive drugs like steroids, a widespread rash with thick scaling may result, a variety of scabies called keratotic or Norwegian scabies.

Melanoma

See above (Fig. 22.19).

Upper Extremities

Atopic Eczematous Dermatitis

Description: Atopic dermatitis also known as atopic eczema, is a hereditary and non-contagious skin disease; onset before age 5 years in 90% of cases and some cases it may persist into old age.

Signs/symptoms: Chronic inflammation and pruritus of the skin.

Fig. 22.19 Melanoma

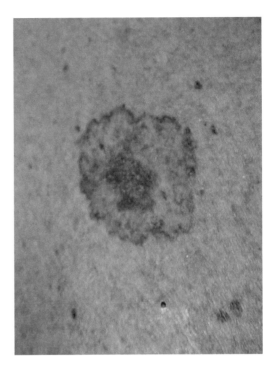

Differential diagnosis: Seborrheic dermatitis, contact dermatitis, nummular
    eczema, scabies, mycosis fungoides, dermatophytosis, stasis dermatitis.
Treatment: Topical corticosteroids, topical immunomodulators (tacrolimus,
    pimecrolimus), emollients.

Skin Tear

Purpura. If a skin tear does occur, non-adherent dressings secured with tubular retention bandages should be used to prevent trauma of the surrounding skin (Fig. 22.20).

Neurotic Excoriations

See Fig. 22.21.

Purpura

With aging, thinning of the dermis leads to increased fragility of the dermal
capillaries, and blood vessels rupture easily with minimal trauma. The resultant

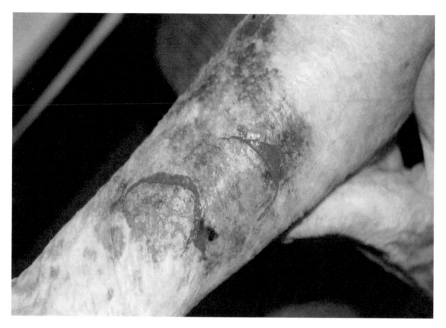

Fig. 22.20 Skin tear

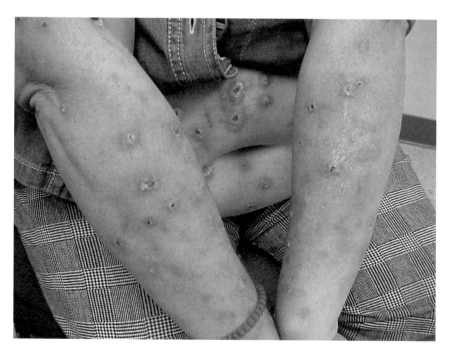

Fig. 22.21 Neurotic excoriations

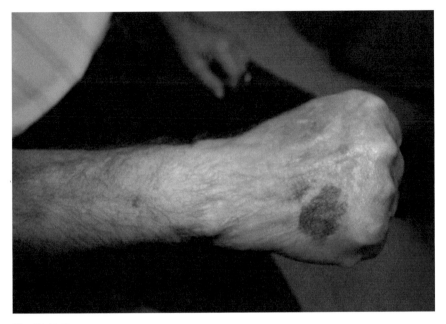

Fig. 22.22 Purpura

extravasation of blood into the surrounding tissue, commonly seen on the dorsal forearm and hands, is referred to as *purpura* or *ecchymosis* (Fig. 22.22).

Treatment: Reassurance that they do not have a bleeding disorder and should be advised to protect their skin against trauma and friction. Long-sleeved shirts reduce shear and friction. Nursing home personnel should be advised that gentle handling of the patient is crucial in the prevention of bruising and skin tears.

Hand

Keratoacanthoma

> *Description*: Smooth dome-shaped papule with central crater (keratinized) (Fig. 22.23).
> *Signs/symptoms*: Usually none. May be tender.
> *Differential diagnosis*: SCC, moluscum contagiosum, actinic keratosis, verruca vulgaris, cutaneous horn.
> *Treatment*: Surgical excision.

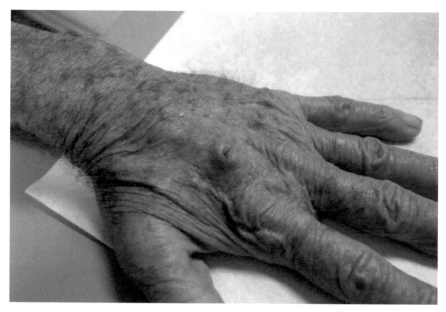

Fig. 22.23 Keratoacanthoma

Pelvis

Candidiasis

Description: Erythematous macules or patches with pustular lesions in fold areas, buttocks, and genital areas. Also can appear as whitish plaques in mucosal membranes and genital areas [1, 2, 4] (Fig. 22.24).
Signs/symptoms: Pruritus, burning, pain [1, 2].
Differential diagnosis: Condyloma acuminata, leukoplakia, lichen planus, hairy tongue [1].
Treatment: Topical and oral antifungal agents [1, 2].

Tinea Cruris

Description: Primarily occurs in men, often obese, prominent in warmer climates.
Signs/symptoms: Erythema with central clearing and an advanced scaly border in the inguinal creases. Also occurs on the medial thighs, lower abdomen, pubic area.
Differential diagnosis: Erythrasma, candidal intertrigo, psoriasis (potassium hydroxide preparation to detect for fungus).
Treatment: Topical antifungal agents.

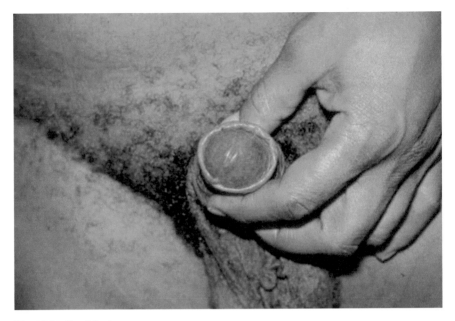

Fig. 22.24 Candidiasis

Buttocks

Pressure Ulcer

See Fig. 22.25.

Lower Extremities

Bullous Pemphigoid

See Fig. 22.26.

Diabetic Ulcers

See Fig. 22.27.

Melanoma

See above.

Fig. 22.25 Pressure ulcer

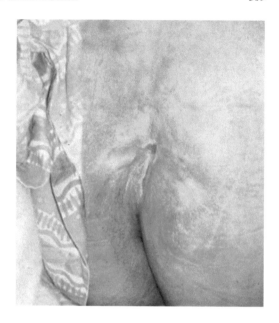

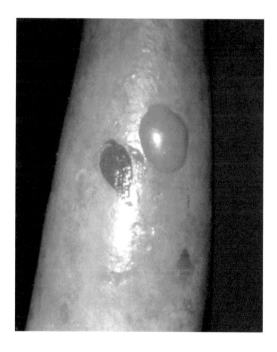

Fig. 22.26 Bullous
pemphigoid

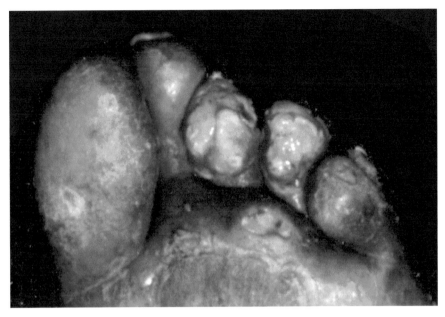

Fig. 22.27 Diabetic ulcers

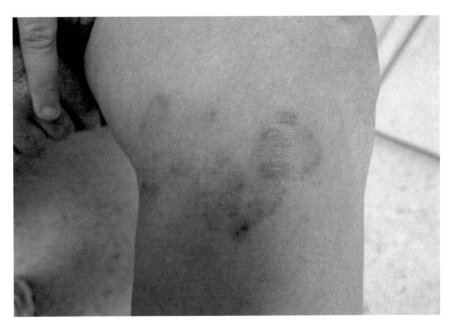

Fig. 22.28 Tinea

Tinea

See Fig. 22.28.

Tinea Pedis

Description: Tinea pedis is an inflammatory dermatophyte infection characterized by vesicles with surrounding erythema in the instep, toe webs, and soles
of the feet. The diagnosis is confirmed by KOH prep, but this can be falsely
negative (Fig. 22.29).

Signs/symptoms: Chronic pruritic scaling of the feet. Variants include interdigital (maceration), mocassin (hyperkeratotic) pattern, vesicular, or ulcerative.

Differential diagnosis: Dyshidrotic eczema, psoriasis, candidiasis, xerosis, contact dermatitis [1, 2, 4, 7].

Treatment: Topical clotrimazole cream, terbinafine cream, oral griseofulvin 500
mg twice a day or ketoconazole (Nizoral tablets) 200 mg daily is usually
effective. Gram-negative infections, often present in chronically wet or macerated areas, must be treated with topical antifungals and appropriate antibiotics [1, 2, 7].

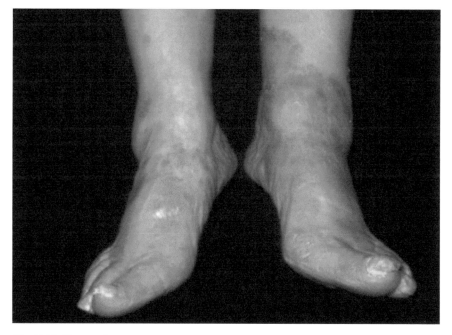

Fig. 22.29 Tinea pedis

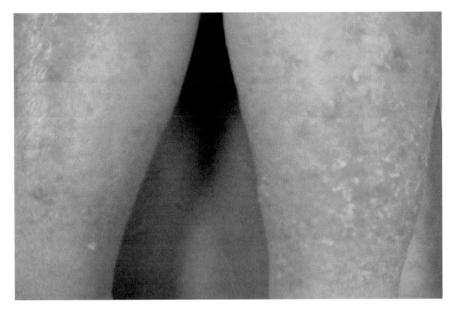

Fig. 22.30 Xerosis

Xerosis

Description: The condition is characterized by pruritic, dry, cracked, and fissured skin with scaling. Xerosis occurs most often on the legs of elderly patients. These skin cracks or fissures result from epidermal water loss (Fig. 22.30).

Signs/symptoms: The skin splits and cracks deeply enough to disrupt dermal capillaries, and bleeding fissures may occur. Itching or pruritis occurs leading to secondary lesions. Scratching and rubbing activities produce excoriations, an inflammatory response, lichen simplex chronicus, and even edematous patches.

Differential diagnosis: stasis dermatitis

Treatment: Emollients at least BID, alpha-hydroxy for moderate to severe disease, avoidance of harsh skin cleansers, ammonium lactate 12% lotion.

Stasis Dermatitis

Management: Includes topical agents such as alpha-hydroxy acid moisturizers or steroid cream or ointment (triamcinolone for 10–14 days) (Fig. 22.31).

Stasis Ulcers

See Fig. 22.32.

Fig. 22.31 Stasis dermatitis

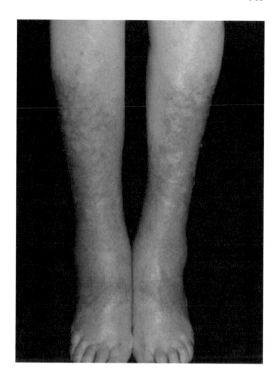

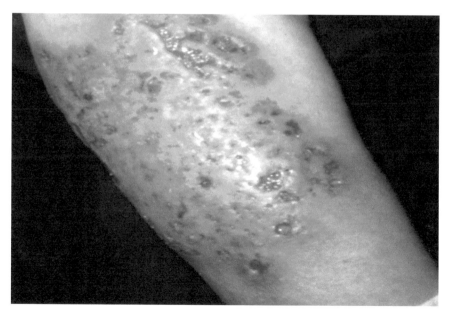

Fig. 22.32 Stasis ulcers

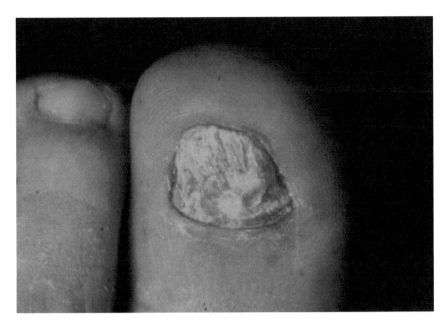

Fig. 22.33 Onychomycosis

Onychomycosis

See Fig. 22.33.

References

1. Fitzpatrick T, Johnson R, Wolff K, Suurmond D. Color Atlas & Synopsis of Clinical Dermatology Common & Serious Diseases, 4th ed. New York: McGraw-Hill, 2001.
2. Habif T. Clinical Dermatology: A Color Guide to Diagnosis and Therapy, 4th ed. St. Louis: Mosby, 2004.
3. Young E, Newcomer V, Kligman A. Geriatric Dermatology: Color Atlas and Practitioner's Guide. Philadelphia: Lea and Febiger, 1993.
4. Marks R. Skin Disease in Old Age, 2nd ed. London: Martin Dunitz, 1999.
5. Norman R, ed. Geriatric Dermatology. Lancaster: Parthenon Publishing, 2001.
6. Thiers B (Consulting Editor), Norman R (Guest Editor). Dermatol. Clin. N. Am. 2004; 22(1).
7. White G. Color Atlas of Regional Dermatology. London: Mosby-Wolfe, 1994.
8. Habif, Thomas. Skin Disease, Diagnosis and Treatment. E-medicine "Epidermal Cysts" http://www.emedicine.com/DERM/topic860.htm Merck Manual-Dermatology "Epidermal cysts".

Chapter 23

Selected Geriatric Dermatology Case Studies

Robert A. Norman, Charles Dewberry, and Megan Bock

Case 1

Name: BC

Ethnicity: Caucasian

Medical Hx: Significant for melanoma in her right arm as well as on the back and on the neck, emphysema, acute bronchitis, and COPD as well as degenerative disc disease.

Social Hx: The patient enjoys gardening. She uses Dial soap.

Family Hx: Significant for heart disease in her mother, breast cancer in her sister, and lung cancer in her brother.

Medications: Xanax, Wellbutrin, Lipitor, Serevent, and Albuterol nebulizer.

Allergies: The patient has allergies to Codeine and Darvocet.

Chief complaint: This 62-year-old female presented to our clinic bringing to our attention a lesion on her nose and one on her left chest.

Physical findings: Physical exam revealed a pleasantly affected female who appeared older than her stated age whose bridge of her nose revealed a flesh-colored, dome-shaped papule approximately 4 mm across. She admitted to a previous cancer surgery of this area but did not know the type of cancer. A brownish-red, variegated verrucous lesion was also noted on the left chest. She had dozens of red scaling and small exophytic red-brown lesions on her arms, legs, neck, and face.

Primary assessment/diagnosis:

1. Possible recurrent squamous cell carcinoma of the nose.
2. Seborrheic keratosis versus squamous cell carcinoma of left chest.
3. Extensive solar elastosis and actinic keratoses.

Treatment and course:

1. The nose papule and the left chest macule were both biopsied.
2. On follow-up, the patient's biopsy sites were well healed. Biopsy results on the nose showed actinic keratosis with nodular solar elastosis with no signs of calcification present. We treated with liquid nitrogen cryotherapy to that area.
3. The patient presented for follow-up of the chest. The biopsy results revealed a squamous cell carcinoma in situ. We have recommended f/u for this to

check for healing. The patient was encouraged to discontinue her smoking habit. In the interim, a second reading of the actinic keratosis with nodular fibrosis of the nose was done (we asked for a second reading) and this revealed a squamous cell carcinoma as well.

4. The patient presented for MOHS procedure. The lesion on the bridge of the nose was chosen as site and this was excised completely using a MOHS procedure and a full thickness skin graft from the leg was used to close the defect. The patient had multiple actinic keratoses and it was difficult to find any donor site that was free of damage.

5. The patient presented for follow-up. The areas were healing rather well, better than expected due to the amount of smoking in the patient and the steroids in her system. The graft was doing fairly well and 50% of the sutures were removed.

6. The remainder of the sutures were removed from the full thickness skin graft on the nose.

7. The patient presented for follow-up. The lateral part of the skin graft was showing some mild necrosis and granulation tissue was oozing out as well with some mild erythema surrounding. We put the patient on Keflex 500 mg twice daily and asked her to continue using good wound care.

8. The patient presented for follow-up. There was excellent healing of the entire skin graft.

9. The patient presented for follow-up on the left chest. Only a small residual erythema with a slightly rough border was noted. We treated with liquid nitrogen cryotherapy to that area.

10. The patient presented for follow-up. The tissue on the nose remained slightly hypertrophic with disproportion of the wound edge approximation. Biopsy was done of an irritated area on the nose graft that revealed an actinic keratosis from the leg donor site that may have interfered with proper healing. The area was anesthetized with lidocaine and a conmed hyfrecator set at low power and a flat bladed curette was used to gently resurface and resculpt the wound margins.

11. The patient presented for follow-up. Excellent approximation of the wound margins was achieved with nearly flush contours and healing nicely. We discussed extensive solar elastosis and actinic keratoses and treatment with 5-Fluorouracil.

Final diagnosis:

1. Atypical actinic keratosis with nodular fibrosis rediagnosed as a squamous cell carcinoma treated with MOHS micrographic surgery.

2. Actinic keratosis from the donor site and wound edge approximation defect treated in the office with a simple thermal dynamic contouring and curette procedure.

3. Extensive solar elastosis and actinic keratoses.

F / U: The patient's full thickness skin graft continued to heal very, very nicely with excellent flush contours and cosmetic results.

Educational relevance: This case was chosen to showcase the atypical actinic keratosis with nodular fibrosis and to highlight the ease of wound margin disappropriation using the simple technique of thermal dynamic contouring and sculpting curettage. The donor site actinic keratosis may have contributed to the delayed healing. In addition, it is important to pursue a diagnosis based on clinical suspicion even when the biopsy report does not reveal significant pathology; the squamous cell carcinoma (most likely recurrent) of the nose treated with MOHS resulted in resolution. The prevention and treatment of further lesions with 5-Fluorouracil was also included.

Ref:

Odom RB, James WD, Berger TG. Andrew's Diseases of the Skin: Clinical Dermatology, 9th ed. WB Sanders, 2000, pp. 804–6.

Bolognia JL, Jorizzo JL, Rapinio RP. Dermatology 1st ed. Mosby, 2003, pp. 873–9.

Freedberg IM, Eisen AZ, Wolff K, Austen KF, Goldsmith LA, Katz ST. Fitzpatrick's Dermatology in Internal Medicine, 5th ed. McGraw-Hill, 1999, pp. 1697–701.

Case 2

Name: SC

Ethnicity: Caucasian

Medical Hx: Significant for bronchitis, arthritis, and a subjective history of "rash."

Family Hx: Negative for heart disease, diabetes, cancer, or arthritis.

Medications: Medications include Naproxen.

Allergies: The patient has no known drug allergies.

Chief complaint: This is a 61-year-old male who presented to our clinic saying he has a rash on his back for ten years.

Physical findings: Physical exam revealed a well-developed, well-nourished, pleasantly affected male who has no malar rash and several erythematous wheals on his back.

Primary assessment/diagnosis: Nummular eczema versus systemic lupus erythematosus.

Treatment and course:

1. On the day of presentation, the patient was thoroughly examined.
2. The patient presented for follow-up with a lesion on the patient's right back. This was in fact biopsied and serum lab results were also requested. The pathology returned to our office showing systemic lupus erythematous. Histologic picture showed hyperkeratosis, follicular plugging, and atrophy, focal liquefaction of the epidermis, and perivascular and perifollicular infiltration of lymphocytes and

histiocytes. Calcium blue stain revealed a copious mucin present in the dermis. Serum lab results showed serum electrolyte panel and metabolic panel within normal limits. The CBC with diff was also within normal limits. The ANA and LE test were positive.

3. The patient presented for follow-up. The patient had contacted a rheumatologist in his network and a bone scan was done the previous week. This time, the patient revealed to us a rash on his stomach as well as dry skin on his right index finger. We reviewed the biopsy report and the lab results with the patient and gave him copies to forward on to his rheumatologist. We gave the patient a prescription for Clobetasol 0.05% cream to apply to the rash and Periactin 4 mg three times per day for the itch.

Final diagnosis: Systemic lupus erythematosus.

F/U: The patient has been referred to a rheumatologist and we will follow up with the patient in 6 months for his cutaneous involvement.

Educational relevance: This case was chosen to showcase the clinical presentation of systemic lupus erythematosus and the appropriate labs and referral to a rheumatology specialist. In the near future (and with the increased use of biologic therapy) dermatologists may be taking more primary care of SLE patients.

Ref:

Odom RB, James WD, Berger TG. Andrew's Diseases of the Skin: Clinical Dermatology, 9th ed. WB Sanders, 2000, pp# 180-185

Bolognia JL, Jorizzo JL, Rapinio RP. Dermatology 1st ed. Mosby, 2003, pp. 1926, 1944, 2005–7, 2056.

Freedberg IM, Eisen AZ, Wolff K, Austen KF, Goldsmith LA, Katz ST. Fitzpatrick's Dermatology in Internal Medicine, 5th ed. McGraw-Hill, 1999, pp. 591–5, 607, 611.

Case 3

Name: JR

Ethnicity: Caucasian

Medical Hx: Significant for hypertension and high cholesterol.

Social Hx: The patient is a postal worker. He uses Coast deodorant soaps, Purex laundry detergent, and V05 hair products.

Family Hx: Significant for diabetes, heart disease, and skin and colon cancer in his father.

Medications: Include blood pressure medications and he was then using Lotrisone.

Allergies: The patient denied any known drug allergies.

Chief complaint: This is a 63-year-old male who presented to our office for a rash on the right areola area for which he was given Lotrisone cream by his primary care physician, which has not improved the lesion to any significant extent.

Physical findings: This 63-year-old male presented with signs of extensive weathering. Otherwise, he was well developed, well nourished, and pleasantly affected.

The right nipple revealed an ill-defined papulosquamous eruption. It was warm to the touch. Also, noted on the patient's left nipple was mild to moderate erythema and scaling. No subcutaneous masses were palpated.

Primary assessment/diagnosis:

1. Nummular eczema of the nipple.
2. Ruled out neoplastic process.

Treatment and course: The patient presented to our office with a non-pruritic papulosquamous eruption on the right nipple as well as a lesser severity similar lesion on the left nipple. The right nipple was biopsied to rule out neoplastic process versus eczematous process. He was given a prescription for Triamcinolone 0.1% cream to apply to the area.

Final diagnosis: Biopsy revealed psoriaform dermatitis.

F/U: The patient was lost to follow-up. The biopsy results of psoriaform dermatitis was conveyed to the patient via phone message.

Educational relevance: This case was chosen to showcase the incidence of not altogether common nummular eczema of the nipple in a male and the clinical prudence still recommends biopsy of any and all nipple eczemas, even in males. Paget's disease of the breast appears as an eczema-like change on the nipple skin and 90% of women who have Paget's have an underlying breast cancer. The underlying breast cancer may be an invasive breast cancer or ductal carcinoma in situ (DCIS). Paget's usually occurs in women their 50s, and can rarely affect men.

Ref:

Odom RB, James WD, Berger TG. Andrew's Diseases of the Skin: Clinical Dermatology, 9th ed. WB Sanders, 2000, p. 77.

Bolognia JL, Jorizzo JL, Rapinio RP. Dermatology 1st ed. Mosby, 2003, pp. 545, 2348.

Freedberg IM, Eisen AZ, Wolff K, Austen KF, Goldsmith LA, Katz ST. Fitzpatrick's Dermatology in Internal Medicine, 5th ed. McGraw-Hill, 1999, pp. 218–9.

Case 4

Name: IB

Ethnicity: Caucasian

Medical Hx: Blood clots, bone cancer, lung cancer, and breast cancer as well as a mastectomy 17 years ago of the left breast.

Family Hx: Positive for lymphoma cancer in the patient's mother.

Medications: Coumadin and Zoloft.

Allergies: No known drug allergies.

Chief complaint: An 82-year-old female who presented with a dry, scaly spot that itched and burned on the left breast which was present for approximately 2 months.

Physical findings: An 82-year-old female whose appearance was consistent with her stated age whose left chest area was devoid of a breast from a surgical mastectomy 17 years ago. She had a 4 cm × 5 cm, erythematous, scaly patch with obvious excoriations on it.

Primary assessment/diagnosis: Metastatic breast cancer.

Treatment and course:

1. A biopsy using a deep shave technique was taken.
2. The patient presented for follow-up. The biopsy revealed metastatic adenocarcinoma. This was discussed with the patient. A referral and an appointment was made for a local oncologist. The patient was given empathetic reassurance with family members present. The patient was asked to return for follow-up pending an evaluation by her oncologist.

Final diagnosis: Metastatic breast cancer.

F/U: The patient was unable to follow-up and discussion with family member revealed the patient was admitted to the hospital and was undergoing tests for possible radiation therapy and chemotherapy.

Educational relevance: This case was chosen for its relevance to eczematous lesions, can in fact be related to internal neoplasms and not necessarily eczema, tinea, xerosis, or impetigo despite what they look like.

Ref:

Odom RB, James WD, Berger TG. Andrew's Diseases of the Skin: Clinical Dermatology, 9th ed. WB Sanders, 2000, pp. 842–3.

Bolognia JL, Jorizzo JL, Rapinio RP. Dermatology 1st ed. Mosby, 2003, pp. 919–23.

Freedberg IM, Eisen AZ, Wolff K, Austen KF, Goldsmith LA, Katz ST. Fitzpatrick's Dermatology in Internal Medicine, 5th ed. McGraw-Hill, 1999, pp. 713–4.

Case 5

Name: BB

Ethnicity: Caucasian

Medical Hx: Negative.

Social Hx: The patient has been a resident of Florida her entire life. She is a mother with one daughter. She works in the food service industry. She has one dog in the home.

Family Hx: Significant only for diabetes in her grandparents and heart disease in her grandparents.

Medications: Medications include Depo Provera injections and occasional muscle relaxers, which she does not remember the name, as well as occasional Tylenol for headaches.

Allergies: The patient denied any known drug allergies.

Chief complaint: The patient presented with a lesion on her right arm that has been present for approximately 1–2 months.

Physical findings: This is a 64-year-old female who appeared consistent with her stated age whose right upper arm revealed a 1 cm fibrous papule with erythema and obvious excoriation.

Primary assessment/diagnosis: Impetiginized dermatofibroma.

Treatment and course:

1. The area was biopsied using a shave technique. The patient was given a prescription for Tetracycline 500 mg twice daily. The patient was asked to return in 2 weeks.
2. In 2 weeks, the biopsy results revealed a dermatofibroma. The biopsy site was healing well. The patient asked about improving the appearance of her facial skin. A prescription for Retin-A 0.025% cream was given and she was asked to use this every other night. A discussion about glycolic peel was given. We decided to see the patient back in approximately 2 months for follow-up.
3. The patient presented complaining of a left leg lesion stating that her dog scratched it and a rash had appeared. The rash had gone away and reappeared again. It was very painful to the touch. The patient's OB/GYN doctor thought that it was perhaps a herpetic infection and the patient presented to us for evaluation. The left leg also revealed a dermatonal-related erythematous, slightly vesiculated rash. The patient was given a prescription for Famvir 500 mg to take twice daily and Lidocaine Mantle cream was also given for the irritation as well as a prescription for Triamcinolone 0.1%. We decided to see the patient back in 2 weeks.
4. In 2 weeks, the patient presented showing a much improved appearance of the lesion and a diagnosis of HSV was made. A prescription for Acyclovir was given to the patient with refills. The patient was educated about prodromal symptoms and to start a round of Acyclovir the next time this rash appeared.

Final diagnosis: HSV of the lower leg dermatone.

F/U: At this point, the patient has remained free of outbreaks in this area. The patient has not needed to take her Acyclovir. Again, the patient was educated that more than six outbreaks in 1 year would necessitate a suppressive regimen. At this point, it was not needed.

Educational relevance: This case was chosen to showcase the all too familiar complaint of a shingles outbreak in persons previously exposed and also for the need to differentiate between primary outbreak and episodic outbreaks and the need to decipher when to use episodic treatment versus suppressive treatment.

Ref:

Odom RB, James WD, Berger TG. Andrew's Diseases of the Skin: Clinical Dermatology, 9th ed. WB Sanders, 2000, pp. 473–82.

Bolognia JL, Jorizzo JL, Rapinio RP. Dermatology 1st ed. Mosby, 2003, pp. 241, 1468–74.

Freedberg IM, Eisen AZ, Wolff K, Austen KF, Goldsmith LA, Katz ST. Fitzpatrick's Dermatology in Internal Medicine, 5th ed. McGraw-Hill, 1999, pp. 1236–9.

Case 6

Name: KA

Ethnicity: Caucasian

Medical Hx: Significant for diabetes and depression.

Social Hx: The patient works outside in the landscape business and he admits to extensive alcohol use as well as recreational drug use.

Family Hx: Significant for alcoholism in his father. No skin cancer.

Medications: Glucotrol, Glucovance, Prilosec, and Prozac.

Allergies: The patient has no known drug allergies.

Chief complaint: This 65-year-old male presented with a brown spot on his left cheek for the past 1 year. He stated that it has enlarged in the last 3 months as well as a spot on his penis that has no changes.

Physical findings: Caucasian male of obvious significant sun exposure with brown macules in numerous areas of sun exposure. His left cheek revealed a brown spot and a brown, macular, non-variegated lesion on the penis.

Primary assessment/diagnosis: R/O malignant melanoma.

Treatment and course:

1. The spot on the left cheek was recommended for biopsy on follow-up.
2. The spot on the left cheek was biopsied without complications.
3. The patient presented for follow-up and the biopsy showed a pigmented actinic keratosis. The patient was given reassurance and the biopsy site was frozen with liquid nitrogen cryotherapy and the precancerous nature of this lesion was discussed at length with the patient as well as discussion at length of ultraviolet protection including the use of SPF 15 daily, wide-brimmed hat, and avoiding peak hours of sunlight unless wearing long sleeves and pants.
4. The patient presented for a yearly checkup stating that the brown spot on his left antihelix has shown up recently. This small, 4 mm, smooth, brown macule was biopsied.
5. The patient presented for follow-up. The biopsy, however, showed malignant melanoma in situ. The patient was scheduled for excision of this lesion and due to this complicated area, MOHS micrographic surgery was used to minimize the margins.
6. The patient presented for excision. However, some problems were noted in the morning as the patient was obviously intoxicated, although accompanied by his mother. The patient was taken to the surgical suite and under local anesthesia and with the expectation of extra bleeding, the site was excised using 0.5 cm margins.
7. The patient presented for follow-up. Excellent healing of the ear excision and flap reconstruction was noted. A spot on the patient's right cheek and right thigh were also biopsied.
8. The patient presented for follow-up. The biopsy sites had healed well. There was excellent healing of the left ear. Biopsy results revealed compound melanocytic

nevus without signs of atypia. The patient was referred to the University of South Florida Moffit Melanoma Center and given instructions for a 3-month follow-up.

9. The patient presented for follow-up. The ear continued to look exceptionally well. The patient has followed-up with the Moffit Melanoma Center and has been counseled extensively for a biannual complete skin check.

Final diagnosis: Malignant melanoma in situ.

F / U: The patient at that time continued to be free of dysplastic nevus or melanoma and has been adherent with his follow-up.

Educational relevance: This case was chosen to showcase the very benign appearance of melanoma as the original site was non-variegated single color, smooth-bordered, and less than 6 mm. It showed no clinical signs of atypia or abnormality.

Ref:

Odom RB, James WD, Berger TG. Andrew's Diseases of the Skin: Clinical Dermatology, 9th ed. WB Sanders, 2000, pp. 882–90.

Bolognia JL, Jorizzo JL, Rapinio RP. Dermatology 1st ed. Mosby, 2003, pp. 1105–8.

Freedberg IM, Eisen AZ, Wolff K, Austen KF, Goldsmith LA, Katz ST. Fitzpatrick's Dermatology in Internal Medicine, 5th ed. McGraw-Hill, 1999, pp. 1779–815.

Case 7

Name: CC

Ethnicity: Hispanic

Medical Hx: Significant for rosacea and colitis.

Social Hx: The patient works as a crossing guard. She is a former homemaker. She does not have any pets. She does not smoke. She uses Cetaphil and antibacterial soaps. She uses different types of laundry detergents.

Family Hx: Significant for heart disease in her uncle and breast cancer in her aunt.

Medications: MetroGel and Hydrocortisone.

Allergies: The patient has an allergy to Tetracycline.

Chief complaint: This is a 63-year-old female who presented for evaluation of rosacea, which she has had for approximately 10 years.

Physical findings: A 63-year-old, Hispanic female whose face revealed pustular and granulomatous lesions along with telangiectatic matting and overall flushing and blushing of the face. Pathology was superficial vascular findings.

Primary assessment/diagnosis: Granulomatous rosacea.

Treatment and course:

1. We gave the patient a prescription for Elidel and told her to discontinue the use of Hydrocortisone. We also extensively educated the patient on avoiding flare factors such as caffeine, hot water, strong soaps, and most importantly ultraviolet

exposure. We asked the patient to use a very mild cleanser such as Cetaphil. She should continue using the MetroGel and the Elidel as a possible off-label use for her rosacea. We also recommended the use of vascular laser for ablation of the superficial vascular proliferation of the face.

2. The patient presented for follow-up stating no improvement with the Elidel and MetroGel. At that time, we recommended laser for the patient. The patient presented for treatment with a V-beam laser 10-mm spot size, 6 ms, and $7\,J/cm^2$, approximately 200+ pulses. Allegra antihistamine was given as well as instructions for cool compresses over the next 36–48 h.

3. The patient presented for follow-up, although it was too soon to notice any significant improvement. A few granulomatous lesions were noted and the patient was put on Keflex 250 mg as a low dose.

4. The patient presented for follow-up. Physical exam revealed a 30–40% reduction in the erythematous findings. No granulomatous lesions were apparent, although some healing lesions were noted. Then, we gave the patient a prescription for Azithromycin 250 mg two pills once weekly #10. We recommended further laser treatments approximately 8–10 weeks apart.

Final diagnosis: Granulomatous rosacea.

F/U: Unfortunately, the patient's insurance did cover the laser treatment for the rosacea and continued episodic antibiotics were being used to treat that even though improvement was achieved with one treatment. The patient did not present for further laser treatment as the cost was more than she can afford and her insurance will not pay for that and continued episodic antibiotics will be tried as well as avoidance of flare factors and the use of topical Metronidazole as well as topical Sodium Sulfacetamide.

Educational relevance: This case was chosen to showcase the possible definitive effective treatment using vascular ablation by the use of lasers for the definitive treatment of rosacea.

Ref:
Odom RB, James WD, Berger TG. Andrew's Diseases of the Skin: Clinical Dermatology, 9th ed. WB Sanders, 2000, pp. 305.
Bolognia JL, Jorizzo JL, Rapinio RP. Dermatology 1st ed. Mosby, 2003, pp. 790.
Freedberg IM, Eisen AZ, Wolff K, Austen KF, Goldsmith LA, Katz ST. Fitzpatrick's Dermatology in Internal Medicine, 5th ed. McGraw-Hill, 1999, pp. 546–7.

Case 8

Name: RC
Ethnicity: Hispanic
Medical Hx: Significant for hypertension.
Social Hx: The patient works as a mechanic and also sells newspapers on the street corner. Products used are Irish Spring and Herbal Essence.

Family Hx: Negative for diabetes, heart disease, asthma, or cancer.

Medications: Ibuprofen p.r.n.

Allergies: The patient has no known drug allergies.

Chief complaint: This 57-year-old, Hispanic male presented to our clinic complaining of discoloration of the right cheek that began approximately 2 years ago.

Physical findings: A well-developed, well-nourished, pleasantly affected, Hispanic male with obvious signs of weathering. He had a hypopigmented area on the right cheek.

Primary assessment/diagnosis:

1. Actinic rosacea.
2. Hypopigmentation of unknown origin, presumed post-inflammatory.

Treatment and course:

1. The patient presented to our office and a punch biopsy was taken of the hypopigmented area to rule out vitiligo versus tinea. The patient was educated extensively on the use of sunblock.
2. The patient presented for follow-up. Pathology showed findings consistent with post-inflammatory hypopigmentation. The patient was put on a prescription of Acclovate ointment and Elidel to be applied twice daily.
3. The patient presented for follow-up. Little or no improvement was noted by the practitioner or the patient. The pathology was sent for a second opinion to rule out vitiligo. The patient was asked to continue using Acclovate and Elidel. Serum labs were drawn for TSH, ANA, and CBC.

Final diagnosis: Post-inflammatory hypopigmentation with characteristics of vitiligo.

F/U: The patient's area continued to be hypopigmented without resolution. Treatment options including pigment transplant and Relume laser treatment were offered. The patient stated that he was not concerned as long as it was not cancer.

Educational relevance: This case was chosen to showcase the difficulty of determining post-inflammatory hypopigmentation versus vitiligo, especially in a pigmented individual.

Ref:

Odom RB, James WD, Berger TG. Andrew's Diseases of the Skin: Clinical Dermatology, 9th ed. WB Sanders, 2000, pp. 1057–72.

Bolognia JL, Jorizzo JL, Rapinio RP. Dermatology 1st ed. Mosby, 2003, pp. 944–86 and 2116.

Freedberg IM, Eisen AZ, Wolff K, Austen KF, Goldsmith LA, Katz ST. Fitzpatrick's Dermatology in Internal Medicine, 5th ed. McGraw-Hill, 1999, pp. 947–55.

Case 9

Name: JC

Ethnicity: Caucasian

Medical Hx: Significant for hypertension.

Family Hx: Noncontributory.

Medications: Atenolol and Lasix. *Allergies*: No known drug allergies.

Chief complaint: This 82-year-old male presented to our clinic accompanied by his son and daughter who was known to our clinic for a number of integumental concerns. A MOHS surgery was performed on the right ear approximately 1 month prior. At this time, the patient complained of a recent large growth on the right arm that has been growing for approximately the last 3 weeks.

Physical findings: The left ear was healing well from the previous micrographic surgery. The left arm revealed a 3 cm × 4 cm, pedunculated, mushroom-type lesion with atypical features throughout.

Primary assessment/diagnosis: Giant keratoacanthoma.

Treatment and course:

1. The lesion was biopsied to rule out giant keratoacanthoma.
2. The biopsy revealed a giant keratoacanthoma. The patient was also using Effudex on several body areas for his extensive sun damage and these areas appeared red and slightly desquamated, most notably on the scalp and face. We asked the patient to discontinue the use of Effudex there and to start using Effudex on his hands and forearms. We recommended the patient for MOHS micrographic surgery for the giant keratoacanthoma.
3. The patient presented for MOHS micrographic surgery. This was performed and clear margins were obtained and a complex flap closure was performed to provide primary closure.
4. The patient presented for suture removal. The right arm was healing very, very well. The sutures were removed. The patient was encouraged to continue his Effudex treatment. We explained to the patient that a crop rotation modality was in his best interest due to his severe actinic damage. The patient was to pick a body site and treat for 3 weeks with the Effudex and take a 1-week vacation from the treatment. The patient was to then choose another body site and treat for 3 weeks with a subsequent 1-week vacation. We outlined the patient's body site as being head and neck #1, face and ears #2, forearms #3, and chest and back #4.
5. The patient presented for follow-up. The patient had quit using Effudex on the face and started using it on the arms.
6. The patient presented for follow-up. The face had calmed down considerably from the 5-Fluorouracil. The arms revealed a number of red, obviously irritated plaques and macules. The patient was recommended to quit using Effudex there and start using Effudex on the upper back and chest as part of his crop rotation.

Final diagnosis: Giant keratoacanthoma, actinic keratoses

F / U: The patient's MOHS surgery site continued to be well-healed and the patient had been fairly compliant with his Effudex crop rotation modality for control of his severe actinic damage.

Educational relevance: This case was chosen to showcase the clinical presentation of a large, rapidly growing keratoacanthoma.

Ref:

Odom RB, James WD, Berger TG. Andrew's Diseases of the Skin: Clinical Dermatology, 9th ed. WB Sanders, 2000, pp. 816–20 and 836.

Bolognia JL, Jorizzo JL, Rapinio RP. Dermatology 1st ed. Mosby, 2003, pp. 865–71 and 2990.

Freedberg IM, Eisen AZ, Wolff K, Austen KF, Goldsmith LA, Katz ST. Fitzpatrick's Dermatology in Internal Medicine, 5th ed. McGraw-Hill, 1999, pp. 1026, 1675–6, 2333.

Case 10

Name: PE

Ethnicity: Caucasian

Medical Hx: Significant for diabetes, irritable bowel syndrome, lupus, anxiety, depression, and cancer of the colon.

Surgical Hx: Significant for a hemi-cholectomy with primary anastamosis.

Social Hx: The patient is disabled. She enjoys being in the sun.

Family Hx: Hypertension.

Medications: Medications include topical Lidex cream for her lupus flare-ups. She was also using insulin for her diabetes, Xanax for her anxiety, and Zoloft for her depression.

Allergies: She has drug allergies to Cipro and Aspirin.

Chief complaint: A 66-year-old female who presented to our clinic with an irritated lesion on her right helix.

Physical findings: Physical exam revealed a pleasantly affected female of a semi-obese nature whose right helix revealed pearly papules on the helical ridge with erythema and excoriation.

Primary assessment/diagnosis: Actinic keratosis versus neoplasm of the ear versus possible verruca vulgaris versus chondrodermatitis nodularis chronica helicis (CNH). CNH is a common, benign, painful condition of the helix or antihelix of the ear that often affects older individuals. Although the exact cause of CNH is unknown, most authorities believe it is caused by prolonged and excessive pressure.

Treatment and course:

1. The patient presented for a lesion on the right helix. We recommended liquid nitrogen cryotherapy to the site and this was done with three freeze–thaw cycles.
2. The patient presented for follow-up. The right ear lesion had not resolved with the liquid nitrogen cryotherapy and a biopsy of this area was performed.

3. The patient returned for follow-up. The biopsy results revealed CDNH with extension into the cartilage and brisk inflammation also in the histologic picture. We discussed with the patient the recommended treatment for this including liquid nitrogen cryotherapy, ED&C, and wide excision. The patient elected upon wide excision treatment.
4. The patient presented for wide excision of the ear lesion. The lesion was excised using a cold steel excision with a 15 Parker blade down to the level of the cartilage along the helical rim. A bilateral helical advancement was used to provide cosmetic closure.
5. The patient presented for suture removal. Excellent healing was noted at the site and the sutures were removed. The patient was educated to continue good wound care.
6. The patient presented stating that the right ear was hurting. Pathology results from the excision had returned to our office showing margins clear. Physical exam of the ear noted a small apparently cicatrix phenomena along the helical margin. We recommended intralesional injection to that area and a 1/4 cc of Kenalog 10 was injected.
7. The patient presented for follow-up. The right ear showed a small amount of tissue loss along the surgical margin. There was some other cicatrix phenomena happening and the patient stated that it did hurt. We gave the patient a prescription for Zonalon cream and Temovate cream 15 g each to apply to the ear twice daily. We discussed with the patient the etiology of poor healing because of her diabetes as well as the possibility of the intralesional injection causing tissue necrosis.
8. The patient presented for follow-up. At that point, there was excellent healing of the ear. Good cosmetic results had been achieved. The patient was no longer using Zonalon and did not complain of persistent pain in the ear.

Final diagnosis: Chondrodermatitis nodularis chronica helicis (CNH) treated with local excision and repair.

F/U: The patient's ear continued to be pain-free without recurrence of the lesion and since the surgery she has trained herself not to sleep on that side.

Educational relevance: This case was chosen to showcase the not altogether common clinical picture of CDNH usually as small calcified nodules below the skin; however, on this patient the clinical picture revealed almost a friable, pearly papule-type lesion much more consistent with either prurigo nodularis or a basal cell carcinoma as well as the prudence in local excision and repair.

Ref:

Odom RB, James WD, Berger TG. Andrew's Diseases of the Skin: Clinical Dermatology, 9th ed. WB Sanders, 2000, pp. 1057–72.

Bolognia JL, Jorizzo JL, Rapinio RP. Dermatology 1st ed. Mosby, 2003, pp. 34–5, 986–1002.

Freedberg IM, Eisen AZ, Wolff K, Austen KF, Goldsmith LA, Katz ST. Fitzpatrick's Dermatology in Internal Medicine, 5th ed. McGraw-Hill, 1999, pp. 975–1004.

Case 11

Name: RE

Ethnicity: Caucasian

Medical Hx: Significant for diabetes, angina, reflux, asthma, arthritis, carpal tunnel syndrome, and a subjective history of lupus.

Social Hx: Noncontributory.

Family Hx: Positive for skin cancer in her uncle. Positive for diabetes in her parents.

Medications: Medications include Tramadol, Zantac, Albuterol nebulizer, and insulin.

Allergies: The patient stated that she was allergic to a medication, but she was unsure of what it was.

Chief complaint: A 68-year-old female who presented to our clinic complaining of an irritation of both the forearms and chest.

Physical findings: Physical exam revealed a 68-year-old female who appeared somewhat older than her stated age whose forearms and chest revealed an erythematous, cracking, peeling tissue with signs of excoriation.

Primary assessment/diagnosis:

1. Cutaneous lupus.
2. Cellulitis of the forearms.
3. Unknown pruritus.

Treatment and course:

1. The patient's forearm and chest were biopsied. The patient was given a prescription for Bactroban ointment and Triamcinolone ointment to be applied twice daily. She was also put on Zyrtec 10 mg b.i.d. as well as Atarax 10 mg in the evening and Keflex 500 mg b.i.d.
2. The patient presented for follow-up. Biopsy results showed severe solar elastosis with dermal inflammation and PAS stain was negative for mycotic hyphae or spores; nor was there any basement midway thickening and follicular plugging. We discussed with the patient that this was highly unlikely to be a flare of lupus and more likely this was actinic pruritus with impetiginization of secondary cellulitis. The patient stated that she was somewhat better. There was still some erythematous boggy, warm to the touch findings of the forearms. The patient was continued on Keflex 500 mg b.i.d.

Final diagnosis: Actinic pruritus.

F/U: The patient was lost to follow-up.

Educational relevance: This case was chosen to showcase the clinical incidence of actinic pruritus as opposed to polymorphous light eruption.

Ref:

Odom RB, James WD, Berger TG. Andrew's Diseases of the Skin: Clinical Dermatology, 9th ed. WB Sanders, 2000, pp. 37, 49–59. Bolognia JL, Jorizzo JL, Rapinio RP. Dermatology 1st ed. Mosby, 2003, pp. 491–2, 487–90, 1709, 1725.

Freedberg IM, Eisen AZ, Wolff K, Austen KF, Goldsmith LA, Katz ST. Fitzpatrick's Dermatology in Internal Medicine, 5th ed. McGraw-Hill, 1999, pp. 85–109.

Case 12

Name: TH

Ethnicity: Caucasian

Medical Hx: Significant for HIV and currently being treated for numerous warts being resistant to treatment. The patient's current CD-4 count is approximately 100. HIV count is above 200,000 viral particles.

Social Hx: The patient is disabled. He is semi-wheelchair bound. He lives with his partner of 14 years.

Family Hx: Noncontributory.

Medications: Antiviral cocktail as well as Bactrim DS, Neurontin, and various anti-nausea medications.

Allergies: Motrin, Compazine, and Tegretol.

Chief complaint: The patient's verruca on his digits resistant to treatment currently being administered with cryotherapy.

Physical findings: Pleasantly affected, 61-year-old male with somewhat of an emaciated appearance, appearing somewhat older than his stated age with verrucal papules on the digits of his fingers. The patient also had a perianal lesion that he brought to our attention.

Primary assessment/diagnosis:

1. Verruca vulgaris.
2. Advanced HIV disease.
3. Presumed condyloma acuminata of the perianal area.

Treatment and course:

1. The patient was given Effudex 5% to apply to the warts twice per day and a prescription for Aldara for the presumed condyloma acuminata of the perianal area. This was also biopsied.
2. The patient presented for follow-up stating that he had been using the 5-Fluorouracil on his warts, some of which had responded. The patient gave a history of episodic response to the 5-Fluorouracil. The biopsy report of the perianal lesion came back as basal cell carcinoma. We applied Canthacur to the digital wart at that time and referred the patient to Moffitt Cancer Center for treatment of the basal cell carcinoma of the anal verge.
3. The patient presented back to our office stating that he had good results with the Canthacur and wished to continue treatment with the Canthacur for the digital warts. The patient also stated that the carcinoma of the perianal area was being treated with radiation treatments at the Moffitt Cancer Center and the patient

brought to our attention the tissue disruption of the area, which he stated has been diagnosed as radiation burns from Moffitt Cancer Center. The patient also complained of a whitish curd-like buildup in the mouth. The patient was given a swish and swallow prescription of Diflucan for the mouth and we asked him to continue using that. The verrucal papules were treated with cryotherapy, and Canthacur was applied. Triamcinolone 0.1% was given for the radiation burns in the perianal area. This was given in the ointment concentrate as well as a prescription for Silvadene ointment.

4. The patient presented for follow-up and stated that the radiation treatments had been discontinued for the perianal basal cell carcinoma and he still was experiencing significant discomfort in this area as well as lack of sphincter tone and incontinence. The patient brought to our attention that he has had a hip replacement on the right side in the interim since our last visit. He was healing well. He was still wheelchair bound. At this point, we gave the patient a prescription for Triamcinolone 0.1% ointment, Lidocaine 4% ointment, and Silvadene ointment to mix these together and apply twice per day to the area. Due to the emaciation and tissue dystrophy in the area, we had also given the patient a prescription for Regranex in the hope that this will be covered by his insurance company.

5. The patient presented for follow-up. The patient stated that the Regranex was not covered by his insurance company, but he was using the Triamcinolone, Silvadene, and Lidocaine in the area. However, he had not recovered continence of the anal sphincter. He stated that it was slowly getting better and he was no longer wiping off tissue and bloody exudate from the area. Physical exam of the area did in fact reveal improvement of the tissue dystrophy in the perianal area. Several more verrucal-type papules were noted on the patient's fingers and these were treated with Canthacur.

6. The patient presented for follow-up. The patient's recent lab work still revealed his CD-4 count to be less than 150 and his viral load to be more than 50,000. The verrucal papules on the fingers were still evident and these were treated again with Canthacur. The patient's perianal area looked slightly better with no signs of bloody serous exudate, but the tissue still remained somewhat friable and morpheaform in appearance.

7. The patient presented for follow-up. The patient described several new verrucal papules on the fingers. The previously treated sites did show decrease in the size of the verrucal papules. Several of these were treated with Canthacur. The patient was given a prescription for Triamcinolone ointment, Lidocaine 4% ointment, and Silvadene ointment and he was to continue applying these twice daily to the perianal area.

8. The patient presented for follow-up. The verrucal papules on the patient's fingers were significantly decreased in size and only three at this time were found and these were treated with Canthacur. If the warts persist, we will do excisional biopsies to r/o squamous cell carcinoma. The patient's recent lab work showed a CD-4 count of 238 and a viral load of approximately 40,000. The perianal area

continued to be problematic for him, but the overall erythema was significantly decreased. We asked the patient to continue using the Lidocaine ointment and Silvadene ointment without the application of Triamcinolone ointment at this point in time.

Final diagnosis:

1. Radiation burns with incontinence of the perianal area secondary to radiation treatment of neoplastic lesions.
2. Recalcitrant verruca vulgaris of the fingers.
3. Advanced HIV disease.

F/U: The patient continued to use Silvadene and Lidocaine ointment in the perianal area. The inflammation had not returned at the time. Triamcinolone had not been readministered to the area. The verrucal papules continued to show rather quickly and were being treated almost as a maintenance therapy with Canthacur PS.

Educational relevance: This case was chosen to showcase the difficulty in treating patients with advanced HIV disease and also the difficulty in treating radiation burns, especially in a person with advanced HIV disease. The modality of Lidocaine, Silvadene, and Triamcinolone appears to be quite beneficial.

Ref:

Odom RB, James WD, Berger TG. Andrew's Diseases of the Skin: Clinical Dermatology, 9th ed. WB Sanders, 2000, pp. 40–1 and 1082–6.

Bolognia JL, Jorizzo JL, Rapinio RP. Dermatology 1st ed. Mosby, 2003, pp. 466–7, 1505, 2178.

Freedberg IM, Eisen AZ, Wolff K, Austen KF, Goldsmith LA, Katz ST. Fitzpatrick's Dermatology in Internal Medicine, 5th ed. McGraw-Hill, 1999, pp. 2189–92.

Case 13

Name: GH

Ethnicity: African/American

Medical Hx: Significant for subjective psoriasis.

Social Hx: The patient is unemployed.

Family Hx: Negative for psoriasis. Positive for diabetes and hypertension.

Medications: The patient was then on no medications.

Allergies: The patient has no known drug allergies.

Chief complaint: A 68-year-old male who presented to our clinic complaining of psoriasis on his elbow for the past 20 years. He had been given several creams, some of which seem to work and some of which do not.

Physical findings: Physical exam revealed a 68-year-old, African/American male whose appearance was somewhat older than his stated age whose bilateral elbows, knees, and lower back revealed lichenified, scaly plaques.

Primary assessment/diagnosis: Psoriasis.
Treatment and course:

1. We gave the patient a prescription for Clobetasol ointment to apply twice daily to these areas. We also recommended a biopsy of the left elbow.
2. The patient presented for follow-up. The biopsy results revealed findings consistent with psoriasis. We discussed biologic therapy with the patient and gave him a lab slip to check his baseline labs and CXR and we decided to see the patient back in 2 weeks.
3. The patient presented for follow-up. He had had his lab work done, which unfortunately revealed a absolute CD-4 count of 495 and a decreased white blood cell count of 3.5 as well as a low platelet count and a low absolute neutrophil count of 469. The patient was put on Amevive injection and a blood work for HIV was asked for.
4. The patient presented for follow-up. The patient stated that the second Amevive injection was received. The HIV test was negative. The absolute CD-4 count dropped to 450 as of 11/26/03. As of 12/3/03, absolute CD-4 count had dropped to 424. A third Amevive intramuscular injection was given after our discussion with the patient.
5. The patient presented for his fourth Amevive injection. His CD-4 count was 432.
6. The patient presented for his Amevive injection. Blood work had not been returned yet, but the Amevive injection was given and the patient promised to get his lab work done that day. Later on that day, blood work was returned to our office showing absolute CD-4 count down to 316.
7. The patient presented for Amevive injection. His labs revealed a CD-4 count of 296 and the Amevive injection was not given. The patient had not noted any improvement in his psoriasis at that point. We then discussed with the patient that if his CD-4 counts continue to drop we will discontinue the Amevive.
8. The patient had labs drawn which showed a CD-4 count of 277 and the Amevive was discontinued. We asked the patient to repeat his labs in 1 month.
9. His CD-4 count had dropped to 240.
10. The patient presented for follow-up. He still had no improvement with his psoriasis. He had not received his Amevive injections for approximately 6 weeks. His last labs showed a CD-4 count of 240. Discussion ensued for possible placement on Raptiva. He was placed on Raptiva and had a good response (PASI 75) within 6 weeks.

Final diagnosis: Psoriasis of elbows and knees recalcitrant to Amevive and inducing an immune-compromised state of low CD-4 and low absolute neutrophil and low platelet count.

F/U: The patient has followed with us and we have maintained regular correspondence with the patient's primary care physician which shows that the patient has followed-up with his primary care physician and monitoring was done.

Educational relevance: This case was chosen to showcase the difficulty in treating psoriasis even with the new "biologics" and the complication of depressing a patient's immune system with the need for baseline and periodic labs. Also there are rescue therapies and more effective therapies for certain patients.

Ref:

Odom RB, James WD, Berger TG. Andrew's Diseases of the Skin: Clinical Dermatology, 9th ed. WB Sanders, 2000, pp. 218–35.

Bolognia JL, Jorizzo JL, Rapinio RP. Dermatology 1st ed. Mosby, 2003, pp. 495–522.

Freedberg IM, Eisen AZ, Wolff K, Austen KF, Goldsmith LA, Katz ST. Fitzpatrick's Dermatology in Internal Medicine, 5th ed. McGraw-Hill, 1999, pp. 125–46, 2047–50.

Selected Cases on Neurodermatitis (Megan Bock)

It is imperative to understand and recognize neurodermatitis or skin conditions that are psychologically related because it is estimated that at least one-third of individuals presenting to a dermatologist have a skin condition due to a psychologic factor [1]. Authors use many different names to refer to skin conditions that are psychologically related. Some of the names used are neurodermatitis, psychocutaneous diseases, psychodermatologic disorders, psychodermatology, psychosomatic dermatology, and psychocutaneous medicine [1–3]. There are many skin conditions whose underlying cause may be the result of a psychological condition. We will describe various types of psychologically related skin conditions so that you can become knowledgeable about the disorders and can help patients seek the proper treatment that they need. The skin conditions that will be discussed in this section include delusions of parasitosis, dermatitis artefacta, lichen simplex chronicus, neurotic excoriations, prurigo nodularis. It is necessary to understand these conditions because if one tries to treat the presenting skin problem and not the underlying psychological problem then the patient's condition may relapse, remain the same, or get worse (see chapter 17).

Delusions of Parasitosis

Mrs A is a 60-year-old female who presents to you today because she feels as though she is infested with bugs that are constantly biting her. She claims that the bugs are all over her house and that the infestation is so bad she may have to sell her house. Mrs A tells you that this problem has been occurring for weeks. At a quick glance you notice scratch marks on her arms and face but do not see any signs of bites or burrowing. Upon furthering questioning, you find that the patient's medical history is negative and the patient seems to be in perfect health. She is on no medications and has no known allergies. The patient denies use of drugs. The patient says that she keeps her house as clean as possible and takes at least two showers a day since the infestation. She has not been outside except to go from her car into her house or work. The patient claims that the bugs follow her wherever she goes so if she moves she will have to find a way to trick the bugs. The bugs are taking over her life. Upon closer examination, you still see no signs of any type of infestation. So what now?

These patients are most likely suffering from delusions of parasitosis where they truly believe that they are being bitten by insects or parasites that are non-existent. While the patients are delusional about their disorder their other mental functions are usually intact. First, it is important to make sure that the patient really does not have parasites and that the biting sensation is not coming from substance abuse [4,5]. Throughout the encounter with the patient it is important to take the patient seriously and not to immediately mention a psychiatrist [6,7]. The biggest consensus is to treat the patient with pimozide, a neuroleptic. It may be difficult convincing the patient to take it [8].

Dermatitis Artefacta

Miss D is a 64-year-old female who comes to you today because of a claimed rash on her left arm. You notice a few acute lesions that look as though they came from a car cigarette lighter and several older scarred lesions. Miss D tells you that she has had this rash for awhile and cannot get it to go away. The rash is only on her left arm. Besides her "rash," Miss D is in impeccable health. Her history is negative for anything that would bring on a rash. Miss D claims that the rash does itch or burn but she would like it to disappear from her arm. When questioned how she thinks the lesions got there, the patient is bewildered and responds, "If I knew that why would I be coming here?"So now what?

Most likely, this patient has dermatitis artefacta. A condition where patients self-inflict wounds and may not be aware of it. Often the lesions will mimic many disorders and then the diagnosis of dermatitis artefacta becomes a diagnosis of exclusion [4].

This condition most commonly occurs in females although it can occur in either sex. Dermatitis artefacta most commonly surfaces first in late adolescence to early adulthood. Often a patient is under stress or suffering from a personality disorder. They will deny that they caused the lesions. It may not be wise to mention a psychiatrist. The mention of a psychiatrist should be on a case-to-case basis. Psychotropic drugs such as serotonin reuptake inhibitors may be the best treatment. The symptoms should be treated as well. Unfortunately, this condition often reoccurs and therefore prognosis for a cure is poor [9].

Lichen Simplex Chronicus

Mr G is a 65-year-old male who presents to you today because he has an itchy rash on his legs. He said that the problem has been occurring for a couple of weeks now and he would just like the itching to diminish. He says that he is constantly scratching because of the itchiness. Mr D claims that his legs started to itch so he began to scratch and it just keeps getting worse and worse. Aside from a beta-blocker to control blood pressure, Mr G is in great health. Upon examination, you notice eczematous leathery looking plaques on his lower extremities. So now what?

Mr D is most likely suffering from a condition known as lichen simplex chronicus. Some refer to it as neurodermatitis. Most commonly occurring in elderly individuals lichen simplex chronicus looks like an eczematous rash. The condition most often occurs in patients with nervous habits [10]. The treatment method includes instructions about not scratching and symptomatic treatment with topical steroids and moisturizer. Bandages may work well to prohibit scratching. Atarax and doxepin are antipruritic drugs that may be helpful [11]. When linked with obsessive-compulsive disorder lichen simplex chronicus can be treated with selective serotonin reuptake inhibitors (SSRIs) [4]. If well maintained these lesions can permanently disappear.

Neurotic Exoriations

Mrs Q is a 72-year-old female who presents to your office today because of several lesions on her right forearm. She tells you that she had been out in the yard about a week ago and had been bit by some mosquitoes. Now the lesions have become crusted and infected and she wants to make sure that the mosquitoes did not have any kind of infection. As she sits there recalling the incident, you notice she is obsessively picking away at the scabs and she is not even aware of it. The rest of her medical history was not pertinent to her coming in today. So now what?

The lesions on Mrs Q's arm are most likely a result of neurotic excoriations. Neurotic excoriations are simply the obsessive picking of existing lesions. While seen at any age and in any sex, neurotic excoriations are most commonly seen in middle-aged women [4]. Neurotic excoriations can fall into many categories and one article states that there are different types of skin pickers [12]. The different types of pickers are angry, anxious/depressed, body dysmorphic, borderline, delusional, guilty, habit, narcissistic, obsessive-compulsive, and organic. It is suggested that aside from symptomatic treatment, patients receive psychotropic medication depending on the type of picker they are [12].

Prurigo Nodularis

Mrs J is 69-year-old female who presents today with several nodular lesions to her right elbow. She said that the area was once very itchy and now these little nodules have appeared. She tries to, "pick the nodules off" but they keep appearing. Her medical history is impeccable. Upon examination, you notice several keratotic nodules. So now what?

Mrs J most likely has prurigo nodularis. First, you would want to exclude any underlying cause such as a renal failure, keratocanthoma, and nodular scabies [4].

The face, palms, and soles are rarely affected and the sparing of the mid-upper back is referred to as the "butterfly" sign [4]. Prurigo nodularis develops from constant picking or scratching. Once it is determined that the patient has prurigo nodularis there are a couple of options for treatment. Symptomatic treatment includes antipruritics and moisturizers, corticosteroids, cryotherapy, oral histamines and steroids, and phototherapy. Doxepin, which is an antidepressant and antianxiety drug, is said to be helpful.

In conclusion, individuals may present with many different psychologically related skin ailments. It is important to take all patients seriously because they would not be coming to the doctor if they did not feel they had a problem.

References

1. Gupta M, Gupta A. Psychodermatology: an update. J. Am. Acad. Dermatol. 1996; 34(6): 1030–46. Retrieved May 26, 2004 online at http://www.mdconsult.com.
2. Koo J. Psychodermatology: the mind and skin connection. Am. Fam. Phys. 2001; 64(11) 1863–8.
3. Silvan M. Psyche and soma. Psychocutan Med. 2003; 71: 267.
4. Koo J, Han A. Psychocutaneous Diseases. Dermatology. Spain: Mosby, 2003, pp. 111–20.
5. Zanol K, Slaughter J, Hall R. An approach to the treatment of psychogenic parasitosis. Int. J. Dermatol. 1988; 37: 56–63.
6. Alexander J. Arthropods and Human Skin. New York: Springer-Verlag, 1984.
7. Frankel E. Treatment of delusions of parasitosis. J. Am. Acad. Dermatol. 1984; 9: 772–3.
8. Zomer S, De Wit R, Van Bronswijk J. Delusions of parasitosis: a psychiatric disorder to be treated by dermatologists? An analysis of 33 patients. Br. J. Dermatol. 1998; 138: 1030–2.
9. Koblenzer C. Dermatitis artefacta. Clinical features and approaches to treatment. Am. J. Clin. Dermatol. 2000; 1(1): 47–55. Retrieved May 2004 from the online database Ovid Medline at www.nova.edu.
10. Parker, F. Chapter 522—Skin Diseases of General Importance. Goldman: Cecil Textbook of Medicine, 21st ed. Saunders Company, 2000. Retrieved May 2004 online at http://www.mdconsult.com.
11. Rakel RE. Textbook of Family Practice, 6th ed. WB Saunders, 2002. Retrieved May 2004 online at http://www.mdconsult.com.
12. Fried R, Fried S. Picking Apart the Picker: A Clinician's Guide for Management of the Patient Presenting with Excoriations. Psychocutan. Med. 2003; 71: 291–8.

Index

Printed in the United States
By Bookmasters